# Birth Plans
## FOR
# DUMMIES®

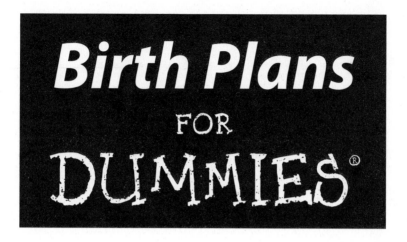

# by Rachel Gurevich and Sharon Perkins, RN

WILEY

John Wiley & Sons, Inc.

**Birth Plans For Dummies®**

Published by
**John Wiley & Sons, Inc.**
111 River St.
Hoboken, NJ 07030-5774
www.wiley.com

Copyright © 2013 by John Wiley & Sons, Inc., Hoboken, New Jersey

Published simultaneously in Canada

For general information on our other products and services, please contact our Customer Care Department within the U.S. at 877-762-2974, outside the U.S. at 317-572-3993, or fax 317-572-4002.

For technical support, please visit www.wiley.com/techsupport.

Wiley publishes in a variety of print and electronic formats and by print-on-demand. Some material included with standard print versions of this book may not be included in e-books or in print-on-demand. If this book refers to media such as a CD or DVD that is not included in the version you purchased, you may download this material at http://booksupport.wiley.com. For more information about Wiley products, visit www.wiley.com.

Library of Congress Control Number: 2012949503

ISBN 978-1-118-31737-2 (pbk); ISBN 978-1-118-43209-9 (ebk); ISBN 978-1-118-43213-6 (ebk); ISBN 978-1-118-43212-9 (ebk)

Manufactured in the United States of America

10 9 8 7 6 5 4 3 2 1

WILEY

# About the Authors

**Rachel Gurevich** is a freelance health writer and author, most notably of *The Doula Advantage: Your Complete Guide to Having an Empowered and Positive Birth with the Help of a Professional Childbirth Assistant* (Three Rivers Press, 2003). Rachel also writes about fertility for About.com, a New York Times Company. Originally from the United States, she currently lives in Israel with her husband and four children, including a set of twins. With three very different births under her belt — a plan-gone-wrong birth, an amazing natural childbirth, and an unwanted but very necessary cesarean-section birth — she understands not only the importance of birth preparation and planning but also the need for flexibility and the difficulty in facing disappointing births. Her website is www.rachelgurevich.com.

**Sharon Perkins** has been an RN for over 25 years, mostly in maternal-child health, and has seen more than her fair share of birth plans. She has also spent her fair share of time on the maternity floor, both while at work and while having five children, although one arrived via plane from Korea. She lives in New Jersey but visits Disney World frequently and loves spending time with her three grandchildren more than just about anything on earth. She has written seven other *For Dummies* books and is still grateful to her very first acquisitions editor for taking a chance on her and coauthor Jackie Thompson over a decade ago.

# Dedication

**From Rachel:** This book is for my mother, Iris Bollinger, and my grandmothers, Blossom Mendlowitz and Jean Bollinger, whose labors never included birthing balls or birth plans, and for the women of their generations, whose lack of birth choices led to a birth revolution and a reclamation of the birthing experience.

**From Sharon:** I dedicate this book to all the nurses and midwives working with women in labor to help them have the best birth experience possible. There is no better job on earth than helping a couple become a family.

# Authors' Acknowledgments

**From Rachel:** I feel honored to have had the privilege to work on this book, on a topic so dear to my heart. I want to thank agent Lauren Ruth, for bringing the project to me, and the entire team at Wiley — most especially acquisitions editor Erin Calligan Mooney, project editor Elizabeth Rea, copy editors Caitie Copple and Amanda Langferman, and technical reviewer Penny Lane — for making this book the best it can be. A very special thanks to Sharon Perkins, my coauthor, who was an excellent "book doula" as I dived into the writing of a *For Dummies* book. I never imagined writing a book with a coauthor could be so much fun, and maybe we'll meet one day in Disney World so we can laugh together, in person!

Writing a book with 2-year-old twins underfoot isn't easy, and I owe thanks to those who supported me, including Jessica A. Naiditch, Dawn Zuckerman, Rachel Rabinowitz, Lindsey S. Daniels, and Tamar Gross. I'd also like to acknowledge the hundreds of women (and a number of men) — the mothers, fathers, and childbirth professionals — who have shared their stories and wisdom with me over the years. I also must thank my children, for providing so much material to draw upon, and most especially thanks to my big kids, Menachem and Eliezer, for helping so much with the twins. Last but not least, I thank my husband Eli, for encouraging me to take on the project and giving up almost all his free time to watch the kids so I could have time to write.

**From Sharon:** This book has been a pleasure to write from beginning to end, thanks to our editorial team at Wiley. As for my coauthor Rachel, it's been so much fun; we've snickered and laughed through much of this book. Even though you live in Israel, it's been like working with a good friend next door.

This book was so easy to write that my husband kept forgetting I was even working on it! For my marvelous children, thanks again for the raw material on motherhood you've given me to draw on over the years. And kudos to my grandchildren, Matthew, Emma, and Jessica, for keeping me in touch with the newest and latest stuff in childrearing.

## Publisher's Acknowledgments

We're proud of this book; please send us your comments at http://dummies.custhelp.com. For other comments, please contact our Customer Care Department within the U.S. at 877-762-2974, outside the U.S. at 317-572-3993, or fax 317-572-4002.

Some of the people who helped bring this book to market include the following:

*Acquisitions, Editorial, and Vertical Websites*

**Project Editor:** Elizabeth Rea

**Acquisitions Editor:** Erin Calligan Mooney

**Copy Editor:** Caitlin Copple

**Assistant Editor:** David Lutton

**Editorial Program Coordinator:** Joe Niesen

**Technical Editor:** Penny Lane, MSN, CNM

**Editorial Manager:** Michelle Hacker

**Editorial Assistant:** Alexa Koschier

**Art Coordinator:** Alicia B. South

**Cover Photos:** ©Johner Images/Alamy

**Cartoons:** Rich Tennant (www.the5thwave.com)

*Composition Services*

**Project Coordinator:** Kristie Rees

**Layout and Graphics:** Jennifer Creasey, Joyce Haughey

**Proofreaders:** Melissa Cossell, Joni Heredia Language Services

**Indexer:** Sharon Shock

**Illustrator:** Kathryn Born

**Publishing and Editorial for Consumer Dummies**

**Kathleen Nebenhaus,** Vice President and Executive Publisher

**David Palmer,** Associate Publisher

**Kristin Ferguson-Wagstaffe,** Product Development Director

**Publishing for Technology Dummies**

**Andy Cummings,** Vice President and Publisher

**Composition Services**

**Debbie Stailey,** Director of Composition Services

# Contents at a Glance

# Table of Contents

## Part II: Choosing Your Birth Team, Birth Place, and Guests .................................................................... 39

### Chapter 3: OB-GYN, Family Practitioners, Midwives, Oh My! ....... 41

### Chapter 4: Leaving Home for a Hospital or Birth Center ........... 53

# Introduction

. . . . . . . . . . . . . . . . . . . . . . . . . . . . . . . . . . . . . . . . . . . . . . . . . . . . . .

Congratulations on one of the most exciting times of your life: pregnancy and the birth of your baby. Like for any big event, you need to do some advance planning if you want birth to go smoothly. A birth plan not only helps you to cope during labor and delivery; it also helps you think clearly and logically about the kind of birth you want and what that requires. This book helps by giving you the information you need to make your baby's birth a time to remember — for all the right reasons.

## About This Book

This book provides both a broad and focused look at childbirth. We explain how it's changing, what your options are, and how to best get your way on issues that may be very important to you, such as nursing your baby immediately after delivery. In general, hospital deliveries are designed for the convenience of the staff, not you. However, this situation is changing as hospitals realize that pregnant women have choices — including delivering outside the hospital in more hospitable settings.

The only way to create a viable birth plan is to fully understand what normally happens during childbirth, including what interventions will happen routinely unless you object to them, and what your alternatives are. Key to having the type of birth you want is choosing the right medical practitioner, so we show you how make that decision as well.

The main point of this book is to help you write a birth plan that meets all your needs and covers all your essential birth requests. In each chapter, we review the information you should include in your birth plan and guide you through the process of making choices between various birth options.

We promise you: *For Dummies* books are not really for dummies. You made a very wise choice in picking up this book because it contains all you need to know about writing a birth plan that not only addresses the important issues but also does it in a way that maximizes your chances that other people will read it and try to follow it.

# Conventions Used in This Book

One problem with discussing people who can be of either sex — such as your medical practitioner, your partner, or your baby — is that we don't know if they're male or female. In the case of the baby, you may not know that yet yourself! So we alternate between using *he* and *she*. Because both your coauthors have more boys than girls in our own families, you may find that we slip up and use *he* slightly more than *she*.

Because we also don't know if your medical practitioner is a doctor or midwife, or whether you have a pediatrician or nurse practitioner for the baby, we use the term *medical practitioner* when we talk about anyone medical. We also use the term *partner* when referring to your spouse or significant other, because that person really is your partner in matters of childbirth! Sometimes we use the term *labor partner,* which simply refers to whomever is supporting you through the birth. It could be your significant other, a friend, or even a doula.

In more practical matters, we use *italic* font to highlight new terms, and we follow each one with a clear definition. **Boldface** font indicates keywords or actions in numbered steps.

# What You're Not to Read

We hate to tell you to skip any of this book, not just because we think it's brilliant but also because we think every word is essential. The truth is, however, that it's probably not. Some sections may not interest you or be applicable to the type of birth you want. Feel free to skip anything that doesn't seem relevant to you.

# Foolish Assumptions

We assume you're reading this book because you're pregnant or hope to be and you have definite ideas about how you want to give birth. Or maybe you have no idea about how'd you'd like to give birth and realize you'd better start figuring it out, because your pregnancy is moving right along. Or perhaps you've heard your friends and relatives tell horror stories of birth and want something better for yourself. You may even be an expectant dad bewildered by the idea of why you need a birth plan in the first place. Whatever your reason for picking up this book, we guarantee you'll come to understand quite a bit about childbirth — and about yourself.

# Icons Used in This Book

Although we consider this book essential in every word (because we wouldn't have written it if we didn't), some information is especially important. Because we don't want you to miss this information, it's marked with an icon.

The Remember icon sits next to information we hope stays in your head for more than a few minutes, although we understand that pregnancy interferes with your ability to fully concentrate.

This icon gives insider info that you may otherwise take years to figure out on your own. One of your authors is an RN with lots of labor and delivery experience, and we're both women's health writers and moms ourselves, so we know this info will benefit you. We learned it the hard way, so you don't have to.

The Try It icon highlights opportunities to practice comfort or movement techniques for labor. If you practice before labor begins, you'll be much more likely to use the techniques effectively. So jump in and try them!

We warn only when something may be harmful or risky, so take heed of these icons.

# Where to Go from Here

From here, you can go anywhere you'd like in this book. If you're extremely methodical, start at the beginning and plod right through to the end. By the time you get there, you'll have a very good idea of what you want your birth plan to include, and actually writing it down will be a breeze. But if you're just days — or hours — away from labor and need some information fast, feel free to skip to the part you need most at the moment. If one chapter jumps out at you because it discusses an issue you're currently grappling with, go there. Dummies books are modular, meaning that each chapter stands on its own, so you don't need to read the chapter before or after to understand the content in a chapter.

# Part I
# Labor and Birth-
# Plan Basics

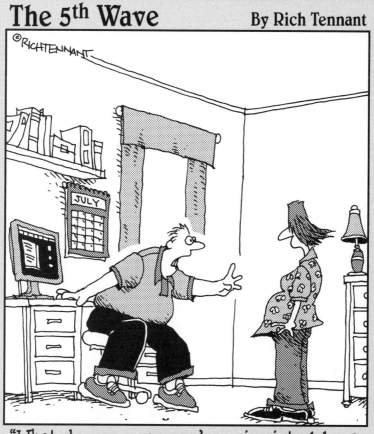

The 5th Wave                    By Rich Tennant

"What do you mean you're going into labor?
Labor Day isn't until September first!"

# In this part . . .

Writing your birth plan requires some knowledge of what birth is all about. Because you may not have experienced birth for yourself yet, this part tells you everything you need to know about labor and delivery to get started on creating your own birth plan. The whole birth process can be overwhelming, with a lot of information to absorb, but we make it easily digestible by breaking it down into sections that address your most pressing concerns.

# Chapter 1

## Creating a Birth Plan: What It's All About

### In This Chapter

▶ Understanding the basic idea of a birth plan

▶ Considering all your options

▶ Planning early — before contractions begin!

▶ Making informed choices

▶ Steering clear of birth-plan snafus

**Y**ou may be wondering how anyone can "plan" birth. Isn't that like trying to plan a rain storm? It'll rain whenever and for as long as it's going to rain regardless of anyone's plans! Although you obviously can't plan every aspect of what will happen when you give birth, you actually have many options. Creating a birth plan gives you an opportunity to research and consider the many aspects of childbirth that *can* be planned, many of which you may not have known about otherwise. After your plan is put together, you can use it to communicate your wishes to your birth team.

In this chapter, we introduce you to birth plans and their benefits, give a general overview of birth and postpartum options, explain how you can make informed decisions, and provide tips on avoiding common birth-plan pitfalls.

## What's a Birth Plan? And Why Would You Want One?

Put simply, a birth plan is a document you create to communicate your wishes and requests to your medical practitioner, the birth team, and your support team (whether that's your partner, a doula, or someone else). You write the plan months before labor begins, when you have time to research and think through your options — preferably before contractions make concentrating difficult! Planning ahead also allows you to switch medical practitioners if your current doctor or midwife isn't on board with your plans.

Despite the name, a birth plan also includes your wishes for the immediate postpartum period, like how you intend to feed your baby and where you want her to sleep if you're giving birth in a hospital. Birth plans also cover the fun options, like who will announce the baby's gender and who cuts the cord. In this section, we explain the reasons you should consider writing a birth plan.

## Making informed choices with a clear head

You may wonder why you should bother considering all the many options for dealing with events that may not even happen during your birth. The reason is simple — thinking straight is much easier when you're not in labor. And unless you bring your laptop into the labor room, researching your choices is difficult when you're actually in the trenches, so to speak.

Technically, whenever your medical practitioner recommends a birth intervention — like *induction,* or attempting to initiate active labor — he should also tell you the potential risks and benefits. In an ideal world, you would also be given alternative options to consider. For example, on the subject of induction, your doctor could explain the choices of giving you oxytocin (Pitocin) intravenously, trying something natural first, or taking a "wait and see" approach before augmenting labor. If he thoroughly explains all three options, you can give true informed consent, which means agreeing to a procedure only after understanding what's involved.

In practice, informed consent for many procedures is covered extremely quickly, way too fast for you to process the information and make a really informed decision. Frequently, procedures are not explained at all, especially if they are routine (which doesn't necessarily mean risk free), or the procedure is presented as if you have no other options. Even if you have an amazing medical practitioner who really explains your risks and alternatives, you may have difficultly thinking through decisions when you're in the middle of labor.

Creating your birth plan allows you to research your options when you're feeling calm and collected. Writing a plan doesn't mean you may not have to make difficult decisions in the midst of labor — as we always say, birth isn't completely plan-friendly — but at least for straightforward issues, you'll be ready.

Birth plans aren't only about interventions, though. We go into more detail on those options throughout this book and in this chapter, in the section "Your Birth-Plan Options: An Overview."

# Visualizing your ideal birth

Everyone's ideal image of birth is different. One mother may consider the perfect birth to be in a well-equipped hospital with an immediate epidural, and another mother may consider her perfect birth to be at home, with no drugs, and in a birthing pool. There's nothing necessarily right or wrong about these different visions (although most people think their ideal birth is the best one!). Every birth choice has its risks and benefits, but many birth choices have more to do with comfort and personal philosophy than statistics.

Don't panic if you're thinking, "But I have no idea what I want. I don't even know what my options are!" Lots of moms and dads have no idea what they want at the beginning of their pregnancy. In fact, their "ideal birth" may change from pregnancy to pregnancy. You don't need to know all your options right now. If you did, you wouldn't need this book! As you find out more about birth and about birth plans, you'll get a better idea of what you want. For a general overview of your options, skip ahead to the section "Your Birth-Plan Options: An Overview."

# Putting what you want on paper for your care providers

A written birth plan helps you communicate your concerns and wishes to your medical practitioner. Discussing your plans for childbirth before you go into labor is essential, and having a written plan in hand can be a huge help.

Never assume your medical practitioner's idea of the perfect birth is similar to your own. Even if your chosen care provider shares your birth philosophy, you should still write down your wishes to prevent misunderstandings.

If you're giving birth in the hospital, you have very little control over which nurse you get, and you get very little time to discuss your birth plans with her. Most nurses want their patients to have a healthy and positive birth, and a written birth plan makes it easier for them to provide you with what you want.

Just writing your plan down won't magically make your birth wishes a reality. Although we discuss many birth options throughout this book, not every option is available in every birth location or with every medical practitioner. Even if the option is available, you still need to advocate for yourself beyond handing your nurse, midwife, or doctor a written birth plan. See Chapter 18 on writing a plan that's assertive without being aggressive, and turn to Chapter 19 for more on advocating for your birth.

# Your Birth-Plan Options: An Overview

We mention birth-plan options a lot in this chapter, but maybe you're wondering what those options actually are. We discuss many birth possibilities in Chapter 18 as well as throughout this book. For now, here's a list of the basics:

- **Where do you want to give birth?** You may give birth at home, in a hospital, or at a birth center. You also should consider which hospital or birth center to choose. In Chapter 4, we explain how to choose a hospital or birth center, and in Chapter 5, we talk about choosing a home birth.

- **What kind of practitioner do you envision?** You may decide on an obstetrician or a midwife. You may or may not want to stick with your current gynecologist or midwife. In Chapter 3, we give you tips on choosing your medical practitioner.

- **Who will support and advocate for you during labor and delivery?** Your significant other is not the only option for labor support. You may consider hiring a doula to work with your partner or as your sole support. You may also choose a friend or family member for this role. In Chapter 6, we explain what makes a good birthing buddy, and in Chapter 3, we tell you how to hire a doula. Chapter 19 provides guidance on how dads, doulas, and friends can support and advocate for you.

- **Whom do you want to invite to the birth?** You can invite friends and family members to the birth, either to wait down the hall or be by your side in the delivery room. You may even consider including your older children at the birth. Or you and your partner can be alone, inviting family after the baby arrives. In Chapter 6, we talk about who to invite and who *not* to invite to the birth.

- **Do you want a natural childbirth?** Women choose natural childbirth for a number of reasons, from concerns about epidural risks to wanting a "natural experience." Whether you're absolutely determined to give birth without pain drugs or you're just considering it, we discuss childbirth methods in Chapter 7 and delve into natural soothing techniques in Chapter 8. If you decide to use pain medications, you have a number of pain-relief options, from epidurals to walking epidurals to IV narcotics. In Chapter 11, we explain their pros and cons.

- **What comfort techniques will you try?** Pain drugs are only one way to get relief from labor pains. To name just a few, you can use massage, hydrotherapy, or hypnosis. Even if you plan an epidural, you probably won't be able to get one right away, so having an arsenal of comfort techniques is important. In Chapter 8, we list many natural soothing methods for you to try during labor.

✔ **What birthing tools or props do you want to use?** Birthing props and comfort tools are not only fun but also extremely helpful! You may decide to use a birthing pool, a squat bar, a birth ball, or massage tools. Even your music choices can be important for the birth. For more on birth tools and props, see Chapter 8.

✔ **How do you expect to stay active during labor?** If you assumed you'd be lying in bed for the entire labor, think again! Many positions and movements can be helpful during labor, and remaining active has lots of benefits. Turn to Chapter 9 for more on labor positions and movement.

✔ **Will you accept an IV for hydration, or do you hope to drink fluids on your own?** IVs are routine in many hospitals, but not all, and you have options. You may even be able to eat and drink lightly. See Chapter 10 for more on nourishing your body during labor.

✔ **What kind of environment do you hope for during delivery?** Perhaps you'd like a meditative environment, with ocean waves playing in the background. Or perhaps you want upbeat music to energize you. Check out Chapters 15 and 18 for more on birth-environment requests.

✔ **What kind of monitoring do you want?** If you're getting an epidural, continuous monitoring is required, but if you're hoping for a natural birth, you may be able to have intermittent monitoring. In Chapter 12, we discuss your monitoring options.

✔ **How do you feel about induction and speeding up labor?** Induction is a controversial topic, especially when done for convenience or when scheduled before your due date. Labor augmentation is another touchy topic, and your medical practitioner plays a big role in your options. In Chapter 13, we discuss the pros and cons to labor augmentation.

✔ **How do you want to push?** Surprise: You don't have to push while lying on your back! In fact, you'll probably have an easier time if you don't. You may even choose to have a water birth. In Chapter 9 we discuss the pros and cons to various pushing positions as well as the pros and cons of water birth.

✔ **How do you envision the delivery of the baby?** Are you hoping to help guide the baby out (with the help of your practitioner)? Do you hope to watch the delivery in a mirror? If you don't know the sex, do you want your medical practitioner to announce it, or do you want your partner to tell you? In Chapter 15, we discuss all these options.

✔ **Do you prefer to receive an episiotomy (surgical incision) or to tear naturally?** Some (but not all) women prefer to tear rather than be cut, and in an emergency, it's not always an option. We discuss the pros and cons to episiotomy in Chapter 13, along with other assisted vaginal-delivery interventions.

✔ **What are your feelings about cesarean section (C-section)?** Some women are fearful of C-section, whereas others actually opt for one (sometimes without medical reason). In the past, after you had a cesarean you always had to have cesarean with subsequent babies, but now many women can try for a vaginal birth after cesarean (VBAC). If you do need a C-section, you have options — yes, even for a cesarean! — like lowering the drape to watch the delivery or breast-feeding on the surgical table. See Chapter 14 for more on cesarean section.

✔ **Who will cut the cord and when? Do you want the baby placed directly on your chest after birth or cleaned up and weighed first?** A number of birth-plan choices are relevant to the moment your baby is born. See Chapter 15 for more on your moment-of-birth options.

✔ **What do you want to do with the placenta?** You even have options regarding the placenta! For the delivery of the placenta, you may request the medical practitioner not use controlled traction and allow a natural delivery of the placenta. In Chapter 13, we explain placenta-related delivery options. You also may request the birth team save the placenta for you so you can make a "placenta print" or bury your placenta in the back yard; see Chapter 22 for more on preserving birth memories.

✔ **Do you plan to take pictures or video of the birth?** Some parents only want pictures after the baby is delivered, but others want photos of the entire birth experience. Flip to Chapters 15 and 22 for photo-taking tips.

✔ **How do you plan to feed your baby?** Will you breast-feed, bottle-feed, or do a little of both? Some bottle-feeding moms face bottle guilt, but breast-feeding isn't always possible or desired. Some hospital routines unintentionally sabotage breast-feeding mothers, but your birth plan can include requests to avoid some potential problems. See Chapter 17 for more on nourishing your baby.

✔ **Where do you want your baby to sleep?** *Full rooming-in* means your baby stays with you around the clock, while *partial rooming-in* means your baby sleeps in the nursery. See Chapter 17 for more on making decisions about where your baby sleeps.

✔ **What drops, shots, and tests do you want for your baby? If you have a baby boy, do you want the hospital to do a circumcision?** Vaccinations are a hot topic in the United States. Some parents decide to forgo all shots, while others accept them all, choose selectively, or delay them. Circumcision is also a hot topic, and parents who decide to snip may or may not want to do so right after the birth or at the hospital. See Chapter 16 for more on the various shots and snips your baby faces.

# Why Planning Must Begin Early in Pregnancy

Although many options exist, everything isn't available in every birth facility or with every medical practitioner. Birth location policies and your medical practitioner's practices have a big effect on your options and on the chances of getting the birth you want. Planning early for the birth gives you time to:

✔ **Interview medical practitioners:** If you start planning early, you'll have more time to consider the right practitioner for you and have time to switch if necessary. In Chapter 3, we discuss choosing a practitioner and what to do if you need to switch at the last moment.

✔ **Tour your chosen birth facility:** You can't make a real decision about where to deliver until you've been there. Tour a couple hospitals or birth centers to evaluate where you'd feel most comfortable. Because where you give birth is often connected to who attends the birth, tour early in your pregnancy in case you need to switch practitioners.

For a home birth, early planning is recommended so you can check your local home-birth laws and find a medical practitioner. Don't make the mistake of thinking all home-birth practitioners share your birth philosophy. You also need to prepare your home, which may include gathering supplies or renting a birthing pool. See Chapter 5 for more on preparing for a home birth.

Are you reading this book late in your pregnancy and thinking you waited too long to start planning? Planning late is always better than never. Also, remember you don't necessarily have to find the "perfect" practitioner or birth location. We're not sure they even exist! As long as you're comfortable with your choices and arrangements, aim for "good enough" instead.

# But I'm Not a Doctor! How Do I Make Smart Choices?

Plenty of mothers-to-be are intimidated at the thought of considering the pros and cons of a medical procedure — especially if they then decide to go against their medical practitioner's protocols or routines. If you feel unqualified to make decisions about childbirth, the good news is you're not the first person to confront all these choices, and you don't have to make them on your own. In this section, we explain how you can educate yourself on your birth options and who you can ask for help when you can't decide what to do.

# Getting an education

If you want to deliver babies, you need to go to medical or midwifery school. If you want to make decisions about your birth plan, medical training is not required! You can get the information you need to make informed choices by taking childbirth-education classes and researching birth on your own.

Childbirth education classes aren't only about teaching natural childbirth methods, though most encourage natural labor and spend a great deal of time on comfort techniques. The rest of class time is spent talking about the mechanics of normal childbirth and the pros and cons of various interventions. In Chapter 7, we help you navigate your education options so you can pick a class that's right for you.

Your education doesn't have to stop there. Reading about birth in books and doing online research can help you write your birth plan. By picking up this book, in fact, you've already armed yourself with plenty of information to make birth-plan decisions (in our humble opinion, of course).

# Consulting the experienced and the wise

Here's more good news about writing your birth plan: You don't have to do it alone! You can ask for advice from all the following people:

- **Your medical practitioner:** Your doctor is not the enemy! Although your medical practitioner has his own concerns regarding your birth choices — including malpractice suits and sometimes his own convenience — he is still an excellent resource. If you don't understand some issues or want more information, ask your doctor or midwife.

- **Your childbirth educator:** Most childbirth instructors are happy to help with birth questions and even help you write your plan. They may be willing to read over what you've put together and make suggestions.

- **Your doula:** Part of a doula's job is to help advocate for your birth choices, and that includes helping you with your birth plan. A doula can also give you inside information on local practitioners and birth locations, which can be a huge help.

- **Other experienced moms and dads:** Anyone who has gone through childbirth can serve as a resource when you're creating your own plan. Friends and relatives can tell you what they wish they had done differently and what was just perfect. They may also be able to give feedback on local medical practitioners and birth locations; just be sure to ask *why* they liked a particular place or person. Remember that everyone visualizes the perfect birth differently and that everyone's circumstances are different.

# Avoiding Potential Birth-Plan Pitfalls

In case you haven't guessed yet, we think birth plans are pretty great advocacy tools, but even we can admit they aren't always perfect. In this section, we discuss some common pitfalls and how to avoid them.

## Navigating through your choices

Considering all the options for your birth can be overwhelming. So many choices to make! If you feel exhausted just thinking about it, remember that you don't have to have an opinion on every aspect of birth. Just because you have options doesn't mean you must specifically choose one or the other.

If you don't have strong feelings about an issue, you can go with whatever your medical practitioner suggests or whatever feels right in the moment. Creating your birth plan should be an energizing experience and a chance to really take charge (as much as possible) of your birth experience. The key is to feel empowered, not overwhelmed, by all your choices.

In your birth plan, be sure to state the issues that are most important to you, even if you think they're obvious. Leave out the issues you don't have an opinion on or don't really care about. See Chapter 18 for more on writing your plan.

## Planning your birth (even if you want an epidural)

Birth plans are not only for natural births. Many aspects of the birth and the immediate postpartum period have nothing to do with using drugs or not. Even within the option of using an epidural, you have choices, like when to start it, whether you want a walking epidural, and whether you want it turned down when it's time to push.

## Remembering that birth is unpredictable

Critics of birth plans say that they set women up for disappointment. If a couple's birth goes badly, they may feel they failed in some way, like their plan wasn't good enough. We think that failing to plan is a worse option than planning and having those plans go awry.

Creating a birth plan isn't about trying to control birth, and it's not about restricting the possibilities of what's considered a positive birth experience. If you keep in mind that your birth plan isn't a contract but more of a flexible guide, you're less likely to feel disappointed if a few little things go differently than planned. In Chapter 20, we discuss changes in plans and how to cope after a traumatic birth experience.

## Standing up for your beliefs

Writing down your birth wishes is only the first step to getting the birth you want. You also need to speak to your practitioner before labor begins if you want him on your side. During the birth itself, you will likely need to work with the nurses and advocate for your plan, especially if your wishes run contrary to the hospital's routines.

In Chapter 19, we explain how you can work with the birth team and advocate for yourself, and in Chapter 21, we discuss how to overcome common birth-plan obstacles.

# Chapter 2

# The Ins and Outs of Labor and Delivery

*T*o make a birth plan, you have to have some idea about what actually happens during birth. Although you may have heard stories about labor and delivery from your family and friends, their experiences may not have been typical. They may also be slightly exaggerated or skewed by faulty memory over time (or a deep-seated need to boast!). In this chapter, we tell you what *really* happens during childbirth so you can make your birth plan using accurate, up-to-date information.

## Getting to the Big Day

When you're pregnant, every abdominal twinge and twitch takes on heightened importance. Count on asking yourself — or your partner — whether "this is it" at least a million times before you deliver. Well, maybe not a million, but many. Sometimes the start of labor isn't easy to recognize, especially if you're a first-time mom. This section tells you how to recognize the roles your reproductive organs play in the onset of labor and explains how to respond to the cues they give that labor is near. Figure 2-1 gives an inside view of your reproductive organs.

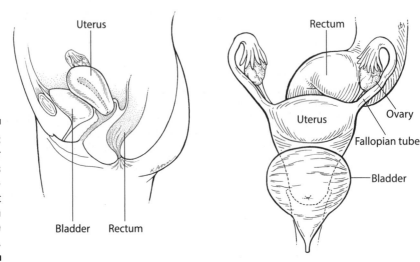

Illustration by Kathryn Born

**Figure 2-1:**
Labor
requires
a coordi-
nated effort
between
reproductive
organs.

## Focusing on the center of operations: The uterus

Your uterus — the muscular, pear-shaped organ that holds your growing baby — is one of the key components of labor. Your uterus consists of *smooth muscle,* which contracts without your voluntary efforts. When the uterine muscle contracts, you can see and feel it hardening through the abdominal wall, just like you'd feel any other tightened muscle.

Uterine contractions pull the cervix upward, first thinning it out and then opening it. True labor contractions start at the top of the uterus and spread downward. After your cervix opens completely, uterine contractions push the baby down — and out!

## Checking out changes in the small but mighty cervix

You can't talk about the actions of the uterus without talking about the cervix, the lowest portion of the uterus and the only part you can actually palpate. When you're not pregnant, the cervix is a tightly closed, firm tissue between 3 and 5 centimeters long. If you insert your fingers into your vagina when you're not pregnant, you can feel the tip of the cervix at the back of the vagina.

During pregnancy, the cervix moves forward and lines up with the opening of the vagina. This movement also happens to some extent when you ovulate in order to give sperm a straight shot. The cervix protects your uterus, ovaries, and fallopian tubes from bacteria that could cause infection.

During most of pregnancy, the cervix stays closed and long, although it softens as the pregnancy progresses. In early pregnancy, the cervix takes on a bluish color known as *Chadwick's sign.* In the days long before home pregnancy tests, the color change of the cervix was one way medical practitioners diagnosed early pregnancy. In the last month, your cervix starts to thin out and may even open slightly, especially if you've given birth before.

Your medical practitioner evaluates your labor progress based on *cervical dilation* (the opening of the cervix) and *effacement* (the medical term for thinning). Your cervix needs to thin out as much as it can, to 100 percent, and to open to 10 centimeters for the baby to pass through; at this point, your practitioner may say that you're "complete," meaning completely dilated. Figure 2-2 shows what your practitioner means when she talks about cervical dilation, also called *dilatation.* (The figure is not to scale.)

In the weeks before delivery, you may pass part of the cervical mucus plug. The mucus plus helps keep bacteria out of the uterus. When your cervix starts to thin and dilate, part of the mucus plug may fall out. This sign is a good indication that your body is getting ready to go into labor, although that may not occur for a few weeks. You may not notice losing your mucus plug, if it comes out over a few days or drops into the commode when you're not looking, so don't worry if you don't see it. During labor, you may notice blood mixed in with the mucus as the cervix opens more and microscopic tears in the cervix cause a small amount of bleeding.

## Finding out the importance of the amniotic sac

Your baby isn't just bumping around inside the uterus; he's floating in the amniotic sac (at least until he becomes too big to float). The amniotic sac, which lies within the uterus, acts as additional protection from infection for your baby. The amniotic fluid inside the sac protects the baby's skin and cushions him from the jarring that occurs when you move around. He swallows amniotic fluid to practice his swallowing skills and urinates into it. The baby also breathes the fluid, which helps expand and mature his lungs. Although that may not sound too appealing, urine is sterile under normal conditions.

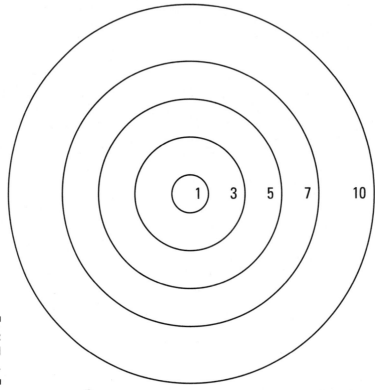

**Figure 2-2:**
Cervical
dilation.

A break in the amniotic sac leaves your baby more vulnerable to infection. Any time you notice clear fluid leaking from your vagina, notify your medical practitioner. Figure 2-3 shows how the amniotic sac develops inside the uterus and protects your baby.

## Preparing yourself for false alarms and Braxton-Hicks contractions

You can expect to experience at least one bout of "false labor." You may even get as far as going to the hospital, if you're birthing there, or calling your midwife, only to be told, "Not yet." The culprit behind most false alarms is Braxton-Hicks contractions. There's a difference, though, between labor contractions and these practice contractions.

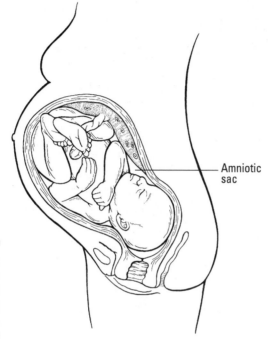

Amniotic
sac

**Figure 2-3:**
The amniotic
sac seals
around your
baby.

*Illustration by Kathryn Born*

Unlike real labor contractions, which start at the top of the uterus and spread downward, Braxton-Hicks contractions are somewhat uncoordinated; the muscles contract all over at the same time. They don't open the cervix much or thin it out like real labor does. Braxton-Hicks contractions also don't come at regular intervals or get stronger and closer together. For example, they don't start out 10 minutes apart, then 8, then 6, as may occur in labor. Bouts of Braxton-Hicks contractions increase in frequency as you get nearer your due date.

Report *any* contractions you feel before 37 weeks to your practitioner, if you have more than four in an hour. Lie on your left side, have something to drink, and call. Don't assume they're just Braxton-Hicks when you're preterm; the contractions in preterm labor may be less intense but still cause your cervix to dilate.

# Will I really know when I'm in labor?

You may fear going to the hospital, thinking you're in labor, and getting sent home, still pregnant. Does it happen a lot? Yes, it does! If you're giving birth at home, at least you won't have a demoralizing trip back home after your midwife checks things out. Most doctors err on the side of caution and send you to the hospital if you sound as if you may be in labor. If getting a reputation as the couple with the most dry runs before actual labor bothers you, keep these pointers in mind:

✔ Real labor contractions don't change or disappear when you lie down, walk around, take a nap, or go shopping.

✔ False labor contractions often occur mostly in your lower abdomen; real labor contractions often but not always start in your back and radiate around the front and also involve the upper abdomen.

✔ Real labor contractions get closer together and more intense.

✔ Real labor contractions normally last 40 to 60 seconds. Fleeting pains that last just a few seconds aren't contractions.

✔ Real labor contractions are often accompanied by an increase in bloody show.

✔ Real labor contractions require you to stop what you're doing. If you can keep talking or walking through contractions, it's either not real labor or it's very early labor.

If your water breaks, call your practitioner whether or not you're having contractions.

## Recognizing signs of early labor

If false labor is common, how can you recognize the real thing? Although every labor is different, a few things don't change from one woman's labor to another. Consider that you may be in real labor if several of the following circumstances apply to you:

✔ Your contractions are becoming more regular — but they don't have to be five minutes apart!

✔ You can't walk or talk during contractions.

✔ You've been having contractions for an hour or more despite changing your position or walking around.

✔ You're having an increased amount of vaginal discharge or a small amount of blood mixed in with mucus.

You can find more about the early stages of labor later in this chapter in the section "Stage 1: What happens in labor."

# I'm Packing My Bag, I'm Ready to Go

If you're giving birth outside your home, the signs of early labor may have you running for your birth bag. You did pack your birth bag, didn't you? Birth outside your home requires lots of stuff, some of which is fairly obvious and some of which you may not have thought of yet.

Labor is no time to start packing a bag, so make sure you've got your things ready to go at least a month before your due date, just in case your little bundle decides to surprise you with an early arrival.

## What's in your birth bag?

The contents of your birth bag may vary from your best friend's, depending on your particular birth plan, but every birth bag should include the following basics:

- A few copies of your birth plan, along with some chocolates to help the nurses warm up to you.

- The real essentials: your health-insurance card and any insurance and hospital paperwork you need. Put these items in an envelope in the bag so they're easy to find. Or you can stick the envelope in the glove compartment of the car so you won't forget it at the last minute.

- A list of people to call, including their phone numbers (or program the numbers into your cellphone).

- A spare cellphone charger. Don't forget to grab your phone on the way to the hospital; if you have an extra charger you don't have to worry about whether it's charged.

- A camera and video cam, along with extra batteries and an extra memory card, if you're going that route.

- An outfit for the baby to come home in. Pick something small — newborns often swim even in newborn clothing. If it's winter, you may also want a few warm receiving blankets.

- Lip balm for dry lips.

- Nursing bras; if you're not planning on nursing, pack supportive bras.

- A robe, slippers, and comfortable old nightgowns you won't mind discarding after delivery. Throw in an oversize t-shirt if you intend to labor in water and don't want to be stark naked in front of everyone.

✔ Makeup — you really may feel the need for it the day after delivery! The hospital will supply shampoo, toothpaste, toothbrush, and soap, but you can pack your own if you prefer your usual brands. Take your hair-brush and a few hairbands or ties to pull your hair out of your face if you have long hair. You may also want to bring deodorant and some nice hand lotion.

✔ A baby book or some other keepsake to record the baby's footprints.

✔ A hand-held personal fan can help you stay cool when things get hot in labor.

✔ A journal, even if you use it just to jot down which breast you started with last feeding.

✔ Books on breast-feeding or newborn care, for both leisurely and frantic browsing. (You're not the only one unsure how to care for that black umbilical cord stump!)

✔ Snacks, including granola bars, crackers, dried fruit, and nuts. Your part-ner can snack during labor, and you'll want them for after the birth. You may also want spare change for vending machines.

✔ Music you want to hear during labor, along with any other comfort tools. See Chapter 8 for more suggestions for soothing your mind and body.

Install the baby car seat before you go into labor; that way, you'll know how it goes in the car and you won't have to fool with it before you leave the hos-pital. Many stores that sell car seats have certified car-seat experts who can install the seat properly and teach you how to do so in the future. Many hospi-tals won't let you leave unless you have an installed car seat for the baby.

## What should you leave at home?

Some items have no place in your birth bag. Leave these things at home in your bureau drawers:

✔ **Clothes you wore pre-pregnancy:** They won't fit right after delivery, and trying them on will just demoralize you, so don't set yourself up for fail-ure. Take your least maternity-looking shirt and pants instead.

✔ **Nice nightgowns:** Unfortunately, they'll simply get ruined if you wear them in the first few days after delivery, when bleeding is heaviest. Hydrogen peroxide will remove any stains if they do get messy.

✔ **Jewelry:** It's at risk of being stolen, sadly, even in a posh hospital. Leave your good earrings and rings at home.

# Taking a Guided Tour through the Basics of Birthing

Your childbirth education classes provide an overview of what to expect during labor and delivery, but the information they teach may be either too simplistic or too far over your head to really sink in. If you take classes fairly early in your pregnancy, you may forget most of what you learned by the time labor finally rolls around. Or labor may seem too far away and abstract until the big day gets closer. (For coverage of childbirth classes, turn to Chapter 7.)

For all these reasons, we give you the basics of what to expect during labor and delivery in this section. Medical personnel divide labor into three stages. Stage 1 labor includes everything up to the pushing stage, which is called Stage 2. (Stage 3 happens after the baby has arrived, and we discuss that part later in this chapter.) Knowing what to expect at each stage helps you create a birth plan that will take you through each stage of labor and delivery.

## Stage 1: What happens in labor

Labor usually starts out slowly and progresses over a number of hours. Often, the early stages of labor move faster when you've already had at least one baby, but labor has lots of variables and this situation may not hold true for you. The baby's position and size can make a difference in the progression of labor. Your birth plan shouldn't need to address too many early-labor details, because hopefully you'll be at home through most of this stage.

### Puttering around in early labor

The early phase of Stage 1 takes the longest. It's the stage in which you may spend several hours — or even as long as a day — trying to figure out whether or not you should go to the hospital.

The early phase of Stage 1 starts when you begin to have regular contractions and ends when you reach 4 centimeters of dilation. The average length of time (which is highly variable from woman to woman) spent in early Stage 1 labor is between 8 and 12 hours. Second and subsequent labors usually progress faster.

Early Stage 1 labor is when most false alarms and unfruitful runs to the hospital occur. If you're having irregular contractions or contractions that are still far apart (ten minutes or more), it's not time to go to the hospital, unless your water breaks. If that happens, call your practitioner, who will probably tell you to head for the hospital, if that's where you're delivering.

Contractions in early labor can be painful, but they're more easily dealt with than the contractions of the active phase of Stage 1. Taking pain medication in the early part of labor can bring the whole process to a halt. If you have an epidural in the early stage of labor, you're more likely to need drugs such as oxytocin to get your labor moving. The more medical interventions you have in labor, the more likely you are to end up having a cesarean birth, which is why trying natural soothing techniques first can be beneficial. Staying home as long as you can, typically until you can't walk or talk through contractions, can also help you avoid too many early interventions. Chapter 11 gives you the rundown on different medications options in labor and their pros and cons, and Chapter 8 describes some natural soothing techniques.

The early phase of Stage 1 is a good time to do the following things:

- ✔ **Utilize the pain relief methods that don't involve medication, such as spending time in a tub, walking, massage, breathing, and birth balls.** (We discuss these options in Chapters 8 and 9.) *Note:* If your water has broken, you may want to talk to your medical practitioner before getting in the bathtub. Although research hasn't found that getting into the tub after your water breaks increases your risk of infection, your doctor still may prefer you not utilize the tub and that you come into the hospital if that's where you're giving birth.

- ✔ **Stay home, if you're leaving home to deliver.**

- ✔ **Get your bed and spa ready if you're birthing at home.**

- ✔ **Alert your partner, midwife, and doula that you're starting labor.** If it's the middle of the night, you can wait until morning before calling your doula and midwife, unless labor starts to get serious before the sun rises.

- ✔ **Get as much rest as possible so you're not worn out when the active phase of labor begins.**

- ✔ **Continue to drink and eat lightly to give you energy for the active part of labor.** See Chapter 10 for more on eating during labor.

### Moving right along in the active phase

The active phase of Stage 1, which lasts from 4 centimeters to 7 or 8 centimeters, is where things really get moving in labor. You normally can't walk or talk during contractions in the active phase of labor. Contractions typically last between 45 seconds to one minute and come every three to five minutes. For this stage of labor, your birth plan should address the following points:

- ✔ **Nourishment, including intravenous fluids:** Some hospitals allow only ice chips and insist on an intravenous infusion. If your hospital is more lenient or if you're giving birth somewhere else, turn to Chapter 10 for info on nourishment during labor.

- ✔ **Medication:** If an epidural is on your birth-plan wish list, this phase is the time to get one. You will need an intravenous infusion if you want an epidural because the medications used can drop your blood pressure if you're not well hydrated. (See Chapter 11 for details on pain meds.)

✔ **Your activity level and how and where you want to give birth:** Note if you want to walk through labor, labor in a birthing tub, or use a birthing ball or other pain-relieving techniques that require you to be out of bed. Continuous monitoring, which is routine in most hospital settings, can limit your movement, so stating your desire to remain active is important. (Chapter 8 covers natural soothing techniques, Chapter 9 covers your movement options in more detail, and Chapter 12 covers monitoring.)

✔ **Vaginal exams:** Because frequent vaginal exams are often the rule in this stage, you may also want to specify who can check you, how often, and when, such as during a contraction or not. (See Chapter 12 for more on cervical checks.)

✔ **Rupture of your membranes:** Intended to speed up your labor, this procedure doesn't always work and may increase the pain you're feeling. (See Chapter 13 for more about artificial rupture of membranes.)

✔ **Use of an internal monitor to measure your baby's heart rate or contractions:** Internal monitors for the baby's heart rate are screwed into your baby's scalp. There's no really nice way to say this, but the wire goes only into the skin and doesn't affect the brain in any way. It's necessary to attach it this way because you can't get a sticky electrode to stay on a baby's wet head. If it's hard to pick up your baby's heart rate or if some question of fetal distress arises, you may want to allow this procedure.

The birth participants (the doctor or midwife, nurses, doula, your partner, or whomever you choose) take an active role in helping you through this stage of labor, which can last between four and eight hours on average. However, coauthor Sharon has seen both primips (women having their first baby) and multips (women who have delivered before) progress very quickly, in an hour or less, after they hit 4 centimeters. Many factors can affect your progress in this stage, including:

✔ **Whether or not you've had an epidural:** It can slow your labor in some cases and speed it up in others.

✔ **Your baby's position:** If your baby's head is facing forward (called a *posterior position*) rather than toward your back, labor often moves more slowly. (See the section "Dealing with your baby's position and labor" later in this chapter for more on the impact of fetal position.)

✔ **The shape of your pelvis:** Every woman's pelvis is shaped slightly differently, which can affect your baby's ability to navigate the turns.

✔ **Your position:** You may dilate faster if you stay upright rather than lying down, because the pressure of the baby's head applied to the cervix helps open it up.

✔ **Your mental state:** If you become anxious or fearful, labor may not progress well. Some women's labors slow down when entering the hospital for this very reason.

The following tips can help you through the active phase of labor:

  ✔ **Use your birth partners to help you get through it.** Some women want their partners to count off the seconds during a contraction; others hate it. You may need a lot of physical contact or may prefer not to be touched. Figure out what works for you and tell the people with you to do it! Chapter 8 includes lots of comfort options, and Chapter 19 talks about being a better support partner.

  ✔ **Change what's not working.** If hee-hee-hoo isn't working for you anymore, try something else. Get out of bed and move around. Experiment with different positions; don't feel locked into using the same technique to get you through the entire labor if it's not working.

  ✔ **Walk around if you can.** The goal of this part of labor is to open the cervix, so take advantage of gravity to push the baby's head against the cervix. Chapter 9 includes more details on movement and positions for labor.

  ✔ **Take medication if it's part of your birth plan.** Pain medication is less likely to slow down labor after you reach the active stage. But narcotics can affect your baby's breathing at delivery if you take them too close to the time he's born, so talk to your practitioner about the optimal timing for narcotics in labor.

  ✔ **Find a mental groove.** Patterned breathing, rocking movements, or vocalizations (like moaning or mantras) during contractions help some women find a rhythm for labor, aiding their relaxation. It also keeps a positive focus on labor.

### Getting through the tumultuous transition

Transition is the last part of Stage 1 labor and lasts from around 7 centimeters to complete dilation, which is 10 centimeters. Transition is often the most difficult part of labor; you may start to feel urges to push, but if you push too soon, the cervix can swell. On the other hand, some practitioners may encourage you to push as your body demands if you feel a strong urge, believing your body knows best. Fighting your body's urges to push while dealing with the strongest contractions of labor makes transition a tough time for many women as well as for their birth partners.

Transition normally lasts from 30 minutes to two hours but can progress much more quickly if you've delivered before. Contractions come every two to three minutes and last 60 to 90 seconds, so you get little breathing time between them.

You may find yourself shocked at the things that come out of your mouth during transition; it's the time when you may use words you didn't know you knew. Flashes of anger, swearing, lashing out at your partner, and feeling overwhelmed with a sea of emotions are all common occurrences during transition. You may shake uncontrollably, vomit, or just feel nauseated. You're most likely to say, "I can't do this anymore!" during this stage — but you can!

Use these tips to get through transition without overly offending your partner, friends, and family:

- ✔ **Warn them ahead of time that you may say things you don't mean.**

- ✔ **Go with what works for you.** You may feel better on all fours, squatting, or spending time in the tub or on the birthing ball. If you're using breathing techniques, you may need to change them in this stage to get through the contractions.

- ✔ **Remember that this stage is usually short.** Even better, it means that you're almost to the finish line of the first stage of labor!

- ✔ **Work through one contraction at a time.** Try to keep your mind in the here and now and don't worry about the next contraction. Stay in the labor rhythm you've established.

### Dealing with your baby's position and labor

Your baby's position can have a big impact on your labor. Around 80 percent of babies go through labor head down, with the face pointing toward the mother's back. This position is called the *occiput anterior* position, and it's the position that gives the baby the most room to maneuver through the pelvis. You can see the occiput anterior position in Figure 2-4a.

The shape of your pelvis can increase the chance that your baby presents in an *occiput posterior* position; see Figure 2-4b. In around 20 percent of cases, the baby's looking forward, with his back to the mother's back, so that he's born "sunny-side up." You and your practitioner may be able to feel the difference before delivery; she may suggest fetal positioning exercises to change the baby's position. You may have the following experiences if you have a posterior baby:

- ✔ Your abdomen may feel less firm because you can't palpate the baby's back, which is towards your back.

- ✔ You may feel lots of kicks and hand and arm movements towards the front of your abdomen.

- ✔ You may feel more backache pains both before and during labor.

- ✔ You may become more constipated.

- ✔ You may leak urine, caused by pressure of the baby's forehead on your bladder.

- ✔ Your practitioner may have more difficulty hearing the fetal heartbeat.

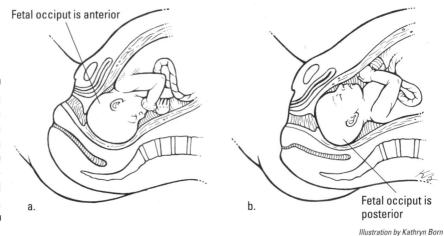

Fetal occiput is anterior

**Figure 2-4:**
The difference between anterior (a) and posterior (b) head positions.

a.     b.

Fetal occiput is posterior

*Illustration by Kathryn Born*

Don't despair if you have a posterior baby. You can take steps before the delivery to help the baby turn. Some babies also turn spontaneously during labor. Your medical practitioner may have suggestions for turning a posterior baby, but these ideas may also help:

- ✔ **Use your maternal influence.** Take a warm, relaxing bath and talk to your baby, telling him to move into the right position while gently massaging your abdomen and visualizing your baby in the correct position. Think it sounds like voodoo? It often works, so don't knock it until you've tried it!

- ✔ **Assume a knee-chest position several times a day for up to 20 minutes at a time.** You can also try using a slant board, which positions your feet above your head, if your practitioner approves.

For some other suggestions on getting your baby to move into a good position for labor and delivery, check out the website www.spinningbabies.com. Talk to your medical practitioner about the techniques the site recommends.

If your baby's *breech,* coming into the world feet or buttocks first, many practitioners prefer to schedule a cesarean section. The art of delivering breech babies has largely been lost in most hospitals today, because of the increased risk of complications to the baby and the increased risk of liability for obstetricians. You can try the same mobilizing techniques to get your breech baby to turn as for a posterior baby.

Your doctor may also schedule a *version,* an attempt to turn the baby before delivery. A version involves the practitioner trying to manipulate the baby's position from the outside of your abdomen, using her hands to gently push the baby into a different position. This procedure is often done under mild anesthesia under ultrasound guidance. It can cause complications, so your practitioner will monitor your baby's heart rate to make sure it doesn't drop during the procedure, which would necessitate an immediate cesarean delivery.

# Stage 2: Pushing at last!

When your cervix opens to the full 10 centimeters, it's time for the big push! If you're not having an epidural, you'll probably start pushing as soon as you get to 10 centimeters or when your body starts feeling the urge. If you have an epidural, your practitioner may let you *labor down,* which means that you let the contractions bring the baby down without pushing. You'll still have to push at the end, but you may push for less time.

Your birth plan can address several pushing issues, including how hard to push and whether or not you want to watch the birth in a mirror. Some moms also want to help "guide" the baby out of the birth canal with their hands.

### Pushing your way to the end

The second stage of labor can last anywhere from two minutes to three hours. Generally, you push longer with your first baby, but your baby's size and position play a part in how long you push as well. You can stipulate how and where you would like to push in your birth plan.

Many women find pushing invigorating because it's active. Because of the pressure you feel during contractions, pushing can feel good. But pushing can also be a little scary and overwhelming; you may be afraid that this humongous baby will never get out of such a little space! These feelings are all quite normal.

In this stage, the way you push may be influenced by the type of childbirth class you took (see Chapter 7), what your practitioners feel is the best way to push, and even what the nurse with you during labor thinks is the best way to push. Some practitioners want you to hold your breath and push as hard and as long as you can, but this method can decrease fetal oxygenation and increase your risk of severe vaginal tears. Others prefer *instinctive pushing* (also called *soft pushing*), which means pushing just as much or as little as your body demands. You can indicate in your birth plan the wish to use instinctive pushing instead of coached pushing. If you have an epidural, you probably won't feel enough urge to push and will have to push when directed. Turning down the epidural near the end of labor can be helpful. Staying upright and using gravity to push gives you the best results; lying flat on your back and trying to push uphill takes longer.

Some hospitals have squatting bars that attach to the bed that you can use to hold onto while squatting and pushing. If you remain in the bed, you can crank up the bed and pull your legs back to open the vaginal canal as much as possible while pushing, though a semi-sitting position may increase your risk of vaginal tears. (We talk more about pushing position options, along with their pros and cons, in Chapter 9.)

Your birth attendants can see the progress you're making as you push when the baby's head comes into view. You won't be able to see without the aid of a mirror, because your still-pregnant stomach gets in the way. You can feel the top of the baby's head with your hand as it appears; it may give you the incentive to keep pushing if you start getting tired.

If you're utilizing a birthing tub for your delivery, some practitioners may prefer that you labor in the tub but get out for the actual delivery. Read up on water births in Chapter 9.

### Hey there, baby!

The actual birth of your baby is the last part of Stage 2 labor. As your baby passes through the birth canal, he needs to make several turns to navigate the bony parts of your pelvis. If you're looking in a mirror while pushing in an upright or semi-siting position, you may see any of the following:

- ✔ If your baby is occiput anterior, his head will appear face down. If he's posterior, he'll be looking up.

- ✔ After his whole head is out, his head will turn to either the right or left. (Most babies turn to the right, a position known as right occiput anterior, or ROA.) He needs to rotate to get the shoulders under the pubic bone.

   Your practitioner may gently pull the baby toward your rear end slightly to get his shoulder under the pubic bone.

- ✔ Because the baby's head is usually his largest part, the rest of his body slips out easily after his head is out and turns.

Some babies have shoulders that are wider than their heads. These babies can get hung up in the birth canal after the head is delivered, a condition called *shoulder dystocia*. Your practitioner may need to take immediate action to get your baby out, including cutting an episiotomy or having you change position to give the baby more space to get the shoulder under the pubic bone. Pulling your legs close to your chest to mimic a squat or changing from one side to the other can also help. Shoulder dystocia is a true medical emergency and can require drastic and rapid action to prevent complications for your baby. Listen carefully to your practitioner's instructions and try to tune out extraneous sounds.

## Planning for a scheduled cesarean

A birth plan can help you even if you know you're having a cesarean delivery. You can address whether you want to go into labor naturally, essentially letting your body decide the delivery day, or whether you want to schedule the date. You can also plan in advance who is with you in the operating room, how you can hold the baby right after birth, and whether the baby stays with you in the recovery room (which has become routine in many hospitals). Chapter 14 has all the details about C-section delivery and your birth plan.

# Making It through the Afterbirth and Aftermath

Everything in your life changes as soon as you meet your baby for the first time. Although the practitioner still has to take care of some medical necessities after the baby's out, such as delivery of the placenta and any surgical repair necessary, your attention may be entirely on your baby. Your birth plan should address the care your baby receives in the first minutes of life, who cuts the umbilical cord, what you want done with the placenta, who announces the sex of the baby, and how soon you initiate breast-feeding. Chapter 13 goes into greater detail on handling the third stage of delivery.

## Stage 3: Tying up loose ends

After your baby's out, your practitioner still has some loose ends to attend to and, in some cases, to literally sew up. One such task is cutting the cord. Some practitioners cut the cord immediately after delivery, whereas others don't cut until the cord stops pulsating, which gives the baby more blood from the placenta. (Chapter 15 discusses delayed cord cutting in more detail.)

The delivery of the placenta usually follows the baby within 5 to 15 minutes. You may feel gentle tugging on the placenta or contractions — and you thought you were done with those! — with the delivery of the placenta. A delay in the arrival of the placenta could mean that you have a placenta accreta, meaning that the placenta is tightly adhered to the uterine wall. Placenta accreta is more common if you've had previous D&Cs, or *dilation and curettage,* a procedure that involves scraping the lining of the uterus. You may have had a D&C with a previous miscarriage for diagnostic purposes or with an abortion. Uterine surgery can also increase your risk. See Chapter 13 for more about placenta accreta.

The uterus needs to contract after delivery to stop bleeding from the site where the placenta was attached. So as soon as the placenta delivers, many practitioners give oxytocin, better known by the brand name Pitocin, to stimulate uterine contractions and reduce the risk of post-partum hemorrhage. Breast-feeding immediately after the delivery can also encourage the uterus to contract. (See Chapter 13 for more detail.)

Several things in the third stage may find a place in your birth plan:

- ✔ Who should cut the cord
- ✔ Whether the cord should be cut immediately or only after it stops pulsating
- ✔ Whether you've made arrangements to bank cord blood for your baby
- ✔ Whether you want to take the placenta home and bury it near a special tree or in a certain area

If you want to save the placenta, take care to include this intention in your birth plan and remind the staff right after delivery, because normally the placenta goes into a container not long after delivery. (See Chapter 15 for the particulars on issues related to the third stage of labor.)

## *Meeting your baby*

Your first meeting with your baby can comprise a big part of a birth plan. If you deliver in a hospital, you may find that a staff member will try to whisk the baby away right after delivery to be dried off, weighed, and measured, with a promise to "bring him back in a few minutes." You, on the other hand, may want to have immediate skin-to-skin contact with the baby and bring him up to the breast to nurse right after delivery, deferring the weighing and measuring ritual until later. If the baby is placed on your tummy skin-to-skin, if allowed time, he may even appear to "crawl" up to the breast to nurse. Amazing but true!

Make these wishes clear in your birth plan. No medical reason requires that the baby be immediately cleaned up and weighed; it's done for staff convenience. Of course, if your baby's having any type of breathing difficulty or doesn't look well, the need for immediate medical care may outweigh the need for bonding.

Most hospitals also place prophylactic eye drops in the baby's eyes to prevent infections picked up in the vaginal tract and give an injection of vitamin K to prevent excessive bleeding. You may need to clarify your wishes regarding these practices in your birth plan. Chapter 16 provides more details.

If you've never seen a newborn, your first meeting could be a bit of a surprise. Real babies look nothing like the ones on TV shows. When first born, they're blue. They gradually pink up in a minute or so but may still be mottled, with bluish hands and feet. Don't be surprised by any of the following characteristics at birth:

- ✔ **Hair all over his back:** Newborns lose this hair in the last few weeks before birth, but if your baby's a little early, he may still be a little hairy.

✔ **Peeling skin:** If your baby's a bit past his due date, he may have peeling skin on his hands and feet. He may also look a little scrawny from loss of subcutaneous fat, which is common in babies born a week or two after their due dates.

✔ **Huge genitals:** Hormones can cause both male and female genitalia to appear out of all proportion to their size. This temporary condition is not necessarily a sign of things to come.

✔ **Wobbliness:** New babies often look like they'll fall apart if you move them. Their head needs constant support and their arms and legs can appear to fly off in different directions. Your baby is actually much more put together and tough than he looks at first glance.

## *Being a new mom in the first few days*

The first day or two of new motherhood may be nothing like you envisioned it. You may be tired from a long labor or heavy blood loss. Your baby may not nurse well, being either too sleepy or too frantic to latch on to the nipple properly, leaving you feeling like a frustrated failure.

And in addition to being on an emotional roller coaster, you have to listen to instructions that the nurses have to give you before you leave the hospital, you may have a roomful of visitors from dawn to dusk, and you have lots of decisions to make about your baby's name, when to have the hospital photographer come in, and whether your baby should have immunizations before going home. Making these decisions ahead of time and addressing them in your birth plan gives you fewer things to worry about at the spur of the moment.

Most hospitals and birth centers today offer *rooming-in,* which means the baby stays with you all day and overnight. In fact, with the new emphasis on customer satisfaction in medical care, hospitals often vie to outdo each other with their décor and amenities for the whole family. Some include a regular bed for your partner; others offer at least a chair that converts into a bed. Most have fairly liberal visiting hours compared to the "visitors from 2–4 and 7–8 only" rules common in hospitals 30 years ago.

Following are some issues to specifically address in your birth plan related to the new-mom stage:

✔ **Feeding your baby:** Note whether you'll be breast-feeding, using formula, or doing a little of both. If you're breast-feeding, include whether you will allow supplemental feedings and under what conditions. (Chapter 17 tells you all you need to know about breast-feeding.) Some hospitals are quick to offer a night feeding of formula so you can sleep or to keep the baby in the nursery, but this can cause problems with breast-feeding. Make your wishes clear about supplemental feedings that are not medically necessary.

✔ **Circumcising:** Decide whether you want your baby boy circumcised and if you want to be present at the time. (We talk about this decision more in Chapter 16.)

✔ **Immunizing:** You should be clear about what immunizations and medications you want your baby to have. (We discuss your options in Chapter 16 in detail.)

✔ **Testing:** Hospitals routinely test newborns for genetic disorders such as PKU. See Chapter 16 for more about what testing is done and how to refuse if you don't want it.

## Dealing with physical changes after birth

If you had a tear or episiotomy repair, you may be quite sore for the first few days. After birth, cramps can also cause pain. When your milk comes in, your breasts become hard and often somewhat painful, especially if you're not nursing. Pain medication can help you out with the discomforts of early motherhood.

Bleeding is often heavy in the first week after delivery. If you engage in too much activity after you go home, you could experience an alarming increase in bleeding. An increase in bleeding is often accompanied by an increase in cramping. Never hesitate to call your doctor or ask the nurses in the hospital about the amount of bleeding you're having.

Your breasts can be a source of considerable discomfort in the first few days of motherhood. Not only do they hurt when your milk comes in, but your nipples may become sore and cracked, especially if your baby isn't latching on properly. Cold cabbage leaves may help relieve engorgement pain, but nipple pain caused by a poor latch needs additional help to heal. Enlist the aid of a lactation consultant (most hospitals today have one) to make sure you have a good latch-on before you go home. (See Chapter 17 for more on breast-feeding.)

## Coping with Postpartum Hormonal Adjustments

Your estrogen and progesterone levels drop very quickly after giving birth, leaving you with emotions that range from wild euphoria and happiness to anxiety, fear, and depression. A new baby in your life also adds to the chaos of the time. In this section, we offer advice on riding the postpartum hormonal roller coaster, recognizing when your moods may need professional attention, and making what should be a happy time in your life a bit less stressful.

## Recognizing baby blues and postpartum depression

You may find yourself swinging between complete happiness with your baby and your new family status to complete despair at ever getting your body or your life back to normal. Crying jags, heightened sensitivity to remarks from family or friends, and a feeling of letdown are common. Around 80 percent of all new moms experience a mild depressive state known as the *baby blues.*

Although these feelings are completely normal as long as they're fleeting, some women become seriously depressed after childbirth. If you're really struggling emotionally, in many cases you won't recognize just how far you've fallen from your normally cheery self. But the people around you will.

If you suffered from depression before you got pregnant, you may experience worse bouts in the first few weeks after delivery. But even if you've been Mary Sunshine all your life, you can still develop clinical depression after delivery. We discuss this risk in more detail in Chapter 20, but be aware that depression can affect anyone, and realize you may be getting too close to the edge and need help if

- ✔ You're unable to carry out normal activities.

- ✔ You find yourself resenting or disliking your baby or thinking that he dislikes you.

- ✔ You sleep too much. Though this situation isn't common for new moms, if you pull the covers over your head at every free moment, you may be deep into depression.

See your doctor or other medical practitioner immediately if you develop these or other symptoms of depression. Sometimes your friends or family may recognize depression symptoms before you do. If they bring the subject up, try not to get defensive; realize they are trying to help. Postpartum depression doesn't make you a bad mom, but it can make being a good mom much harder. Seek help for not only for your benefit but also your baby's benefit.

## Getting back to your un-pregnant self

It takes time for the dust to settle and for your moods and your body to get back to normal after you've given birth. Nothing in your birth plan can prepare you for the utter chaos one small baby can bring into your house. Some babies eat every four hours like clockwork and sleep 20 hours a day in the first few weeks, leaving you plenty of time to do the laundry and clean the kitchen. But other babies cry incessantly, sleep what seems like 20 minutes a day, and want to nurse constantly, leaving you precious little time to do anything other than catch a few winks when you get a chance.

Getting your body back in shape can help both your mental and physical states. You can normally begin exercising within a few weeks after birth, after you stop having heavy *lochia,* the post-pregnancy discharge. You can also boost your mental state by improving your diet as you settle in with your little one. Don't use nursing as an excuse to eat for two: Producing breast milk takes only an extra 300 to 500 calories per day.

Being a new mom can be an isolating experience if all your friends are still working or don't have kids yet. Before delivery, plan ahead with some of these tips to ward off the isolation that can worsen depression:

- **Stagger your visitors.** Everyone wants to see the baby immediately, but that leaves you with an overwhelming number of visitors in the first week and no one to help you after that. Let your partner help out the first week, your mom the next, and your in-laws the next, or whatever schedule works for you.

- **Make mom-friends.** Mom-friends are people in the same boat as you. Childbirth classes can be an excellent source of mom-friends because your babies are around the same age. Look around your neighborhood for people wheeling strollers; you may not have noticed them back when you were leaving for work at 6:30 every morning.

- **Get out of the house.** Just taking a walk around the block or going to the mall can lift your spirits and negate the feeling that the walls are closing in on you. If getting out of the house feels too hard, try making smaller goals.

  When coauthor Rachel was fighting the blues after the birth of her twins, she challenged herself to just get the babies into the stroller outside her apartment. If she got to take a walk around the block with them, that was a bonus! This small step was extremely helpful.

# Part II
# Choosing Your Birth Team, Birth Place, and Guests

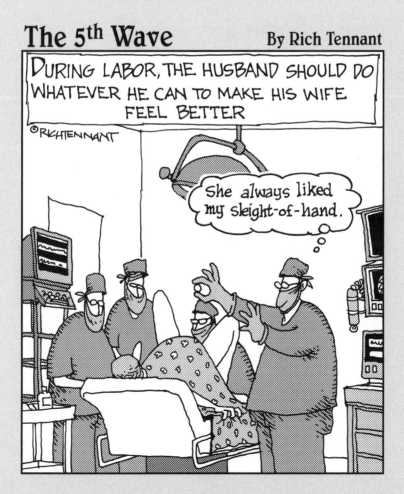

# In this part . . .

The birth of your baby is one of the biggest events of your life. Deciding on the *who* and the *where* are two of the most important parts of planning any big event, and that includes your labor and delivery. In this part, we look not only at who should be at your birth but where to hold the big event. We also help you pick a practitioner who will support your decisions and guide you and your baby safely through the experience of birth.

# Chapter 3

# OB-GYN, Family Practitioners, Midwives, Oh My!

· · · · · · · · · · · · · · · · · · · · · · · · · · · · · · · · · · · · · · ·

· · · · · · · · · · · · · · · · · · · · · · · · · · · · · · · · · · · · · · ·

Choosing the right person to help you through your baby's birth can be easy if you already have a gynecologist you love who also delivers babies. Finding the right person can also be quite difficult, though, if you're looking for someone out of the mainstream, such as a midwife who will do a home delivery. In this chapter, we describe the different options you have, the pros and cons of each, and how your choice of a practitioner can influence all the other decisions you make during pregnancy, including what goes into your birth plan.

# Finding the Right Obstetrician

The primary medial-care provider most women use during pregnancy is an obstetrician/gynecologist. The ideal situation is to have your gynecologist — someone who you already know and, hopefully, trust — be your birth practitioner. This solution isn't always as easy it sounds, though. Many gynecologists stop practicing obstetrics at a certain age, either because they're tired of getting up for deliveries in the middle of the night or because the risk of being sued and the rising costs of medical malpractice have driven them to it.

Even if your gynecologist practices obstetrics, he may not be the best person for the job of guiding you through labor and delivery, for various reasons. In this section, we talk about the pros and cons of staying with the familiar versus finding someone new.

# Enjoying the benefits of sticking with Dr. Familiar

You've gone to Dr. Familiar since you were a teen, and he knows your insides inside out. Although you've never really talked about his philosophical views on pregnancy, childbirth, and breast-feeding, you're pretty sure he practices the type of obstetrics you're looking for: open to patient input, willing to try new things, and not set in a rigid mindset.

If Dr. Familiar fits the bill, you're very fortunate. You know him, he knows you, the office has all your insurance information, and you don't have to interview new candidates. You may already know where he does deliveries. If Dr. Familiar meets all your requirements, there are no drawbacks to sticking with someone you already know and trust.

Most doctors who deliver babies today are trained obstetricians. However, in some parts of the country, some family-medicine doctors or general practitioners still do deliveries. This practice is far less common than it was a few decades ago, due to the high cost of malpractice insurance for doctors who practice obstetrics. Most general practitioners don't have the salaries to support expensive malpractice costs. But if your general practitioner is willing and able to do the delivery and you're very comfortable with him, you can stay with him. General practitioners are not able to do surgery; if you need a cesarean section, he will make arrangements for an obstetrician to perform the surgery.

# Recognizing when the perfect GYN isn't the perfect OB for you

Sometimes the perfect gynecologist isn't the perfect obstetrician for you. If you've been going to your GYN since you were a teenager, his paternalistic "there, there" approach that was reassuring when you were younger may not be what you're looking for in an OB. Why else would you ever think of leaving your trusted GYN for another obstetrician? Let us count the ways!

✔ You have fundamental differences on basic birth issues. These differences can be anything from having a reputation for a high cesarean delivery rate to an insistence on doing childbirth a certain way, such as saying he won't do your delivery if you don't consent to an IV in labor.

✔ He doesn't deliver at the hospital you want to use.

✔ He's a "let me take care of everything" doctor, which you may have appreciated when you were 15, but now you want to feel free to ask questions, make decisions, and have access to all your medical information.

✔ He doesn't take your insurance. Although this problem isn't likely if you're already seeing him for GYN care, you may encounter it if you have to change insurance providers because your old provider doesn't cover obstetrics.

Changing doctors is never easy or fun, especially if you been with your GYN for any amount of time. But it's not unheard of, and your doctor has certainly been through this situation in the past. Most practitioners take it philosophically and move on. Some will want to know why you're changing practitioners and will call to find out; others won't.

## *Asking the right questions*

Whether you're interviewing Dr. Familiar for the new job of baby catcher or interviewing a doctor you've never met before, you need to ask the right questions to determine whether or not he's the right person. Start with this list and add questions that address your particular concerns:

✔ **Where do you deliver?** Many doctors deliver at just one hospital, but some have delivery privileges at more than one hospital. If yours delivers at several hospitals, ask which hospital he utilizes the most. Many doctors do only a few deliveries at one hospital and the lion's share at another, and if your doctor is doing two other deliveries at his preferred hospital the night you go into labor, chances of getting him over to the "other" hospital for your delivery are slim to none. You could end up delivering somewhere you've never been and didn't want to go. You can still go to the hospital of your choice, but you'll be seen essentially as a patient without a doctor and be assigned to whoever is on call — not an ideal situation.

If an epidural is in your birth plan, ask if the hospital has 24-hour anesthesia coverage. Some hospitals have to call in an anesthesiologist during the night to do epidurals, which means you may have to wait.

✔ **Will I see all the partners for prenatal care? Can I choose who I'd like for the delivery?** Because OB is a demanding specialty, most OBs work in group practices. You may love all the partners but one — and fear she'll be the one who's covering when you go into labor. It's hard to ask this question nicely, but ask if there's any way you can avoid having Dr. Uncomfortable deliver, even if she's on call the night you go into labor.

✔ **Who covers for you?** This issue arises if your OB is a solo practitioner without partners to cover for him. Although many women don't think of this at the beginning of pregnancy, doctors do go on vacation and other doctors cover their practices. If you don't know the other doctor by name or by reputation, a visit to his office might be helpful. Ask your doctor if he has extended trips planned for the time frame you plan to deliver in.

✔ **When will you come to the hospital?** If you expect your OB to show up at the hospital with your first contraction, you're probably going to be sorely disappointed. In the middle of the night, most OBs won't come in until the nurses tell them you're in active labor. During the day, your doctor may be seeing patients in his office nearby or even doing surgeries, such as scheduled cesarean deliveries. And in some hospitals, anesthesiologists insist on your OB being in the hospital before they'll give you an epidural, so you'll want to know what timing you can expect.

✔ **What's your cesarean rate?** You can expect a bit of bristling at this question, and most doctors will tell you they do only as many cesarean deliveries as necessary. But the wide variation between practitioners and different parts of the country tell you that's not necessarily true.

✔ **How do you feel about induction?** Along with the rate of cesarean section, the induction rate has also risen. Although being induced doesn't sound like such a bad thing when you're 40 weeks pregnant and thoroughly tired of it, inductions are invasive and increase the risk of complications, including C-sections.

✔ **What are your thoughts about [insert whatever is important to you in labor, such as water birth, walking through labor, unmedicated labor, or no episiotomy]?** Some doctors will tell you that those type of decisions are decided on an individual basis, but his general response toward the question may tell you what you need to know. A good answer is, "I'm willing to try it as long as it doesn't compromise your safety or your baby's." However, practice does make perfect, and you may prefer a doctor who has already had some on-the-job training.

# Do You Need a Specialist?

Specialists can help monitor and manage your condition through pregnancy and ensure a safe delivery. If you're what's called a *high-risk patient,* you may need to see a perinatologist or other specialists in addition to your OB or nurse-midwife. High-risk can mean anything from a history of pregnancy loss to a history of genetic disorders or a multiple pregnancy.

Your age may also put you in the high-risk category. These days, being over age 35 is no longer considered a high-risk factor for delivery, although being over 45 may, in some cases. The older you are, the more likely you are to have chronic health disorders such as high blood pressure or diabetes.

## Working with a perinatologist

Perinatologists are obstetricians with two to three years of further training in complications of pregnancy. Most perinatologists don't deliver babies; they coordinate care and see women who have unusual risk factors related to their own health or their baby's health. Your obstetrician may recommend that you see a perinatologist if your baby appears to have a genetic disorder of if you have health issues that could affect your baby. If you have a medical issue or are carrying multiples, you can initiate an appointment yourself as well.

Following are some issues that may necessitate seeing a perinatologist:

- ✔ Fetal birth defects such as heart defects, gastrointestinal malformations, or problems with the lungs or brain
- ✔ Genetic disorders such as trisomy 13, 17, or 21
- ✔ History of early pregnancy loss or stillbirth
- ✔ Multiple pregnancy, especially if you're carrying triplets or other high-order multiples

A perinatologist can perform advanced ultrasound imaging to diagnose problems not normally seen during pregnancy ultrasounds. He may also perform amniocentesis or other diagnostic procedures. A perinatologist will normally monitor your care more closely than an obstetrician would in pregnancy.

You may see a perinatologist just a few times during your pregnancy, or you may see him as often as your obstetrician, depending on what your risk factors are. Depending on your insurance, you may need a referral from your obstetrician before an initial visit.

## Enlarging your team if you have other health issues

If you have a heart condition, an autoimmune disorder such as systemic lupus erythematosus, diabetes, or severe asthma, you may need specialists in these areas on your team during pregnancy as well. If you routinely see several doctors, coordinating their care is important to make sure you're getting medications that won't harm your baby and to ensure that your doctors aren't duplicating medications. Make sure each doctor knows which others you're seeing and have them send copies of medications, lab results, and any other pertinent information to one another to avoid duplication or medications that act at cross-purposes to one another.

If you have diabetes, especially type 1 diabetes, your blood sugar may fluctuate quite a bit during pregnancy. Your doctor will want to maintain tight control over your levels, because high blood sugar can cause birth defects and *macrosomia,* or extra weight gain in your baby. Macrosomia can cause problems during the delivery and may increase your risk of cesarean. (Although some doctors may suggest scheduling a cesarean if the baby appears large on the ultrasound, you should be able to request a trial of labor first because ultrasound measurements are inaccurate and many big babies can be delivered vaginally.)

Very large babies often have difficulty regulating their blood glucose levels after delivery and may need careful observation and frequent blood glucose tests to avoid low blood sugar levels. If you have diabetes during pregnancy, you may want to write specific instructions in your birth plan for doing blood glucose tests on your baby; for example, you may want to hold your baby during sticks and nurse him right afterward for comfort rather than having blood tests done in the nursery. See Chapter 16 for more on newborn testing.

Autoimmune disorders can also cause problems in pregnancy, including blood clots that can cause early pregnancy loss. Heart conditions can affect your activity level in pregnancy as well as the amount of stress you can tolerate in labor. If you normally see a rheumatologist for autoimmune disease when you're not pregnant or a cardiologist for heart disease, make sure they know you're pregnant and can coordinate your care with your obstetrician and possibly a perinatologist.

# Looking for a Midwife

The word *midwife* may conjure up a picture of a woman in a long skirt with sandals on her feet and a baskets of herbs, but midwives today come in all different types. Some midwives have been trained in hospitals, and others, like direct-entry midwives, learned their skills from other midwives through apprenticeship. Others have no formal training, learned their skills from other midwives, and do mostly home deliveries.

A midwife is more likely than an OB to be supportive if you want to deliver at home or in a home-like setting, though midwives also attend hospital births, and they are also more likely to be open to water birth or other alternative types of birth. A midwife may also be less likely to perform invasive procedures such as cutting an episiotomy or rupturing membranes. Midwives often do intermittent fetal monitoring, as opposed to the routine continuous monitoring done in hospitals. (Research has found continuous monitoring to be unnecessary in low-risk women.) They are also unlikely to require routine intravenous fluids, and this together with the intermittent monitoring allows you to move around more in labor. (See Chapter 9 for why staying active in labor is good for you.)

If those or other alternative delivery situations appeal to you, read on to find out how to locate a midwife who can help you.

## Deciding between different types of midwives

Certified nurse-midwives are RNs (registered nurses) who go back to school for advanced training. They have a minimum of a bachelor's degree in nursing (BSN) or master's degree in nursing (MSN), and they often practice in hospitals, although some also have private practices and do home deliveries. Some deliver in birthing centers, where backup is just a phone call away if your case gets too complicated for them to handle. Certified nurse-midwives, for example, don't do cesarean sections.

The American College of Nurse-Midwives, the national organization for CNMs, believes that home birth is a viable option for women and that it's low risk when a qualified birth attendant such as a CNM is present. The American College of Nurse-Midwives website, www.midwife.org, can help you find a certified nurse-midwife in your area.

In addition to CNMs, two other types of midwives generally deliver at home:

- Lay midwives, who have no certifications and have not passed any tests to practice their art
- Certified professional midwives, who have passed written tests and skill tests to become certified by the North American Registry of Midwives

You can get started on finding a midwife at this website: www.mothers naturally.org/midwives.

If you're planning a birth with a midwife, you will probably develop a much different relationship with her than you would with an obstetrician. You may see her more often, and your appointments may be longer and feel more personal. If you're having a home birth, she may come to your home rather than seeing you in an office.

However, not all midwives offer this kind of personalized care, especially those who work together with OBs in an obstetric practice. A certified nurse-midwife may also practice in a clinic along with other CNMs, and you may not have a choice of who you get for your labor. Just as you'd interview an OB to get a feel for her philosophy, you should do the same when considering a midwife. Don't make the mistake of thinking all midwives share the same philosophies on care and birth.

## *Interviewing midwives*

When looking for a midwife to be with you for your entire labor and delivery, you need to make sure you're comfortable with each other and on the same wavelength. And if you go with a midwife-assisted delivery, particularly if you want to give birth at home, it's wise to ask the midwife you're considering some pointed questions aimed at keeping both you and your baby safe during labor and delivery.

Start with the following questions and add any others that pertain to your situation:

- **How long have you been a midwife?** The longer, the better. Childbirth complications are rare, but when they do happen, you want someone with you who has experience in dealing with different scenarios. Some CNMs have had years of nursing experience in areas of maternal-child health before becoming CNMs, which can provide a helpful knowledge base.

- **How were you trained?** You may feel more confident and reassured if the midwife has formal training and certification. However, many midwives who do home births learned from another unschooled but experienced midwife. Even without formal training, many midwives who learned by working with an older midwife often have great skills.

- **What's your philosophy of childbirth?** Although this question sounds a bit hippy-dippy, it's important. Most midwives have a strong belief in natural childbirth and that women's bodies know how to give birth. At the same time, a good midwife also recognizes that life-threatening complications that require immediate intervention — often medical intervention — can occur during or after labor.

- **Are you licensed in this state?** A lay midwife who is not licensed in your state could be prosecuted for practicing medicine or midwifery without a license if something goes wrong. A licensed CNM has the background and training to provide safe care for you and your baby without her — or you! — worrying that she's breaking the law during your birth.

✔ **What's your backup plan?** Every midwife should have one. If you're delivering at home with a lay midwife and complications require you need to go to the hospital, she probably won't be able to go with you, except as a friend. Does she have a physician willing to take her cases, or will you need to go through the emergency room and take whoever you get? A CNM can transfer your care to the obstetrician on-call or to an obstetrician she collaborates with, as one practitioner to another.

✔ **When would you suggest going to the hospital?** A midwife who hasn't planned details like this hasn't done enough deliveries. Of course, if your midwife delivers in a hospital, you don't need to ask this question.

✔ **What supplies do you carry and what emergencies can you handle?** A midwife should have basic supplies in her bag, such as oxytocin in case of postpartum hemorrhage, suction equipment for the baby, and possibly suturing equipment. CNMs carry a small portable oxygen tank and bag and mask for the baby, along with a full complement of resuscitation and monitoring equipment. Lay midwives may not. Lack of equipment or experience in emergency resuscitation is very risky for you and your baby.

✔ **What would you do if two of your clients went into labor at the same time?** Hopefully, she has a backup partner to assist until she can get to the second labor. Get to know the backup partner, just in case she shows up for your delivery.

✔ **What are your fees?** Home birth with a lay midwife isn't usually covered by insurance, so you will most likely be paying these costs out of pocket. However, most insurances, including Medicaid, will cover a CNM's "global care" costs, which includes prenatal care and attending the birth whether at home, in a hospital, or in a birthing center. If the CNM you choose is out-of-network and other CNMs are available in your area who are in-network, be aware that you may have to fight to get reimbursed. Ask your midwife about her clients' past experiences with getting fees covered with your particular insurance provider.

When choosing a midwife, your feelings may have as much to do with your choice as the person's qualifications. If you're not comfortable with a midwife at the beginning or if you don't have the same philosophies, don't try to work it out or think that things will get better as you go through pregnancy. Find someone else before you get too far into your pregnancy to be comfortable changing practitioners.

If you want a home delivery, you may be very limited to just a few midwives in your area. After talking to midwives that do home deliveries, make sure you do the following:

✔ Ask for references, no matter what type of midwife you're considering.

✔ Contact at least three references to get a balanced view. Interview moms who have already delivered so you can get a picture of their complete experience with a particular midwife.

✔ Verify the midwife's licensure via the State Board of Nursing or State Board of Midwifery.

# Deciding on a Doula

The word *doula* comes from a Greek word meaning "a woman who serves." A doula is not a medical practitioner; she provides emotional and physical support throughout labor. Doulas are a fairly new addition to a woman's labor team in the United States, although the tradition of women helping other women through labor goes back centuries. In some cases, doulas take the place of relatives who would have, in times gone by, assisted during childbirth. With the advent of hospital births, especially the over-medicated, drugged-up births that women went through alone in the 1940s through 1960s, the art of assisting friends and relatives through labor has been completely lost in the U.S.

## What does a doula do?

Doulas don't just assist during labor; they can also help you prepare for labor, providing you with information and resources. They also help you in the immediate postpartum period, helping you get started with breast-feeding and referring you to additional professionals if necessary. (If you want daily support after the baby is born, you can look for a postpartum doula, which is different than a labor doula, whose main focus is on childbirth. See Chapter 5 for more on postpartum doulas.)

Doulas have benefits that go beyond the support they give before, during, and after labor. Studies show that women who use doulas are more likely to have a positive birth experience, have a reduced need for pain medications, have shorter labors with fewer complications for mom and baby, are less likely to have a cesarean section, and are also more likely to succeed with breast-feeding.

A doula can help you in the following ways:

✔ Assessing all your labor options and creating your birth plan

✔ Supporting you and your partner before, during, and after labor and delivery

✔ Advocating for your birth plan, sometimes speaking with the birth team directly if necessary (but usually just helping you or your partner speak up and be heard by staff)

✔ Helping you establish breast-feeding and serving as a source of information about routine baby care and typical issues that arise after delivery

✔ Offering pregnancy and birthing extras, like helping you create a belly cast made with plaster during your pregnancy, or taking photos or video during the birth itself

Anyone can call themselves a doula. Interview multiple candidates to make sure you find someone whose personality meshes with both yours and your partner's, and ensure that she's certified by one of the national doula certification organizations like Doulas of North America (DONA), Childbirth and Postpartum Association (CAPPA), or International Childbirth Education Association (ICEA). In this day and age, a background check is also prudent. For more information about hiring a doula, visit www.dona.org.

## Will Dad feel left out?

You may worry about whether Dad will feel like a fifth wheel if you use a doula. Most doulas go out of their way to make sure that the father is a participant in every aspect of the childbearing process, if that's what you and he desire. Not all partners want to be fully involved in all aspects of childbirth! Having a doula there to provide some help and pointers may actually make your partner more confident about his role in labor and delivery and more comfortable handling his newborn.

During labor, knowing your doula is there gives your partner the freedom to leave the room for a few minutes or get something to eat without worrying that you're going to need something. Providing labor support can also be physically intense, and having someone else to massage your back while he takes a breather can really help.

# Switching Medical-Care Providers Late in Your Pregnancy

Sometimes you don't find out until delivery time is close that your medical practitioner has decidedly different views than yours on how labor and delivery should happen. Maybe the doctor who said "We'll work all that out" at the beginning of your pregnancy now says that it's his way or the highway, or that a hospital policy can't be changed. You're probably upset, almost certainly angry, and possibly quite unsure about whether or not to change practitioners midstream.

If you or your partner change jobs unexpectedly at the end of your pregnancy, you may also find yourself needing to change medical practitioners due to the change in your insurance. This switch can be especially upsetting if you've established a good rapport with your current medical provider and have already ironed out all the details of your birth plan with him.

Doctors do take new patients at the end of pregnancy, but it's usually because of insurance issues or because a patient has moved from another area. If you're making a voluntary switch, you may have to present your case well to avoid being labeled a "difficult patient." Doctors do know each other, and although they're not going to discuss your case on the squash court (you hope), they do know enough about each other to know who is a solid practitioner and who isn't. If the doctor you leave is seen as a reasonable doctor who practices sound medicine, expect some questions on exactly why you're changing practices.

Doctors are more familiar with informed patients today than they were a few decades ago and are more likely to understand "irreconcilable differences" than they may have been just a few years ago. On the other hand, many doctors view patients with their own opinions on birthing options as being possibly more trouble than they want to take on. It's up to you to convince them that you're not a troublemaker; you just have a certain view of your labor and would like to make it a reality, if at all possible.

 Building a relationship with a new medical provider takes time, and accelerating a relationship that normally builds over nine months into the last month of pregnancy is difficult. Choose a small or solo practice if at all possible, because you'll have trouble getting to know a large number of practice partners over just a few weeks or months.

# Chapter 4

# Leaving Home for a Hospital or Birth Center

## In This Chapter

▶ Weighing the advantages and disadvantages of giving birth in the hospital

▶ Deciding whether a birthing center is the better option for you

*W*hen you tell people you're pregnant, one of the first questions they may ask is, "Which hospital are you going to deliver at?" In many cases, people assume in the United States that if you're having a baby, you're having it in the hospital. However, this situation isn't the norm in many other industrialized countries, including many with much better delivery statistics and fewer complications than the U.S.

In this chapter, we look at how the hospital became the delivery place of choice for many women, how hospitals use their delivery units to enhance their reputations and bottom line, and why you may want to consider — or not consider — delivering there. We also look at the advantages and disadvantages of birthing centers over hospitals.

## Deciding on a Hospital Delivery

Many American women never give alternative birthing locations a second thought. Having a baby means packing your overnight bag — because that's about how long you get to stay there these days — and making the drive to the hospital. There's nothing wrong with delivering in the hospital, and in fact it has many advantages. But if you want a noninterventional labor and delivery at a hospital, your birth plan will need to reflect your desires more than if you deliver at a birth center or at home, where your desires may mesh better with the birthing philosophies of the staff.

# Why most Americans deliver in the hospital

In many countries, women still deliver at home or in designated birthing centers rather than in hospitals. Why has going to the hospital become the American way of birth? Many factors have contributed, and not all have their basis in maternal or infant safety. Doctor preference and tradition have more to do with the switch from home to hospital for delivery than safety issues, although when an emergency arises, lifesaving treatments are often more available in the hospital than at home.

On the plus side, obstetricians — who mostly practice in hospitals, although a tiny minority may do home births — are well trained to handle any emergencies that may occur during birth and to perform life-saving surgery quickly if needed.

Your comfort level with hospital birth may also influence your decision to give birth there; if your friends and family have all had hospital births, it may seems like the logical choice to you.

## Seeing why your doctor prefers it

Understanding why doctors prefer their patients to deliver in the hospital isn't difficult. If you were a doctor, that's what you would want to do, too, for the following reasons:

- **The hospital provides a central location for all her patients.** Doctors today don't have time to run from one home to another to sit with laboring women and do deliveries. Having everyone in one place makes your doc's job simpler and allows her to do more deliveries.

- **The hospital allows her to use the nurses, medical interns, and residents as her backup system.** If you've already had a baby, you know that the typical obstetrician makes her appearance about three minutes before your baby emerges. That's an exaggeration, but not by much. Doctors rely heavily on the nurses and doctors in training to monitor their patients and keep them informed on what's going on so they can go do other things — like work their office hours.

- **The hospital may provide immediate access to emergency services such as an operating room and anesthesiologists.** Although not all hospitals have in-house anesthesiologists available at night, many do. Doctors, especially obstetricians, don't want to be sued. They pay very large malpractice insurance premiums because they practice in a very high-risk specialty. To minimize the risk of anything going wrong that could result in a lawsuit, an obstetrician wants all the help she can get at her fingertips.

### *Figuring out your comfort level*

The other reason why hospitals remain the most common delivery site in the United States is familiarity. Most likely, your mom and maybe her mom delivered babies in the hospital, although the generation before that was more often born at home. You've probably been to the hospital to visit friends who have had babies, although with hospital stays shortened to 24 hours in many places, these visits may become less common with the next generation — there simply isn't time!

Because familiarity breeds comfort, in many cases, the hospital may seem like a logical place to have your baby. You may also fear the thought of delivering outside the hospital because it's an unknown scenario, unless you have friends who have delivered at home with midwives. Your grandmother and other older relatives can also add to the fear factor; nearly everyone from a generation or two ago has a horror story about a relative who died in childbirth or whose baby had lifelong problems after a home delivery. Even if the home delivery wasn't the cause — and it in all likelihood was not — perceptions are hard to change.

Although complications can arise at home as well as in the hospital, remember that many of the complications from 60 years ago occurred more because of a lack of monitoring tools, obstetrical knowledge, and antibiotics than from problems caused by delivering at home. Midwives were often not used; a female relative would come for the delivery, but her prior experience was usually limited to helping at a few family home deliveries.

If delivering outside the hospital intrigues you but also makes you nervous, talk to as many women as you can who have had home deliveries. Talk to different midwives and question them thoroughly about how they handle emergencies. (See Chapter 3 for more questions to ask a midwife you're considering using for a delivery.) Talk to your partner, too; in some cases, he may be more uncomfortable with the idea of delivering at home than you are. Research birthing centers in your area, if there are any. Check out www.birthcenters.org to find a center in your area.

Childbirth is no time to be uncomfortable with the place you're delivering. Taking fears about your delivery location into labor with you may make your labor more difficult. If the thought of developing complications that can't be handled rapidly outside the hospital keeps you awake at night, the hospital may be the best place for you to have your baby. And you'll be in good company; most American women do deliver in hospitals — and most never even consider delivering anywhere else. See Chapter 5 for more on the pros and cons of home delivery.

# Determining the pros and cons of hospital delivery

Hospitals are generally safe and familiar places to have a baby, although you're certainly more likely to have a cesarean section, undergo labor induction or augmentation with oxytocin, or develop an infection in the hospital than out of it. Many of the complications that occur in labor would occur whether you delivered at home or in the hospital, although hospital interventions such as labor induction or epidural anesthesia can increase the risk of some complications. Both hospital and home or birthing-center deliveries have pros and cons.

## Sorting out safety statistics

You may be concerned that some studies report that home birth is safer than delivering in the hospital. If there's one thing that everyone agrees on when it comes to statistics, it's that they can — and often are — easily misinterpreted.

Statistics show that home birth, when attended by a trained midwife or doctor, is generally quite safe — as safe or safer, in some instances, as delivering in the hospital. However, because home births, which comprise just 1 percent of all births in the United States according to 2009 CDC statistics, are less likely to involve teen or high-risk moms, comparing statistics for the two groups in terms of safety is complex. Home birth is extremely safe if you use a trained certified nurse-midwife. Hospital birth is also safe, particularly if you carefully choose your medical practitioner.

## Weighing the conveniences

When you deliver at the hospital, all you have to do is show up, although the trip to the hospital can be a hair-raising experience if you're uncomfortable. The hospital provides you with a place to labor, a clean-up crew, and all the emergency equipment you or your baby may (but hopefully won't) need. (However, some smaller hospitals may not have the facilities a very sick mom or newborn needs, which means you may have to be transported elsewhere, even if you're at the hospital. This situation is rare, though.)

The hospital also supplies clothing for you — although its appeal is certainly limited — and for your baby, including diapers. This location can also have the following advantages:

- **Access to pain medication:** Epidurals and a variety of pain killers are on hand.
- **The ability to perform a cesarean section:** If C-section is necessary, you won't have to transfer from home to the hospital.

✔ **A nursery for the baby to stay in overnight:** Although most hospitals now provide rooming-in — ideal if you're breast-feeding — if you're bottle-feeding, you may prefer a good night's sleep before you go home.

✔ **A place to labor without worrying about what your other children will hear or see:** Most moms (but not all!) prefer to labor without their other children there. If you're in the hospital, your children can stay at home in familiar surroundings.

✔ **Most American women deliver in the hospital:** Delivering outside the hospital may make you feel uncomfortable if you don't know anyone who has given birth at home.

### *Determining the disadvantages*

Hospitals are designed to treat sick people, not healthy ones. Because most pregnant women aren't sick, the rules and regulations that hospitals apply to other patients often don't work for pregnant women. But the hospital applies them nonetheless, insisting on visiting rules and imposing eating and drinking restrictions.

In the last few decades, hospitals have made a concerted effort to change the way they treat pregnant women. (Be thankful that the days of receiving an enema the minute you hit the labor floor are long gone!) But consumer demand, not the hospital's sudden sensitivity to the issues of laboring women, has driven the change.

The obstetrician you pick can make a big difference in the type of hospital experience you have. Her attitude about childbirth will affect the procedures you undergo in the hospital.

Most obstetricians know, intellectually, that pregnancy is not a disease. But they often treat it as one for the following reasons:

✔ They're trained to think of pregnancy as a condition where things can go wrong at any time. Any OB who has practiced any length of time has had at least one case that reinforces the fact that things can and do go wrong in the blink of an eye in labor.

✔ Older OBs were trained under the assumption that women didn't know what was good for them.

✔ They're trained — or learn very quickly in private practice — that obstetrics is the branch of medicine most likely to be sued if any complications at all occur in mom or baby. This fact makes OBs very quick to jump into the OR at the first sign of trouble during labor.

The hospital can be an isolating and lonely place to have your baby. Pretty curtains don't make the hospital feel any more like home when you feel alone and scared. On the other hand, with more liberal visiting policies than in years past, a hospital delivery can also seem like party central — which can also be a disadvantage at times.

Hospital nurses often have more than one laboring patient and not enough time to sit with you during your labor. Watching your labor on a fetal monitor from the nurse's station doesn't provide the same quality of care as having trained personnel with you continuously. You may feel like little more than a number if you arrive in labor on the night of a full moon, when half the pregnant women in the city also decided to go into labor.

Your doctor may be busy in another delivery room or running her office down the street until just before you're ready to deliver, so she generally isn't around to keep you company and tell you what's happening, either.

After your baby is born, the hospital may have barriers to parenting the way you want. If you're determined to breast-feed and room-in but the hospital has routine separation policies or tries to sneak an unnecessary bottle of formula to your baby, you may feel frustrated and upset. Of course, your birth plan can insist on rooming-in and no supplements, but as a postpartum mother, arguing with staff is probably not something you'd like to waste energy on.

Sleeping can also be uncomfortable in a hospital. There's noise in the hallways, nurses come in for vital sign checks in the middle of the night, and the bed may not be as cozy as your bed at home. If you plan to co-sleep with your baby, the hospital bed might not be set up safely to do so, although some units now feature full-sized postpartum beds. They may mean even less sleep if you're breast-feeding.

If you prefer to deliver in the hospital but want to go home as soon as possible after, speak to your obstetrician and your chosen pediatrician about the possibility of early discharge (ideally before labor begins). As long as you and your baby are doing well, some hospitals will allow you to go home within 12 hours of birth. Before you give birth, talk to your doctor about how soon you can leave, and put your preference in your birth plan.

The whole purpose of your birth plan is to make your birth *yours* as much as possible in a setting that doesn't value originality or deviation from the standard procedure. Don't expect the nurses to embrace your birth plan or even follow it without gentle and positive coercion from you, your partner, or your doula.

But having a birth plan does clarify your wishes and may make it easier to navigate the sometimes choppy waters of informed hospital birth, especially if you've discussed your wishes with your doctor and the hospital before D Day. A proactive partner or a doula who isn't as emotionally invested in the outcome and who can present your wishes in an unemotional way also helps when you're uncomfortable and less able to reinforce what's in your birth plan.

# Picking a hospital

If you live in a rural and isolated area, your hospital choices may be extremely limited. If you live near a large city or in a populated suburban area, you probably have three or four choices within a 30 mile radius. Many factors influence your choice of hospitals, not the least of which is your doctor's preference.

## Who really picks the hospital, you or your doctor?

If you already have an obstetrician picked out, your choice of hospitals has probably already been made for you. Although some doctors deliver at more than one hospital, they probably do most of their deliveries at one of them (probably the one that's nearest to their office).

Doctors can't just go anywhere to do their deliveries and surgeries; they need to have privileges at the hospital. A doctor in good standing with the medical community usually doesn't have any difficulty getting permission to deliver at a new hospital, but it isn't worth her time to do so for only a handful of patients. A busy OB may have three or four patients (or more!) in labor at the same time. Obviously, keeping all her eggs in one basket makes more sense than running from one hospital to another to do deliveries.

## Making the right choice

The hospital labor-and-delivery suite décor is the last thing you should consider when choosing a hospital to have your baby — but it isn't, and hospitals know it. You may not consider yourself shallow enough to fall for painted rocking chairs, pastel bedspreads, and adorable wallpaper borders, but when those pregnancy hormones have you honing in on anything and everything that appeals to your maternal instincts, you are. Little lambs gamboling on a wallpaper border may not send you into ecstasies at any other time of your life, but during pregnancy, they look like the epitome of adorable.

Because pregnant women do look at the room decorations when assessing hospitals, most hospitals have banished the sterile walls, linoleum floors, and metal bars common to maternity wards 50 years ago in favor of wood floors and more modern furniture, along with appealing curtains. Although an attractive setting does have more appeal for baby birthing than a sterile room, keep the décor in perspective and remember that you probably won't even notice your surroundings when you're in active labor. And a fetal monitor in a wooden cabinet rather than on a metal stand is still a fetal monitor.

So if the furnishings shouldn't guide your choice, what should? Here's a list to start:

- ✔ **How many deliveries does the hospital do per year?** Deciding what answer you're looking for is tricky. Busy hospitals can sometimes feel like a baby factory, but they generally have level III neonatal intensive care units that can treat very sick babies without transferring them to another hospital.

- ✔ **What's the hospital's overall cesarean-section rate?** Local newspapers often print this information, but it may not be all that relevant in your case, because one doctor with a high rate can skew the statistics.

- ✔ **What type of nursery does the hospital have?** The choices range from level I to level III, with level I the most basic and level III able to handle the most complex problems. If you know your baby is going to have problems at birth or if you have serious health problems, choose a hospital with a level III nursery.

- ✔ **What are the hospital's policies on visiting hours, number of people in the delivery room, and other issues are important to you?** Hospitals used to have visiting hours only twice a day for one hour at a time. Hospital hours are much more liberal now, which can be a blessing — or a curse, if you want to be alone with your partner after the delivery.

- ✔ **Does the hospital have private rooms?** Probably no hospitals in the United States still have communal labor rooms (once very common) but not all offer private rooms after the delivery, a time when you really need your rest and private space to get to know your baby before the hospital kicks you out the door. More hospitals have gone to all-private rooms throughout the hospital, but ask. Almost nothing can make your postdelivery time in the hospital more miserable than a rotten roommate or her immediate family of 100, all of whom plan to stay at the hospital with her all day until she goes home.

- ✔ **Can you talk to the hospital liaison or patient advocate before your delivery?** If your birth plan includes items that you know will be out of the mainstream for the hospital, ask to talk to the person who advocates for patients. Hospitals don't like to bend their rules, but they will as long as the deviation doesn't interfere too much with their routine or if it brings them good publicity or good will. If your doctor is okay with something but it's against hospital rules, discuss it with someone (and get official permission in writing) before you go into labor.

### Checking out natural birthing wings

Some hospitals have attempted to cut into the natural-birth market by offering wings or, in more cases, single birthing rooms, that cater to natural delivery. You may find a large tub, a birthing ball, a rocking chair, and a squat bar attached to the bed in these rooms. Most have a large bed so your partner can stay with you and possibly even a separate room for family and friends.

In the 1980s, hospitals started incorporating rooms that women could both labor and deliver in. At the time, this exciting concept eliminated the push across the hallway to the delivery room on a stretcher, open gown flapping in the breeze. Doctors and nurses had to assess the timing of deliveries carefully, to avoid tying up the delivery room for too long, because most units had just one or two. Therefore, going to the delivery room was usually a chaotic move that involved shifting yourself from bed to delivery table at the worst possible moment of labor.

Today, most hospitals have labor-delivery-recovery (LDR) rooms, where you labor, deliver, and recover in the same room. After an hour or so, you move to a postpartum room for the rest of your stay. Some hospitals have gone a step further and keep you in the same room for your entire hospital stay, called LDRPs which means that not only will you have a large, private room but that you won't have to change rooms after you settle in.

# Choosing a Birth Center

Birth centers are the middle ground between delivering in the traditional hospital setting and delivering at home. They're a compromise — in some ways a good one, in others not, depending on what type of birth you hope to have.

On the plus side, birth centers are often either attached to a traditional hospital or have a working relationship with one nearby. This arrangement helps ensure that any emergency care you need is not too far away. On the negative side, a birth center is still not the same as having your baby at home in a familiar setting and with complete freedom to do whatever you want to do in labor without asking medical personnel.

A birth center specializes in natural, noninterventional births. In most of them, you can't get an epidural in labor. If your birth plan includes an epidural on demand, a birth center is not for you. Birth centers don't do cesarean sections, so if your baby is in an unusual position or if you develop complications that necessitate immediate delivery, a birth center is also not for you. In most cases, birth-center practitioners try to avoid doing episiotomies and other invasive procedures.

## Weighing the differences between different types of birth centers

Some birth centers aren't all that different from hospital labor and delivery units. (Some hospitals even call their regular labor and delivery wings *birth centers,* which really is false advertising.) Birth centers may be more likely to have birthing tubs and other birth tools, and they're more likely to employ midwives for delivery. When you're thinking about using a birth center, weighing the differences between different types of units can help make your decision on where to give birth easier. Consider the following facts about birth centers:

- **A birth center attached to a hospital can provide the same access to emergency services that a hospital can.** And if your baby needs to stay in the neonatal intensive care unit, you'll be close by.

- **At a freestanding birth center, if your baby needs specialized care, he will be taken to a hospital.** In some cases, both mom and baby can be transferred to the hospital. It's also possible that the birth center will release you quickly after the birth so you can go spend time with your baby, as long as your own medical condition is stable.

## Determining whether a birth center is right for you

If you know you want a noninterventional type of labor and delivery, look into birth centers near you. Don't hesitate to ask birth-center practitioners, who may be doctors or midwives, the same types of questions you would ask a potential obstetrician or other medical practitioner. Following are some the things you want to know:

- **Are you an accredited birthing center?** The American Association of Birth Centers sets the standards for accreditation, which include having licensed personnel and at least two people trained in CPR and newborn resuscitation at every delivery.

- **What is your emergency backup plan?** Find out where you go if you or your baby develop complications and how fast the usual response time is.

- **How often do you transfer women to the hospital because of complications?** Complications arise in some labors, no matter where they occur. "Never" is not a good answer in this case; it indicates that the center takes too many risks by not prudently sending women elsewhere for their safety or their baby's. The American Pregnancy Association suggests between 7 to 10 percent as a reasonable answer.

✔ **Will I see one midwife or doctor for pregnancy and birth or will I see everyone in a group?** Although seeing just one or two practitioners is preferable, you may rotate through a group of midwives, depending on who's on call or in clinic that day.

✔ **How often do you do episiotomies rather than letting a woman tear naturally?** Less than 10 percent of the time is a good answer in this case also.

✔ **Do you have any restrictions on how or where I labor or give birth?** If you want to give birth in water, ask about the policies on water birth and on the training that personnel receive.

✔ **Who can be present when I give birth? Do you have a restrictive policy on having my other children in the room?** Some centers allow the baby's siblings only if you have a designated person with them who will take them from the room as necessary.

✔ **What type of monitoring do you use and how often will I need to be monitored?** Electronic fetal monitoring is not normally a done at birthing centers. Midwives check fetal heart tones with a hand-held Doppler ultrasound during and after contractions every hour or so for a few minutes.

✔ **Can I receive any type of pain medication?** It's nice to know what's available in case you decide you need something. Although you probably won't have access to an epidural, intravenous narcotics may be available at a birth center.

✔ **What type of emergency equipment do you have available?** Some centers have little more than oxygen available, but they should have personnel who can ventilate your baby with a bag and mask until the emergency crew arrives.

✔ **Is your staff trained in CPR, neonatal resuscitation, or advanced cardiac life support?** These courses, all devised by the American Heart Association, teach medical personnel the initial steps to take if you or your baby stops breathing or he has problems with his heartbeat. You want personnel trained in all advanced life-support courses for you and your baby, including the ability to place a breathing tube for your baby if needed.

## Recognizing when a birth center won't work for you

In some circumstances, you shouldn't even consider giving birth at a birth center. In most of these cases, you won't be accepted as a patient there, anyway, because of increased risk to you or your baby. Following are some conditions that would make a birth center a poor choice for giving birth:

✔ **If you're having twins, triplets, or more:** When you're carrying multiples, you have an increased risk of needing a cesarean. Even if you have twins who are both head down, in proper position for a vaginal delivery, the second baby can shift position after delivery of the first. Coauthor Sharon has seen cases where the first twin delivered vaginally but the second baby turned sideways and needed cesarean delivery. In these cases, you typically have little time to get the second baby out safely. The hospital is a safer place to be.

✔ **If you have health issues such as severe diabetes or pregnancy complications such as pregnancy-induced hypertension:** Both you and your baby need very close monitoring and may need intensive care treatment.

✔ **If your baby is being born prematurely, before 37 weeks of pregnancy:** Although many premature babies do well, and those born at 36 or so weeks need no intervention, others need oxygen or ventilation, have trouble maintaining their temperatures, or can't feed properly.

✔ **If your baby has a known congenital condition that could necessitate immediate resuscitation:** If your baby has a congenital heart defect, chromosomal abnormalities, lung defects, or other conditions that could affect his ability to survive without medical intervention, obviously a birth center isn't a good choice.

# Chapter 5

# Home Sweet Home Birth

. . . . . . . . . . . . . . . . . . . . . . . . . . . . . . . . . . . . . . . . . . .

## In This Chapter

▶ Weighing the pros and cons of home birth

▶ Hiring your home-birth team

▶ Gathering supplies and preparing your family for the big day

▶ Making sure you have support lined up for afterward

. . . . . . . . . . . . . . . . . . . . . . . . . . . . . . . . . . . . . . . . . . .

*H*ome birth, fairly common just 70 years ago, has been reemerging as a viable option for women with low-risk pregnancies. In fact, approximately 30,000 women — about 1 out of 140 — choose home birth in the United States each year. In Canada, about 1 in 100 births takes place outside of a hospital, and in the United Kingdom, 2 in 100 births take place at home. The Netherlands has the highest rate of home births in the world, with 29 percent of all deliveries being planned home births. One big advantage to home birth is that your birth-plan wishes are much more likely to be granted. In this chapter, we discuss the advantages of home birth, the potential risks, and the practical matters, like hiring your support team and preparing your family and home.

## Choosing a Home Birth

If a friend or family member has given birth at home, you may already know you'd like a home birth, too. Advocates of home birth are usually quite vocal about their experiences and the research they've done, so you may feel like you've already taken Home Birth 101! However, if you're the first among your friends to go this route, or you're just not sure yet if it's for you, considering the advantages and disadvantages to home birth is an important part of making your decision. In this section, we lay out the pros and cons of home birth and provide some questions to consider when evaluating if home birth is for you.

# Considering the advantages and potential risks

When considering the advantages and risks of home birth, checking out the research is essential. Before you begin your own research digging, keep in mind that studies can be biased, and comparing hospital births with home births has been difficult. Some studies that found home birth dangerous included unplanned home births (women who never intended to give birth at home and just accidently delivered in the car or in their bathroom), which isn't at all the same as a planned home birth with a midwife. Other studies that have found hospital births more dangerous than home may not be taking into consideration that hospitals often handle complicated pregnancies and sick babies as well as women with little prenatal care. On the other hand, women who choose home births are generally highly educated, receive good prenatal care, and have low-risk pregnancies.

Thankfully, some studies have carefully looked at home birth and hospital births while including only planned home births and comparing low-risk women delivering at the hospital with low-risk women delivering at home. In this section, we lay out these studies for your consideration as you decide whether home birth delivery is for you.

## Advantages to home birth

According to many research studies, women with low-risk pregnancies who give birth at home have lower rates of episiotomy, severe perennial tears, hemorrhage, and infection than women delivering in a hospital. This difference is likely due to the lower rates of intervention, because women giving birth at home are also less likely to have assisted vaginal deliveries (involving vacuum or forceps, for example), cesarean sections, labor augmentation to induce or speed up labor, or epidurals.

For babies, home birth has been found to have lower rates of prematurity and low birth weight and less need for assisted newborn ventilation. A possible reason is that home birth is usually ruled out for high-risk pregnancies and labor that begins before 37 weeks, so babies at risk are more likely to be born in a hospital. Another possible reason is that interventions more likely to occur in a hospital — like induction (without strong medical reason) — may increase the risk of these outcomes in hospitals.

The rates of *perinatal mortality,* which means the death of a baby either during birth or up to seven days after, are similar for home births and hospital births. According to a study published in 2009 in the *Canadian Medical Association Journal* (CMAJ), the rate of perinatal death was 0.35 per 1,000 for planned home births with a registered midwife, compared to 0.57 per 1,000 for hospital births with a registered midwife.

# The legality of home birth

Home birth is legal throughout Canada, Australia, the United Kingdom, and the United States. However, in the U.S., laws regarding who can attend a home birth vary from state to state. Although almost every state permits certified nurse midwives (CNMs) to attend home births, almost half forbid lay midwives from attending home deliveries, and others require special licensure for certified professional midwives.

Because CNMs are sometimes difficult to find, you may be tempted to hire a midwife who is practicing illegally. Keep in mind that should an emergency occur, an illegally practicing midwife may hesitate to transfer you quickly or may even abandon you in the middle of labor for fear of legal repercussions.

At home, your birth plan is more likely to be respected, as you don't need to fight hospital protocol. Medical practitioners who attend home births are usually more open to following their client's requests, though you should still speak to your midwife about your birth wishes before labor begins because not every midwife is open to all natural birthing options. For example, some may absolutely not be willing to do a water birth. Others may be more hands-on than you hoped for.

Home birth has practical advantages as well, including the fact that the only restrictions on friends and family attending are the restrictions you impose yourself. Home birth certainly feels more homey, and remaining in familiar surroundings can be comforting. You have access to whatever food and drink you want, you can moan and groan without worrying about patients in the next room, and all your comfort tools are handy (assuming you gathered them before birth began).

Remaining with your baby around the clock after birth is also easier, because you don't need to deal with required nursery visits or hospital policies that separate mother and baby (though many hospitals today keep mother and child together as much as possible). Maintaining constant contact between mother and baby increases your chances for successful breast-feeding. See Chapter 17 for more on this topic. You'll also have more privacy and probably quieter surroundings, giving you and your baby space and time to bond.

## Disadvantages and risks of home birth

Needing to transfer to a hospital in the midst of labor, or even during the delivery itself, is a potential disadvantage of home birth. About 12 percent of mothers require transfer to a hospital. The process may be relatively smooth or may be traumatic, depending on the reason for transfer. At the hospital, unless your midwife has privileges or works alongside a specific obstetrician, you'll likely be under the care of whomever is available, and that doctor may or may not be pleasant, knowing you're a home-birth transfer.

According to a 2010 study from the *American Journal of Obstetrics and Gynecology,* infant deaths between day 7 and day 28 of life were found to be higher for home-birth babies than for hospital-born babies. The rate was double for babies in general, and almost triple for babies with special needs or birth defects. This study has been criticized, however, for including data from unplanned home births, which may have skewed the results. The overall risk was still relatively low: Of the 16,000 home births studied, only 0.20 percent of the births involved infant death. That percent is about 1 in 500 (compared to 1 in 1,000 of the hospital births reviewed).

Although rare, some emergencies require immediate interventions only available in the hospital. Mothers and babies have died during or as a result of home-birth emergencies. In most (but not all) situations, the death would have occurred at a hospital as well or was found to be the result of negligence of the attending midwife. Women who choose home birth acknowledge this risk and accept it as a possibility.

Legal issues may make home birth less safe in some areas. Some state laws may make it difficult or even illegal for midwives to attend home births, decreasing your options for a childbirth attendants. Some states limit certified professional midwives' access to certain medical supplies required for safe home birth, like oxygen or oxytocin.

Home delivery also has some practical disadvantages. If you change your mind about pain medication, you need to transfer to the hospital, because you can't get an epidural at home. Birth can be messy, and someone will need to clean up afterward, though usually the midwife team handles this task. If you have other kids, someone needs to care for them, either away from home or at your home. And because you won't have nurses or staff around to assist you, you also must find support for yourself and your family in the early postpartum days.

## *Evaluating whether home birth is for you*

Consider these questions as you evaluate whether home birth is right for you and your family:

✔ **Are you certain you want a natural childbirth?** Epidurals are not available at home, and although you can transfer to the hospital if you change your mind, doing so while you're in labor isn't ideal.

✔ **Are you relatively healthy, and is your pregnancy considered low risk?** Everyone defines low risk differently, and the midwives available in your area may disagree with each other or have different skill sets. For example, one midwife may refuse to attend a home birth for twins, whereas another will be comfortable with it. Keep in mind that the more complex your pregnancy is, the higher the risk of something going wrong.

# Why women choose home birth

Women choose to give birth at home for a variety of reasons. In 2009, the *Journal of Midwifery and Women's Health* published a study that surveyed 160 women, asking them why they chose home birth. Following were the most common reasons cited:

✔ **Feeling safer:** One of the most commonly cited reasons, home birth may feel (or actually be!) safer because unnecessary interventions and surgeries — like "failure-to-progress" C-sections — are less likely to take place.

✔ **Wanting to avoiding unnecessary interventions:** At a home birth, routine interventions are significantly less likely to occur, because most midwives embrace a more natural approach to childbirth and are less likely to intervene unless absolutely necessary.

✔ **Having experienced a negative hospital birth:** Women who have experienced a traumatic hospital birth, especially one that included interventions or surgery that seemed unnecessary or pushed upon them, may decide to give birth at home for subsequent children.

✔ **Desiring more control:** At home, you can move as you like, moan as you like, wear what you like, and eat and drink as you like. Maintaining a sense of control may also help a woman feel safer, leading to an easier labor. (See Chapter 8 for more on tapping into the power of your mind.)

✔ **Wanting a more comfortable environment:** When comparing the cold, unfamiliar rooms and halls of a hospital to the cozy familiar walls of your house, there's just no place like home!

✔ **Trusting their bodies and the birth process:** Many women who choose home birth believe that their bodies know instinctively how to give birth, and they believe the interventions and outside control imposed by many hospitals interfere with this natural birth process.

✔ **Are you within reasonable distance of a hospital?** If an emergency did occur, how long would it take an ambulance to get to your home and transfer you to the hospital? If you're expecting in the winter, do you live in a place where weather may complicate an emergency transfer?

✔ **Are you prepared to deal with negative reactions to your choice to delivery at home?** Friends and family may or may not be supportive. If you're transferred to the hospital, doctors and nurses may also react strongly to your choice, even if everything goes smoothly in the end. Can you channel your inner rebel?

✔ **Do you and your partner agree on home birth?** Although the dad-to-be may not get the final say in where you deliver, you'll feel better if any disagreements are resolved before labor begins.

✔ **Are you willing to take responsibility for your health and your baby's?** Home birth requires proactivity — including preparing your home for the birth and postpartum period — and involves some risk. Home-birth advocates often say that hospital births also involve preparation and risk, and this is true, but at home your responsibilities are greater.

If you like the idea of a home birth but aren't completely sure it's right for you, you may want to consider a birth center. Birth centers offer some of the benefits of home birth, including less intervention and a positive attitude toward natural childbirth. See Chapter 4 for more on finding and using a birth center.

# Hiring the Baby Catcher: Birth Attendants for Home Birth

In the hospital, the majority of your birth attendants are people you have never met and have little choice over. The only person you may know is your doctor, and if the doctor you chose is part of a large group of obstetricians working together, you may get someone else from the group who you've only met once before the birth. With home birth, the opposite is true. Whoever is there is not only someone you chose but also hopefully someone you have spent time getting to know. In this section, we talk about hiring your home-birth team.

One home-birth movement encourages women to give birth without a midwife or doctor present, called *unassisted childbirth* or *free birthing*. Proponents who declare the practice to be safe reference home-birth studies, but midwives attending home births make choices and take actions that save mothers' and babies' lives. Childbirth without a trained professional is extremely risky.

## Finding a home-birth midwife or doctor

The vast majority of home births are attended by midwives. Doctors also may attend a home birth, though this practice is rare, with less than 5 percent of births outside of hospitals in the U.S. attended by doctors. There are three kinds of midwives: lay midwives, certified professional midwives, and certified nurse-midwives. You can read about the differences between these midwives and find out how to hire a midwife in Chapter 3.

Most midwives attending home births are lay midwives or certified professional midwives, even though the majority of states only allow certified nurse-midwives to legally attend home births. However, Nebraska and Alabama are the exception, where home birth is legal but certified nurse-midwives are not legally permitted to attend them. Finding a midwife may be easy if home birth is popular in your area and the laws are favorable, but in areas that require certified nurse-midwives to attend home births, finding a birth attendant for your home birth may be tricky.

In some states, laws regulating home birth may also limit the medical supplies a certified professional midwife is permitted to carry. (Certified nurse-midwives are not limited in this way.) Not having these essentials can make home birth riskier. Be sure to ask any midwife you interview if she carries oxytocin, oxygen, intubation equipment, antibiotics, IV fluids, and vitamin K with her to deliveries, and if she doesn't, how she plans to handle a situation that requires them.

To begin your search, ask local childbirth professionals (like childbirth education instructors or local doulas) about home-birth attendants they know and suggest. Being plugged into the birthing community, they often hear stories about certain midwives and doctors, so they can steer you toward the better care providers.

You can also use midwife databases online such as www.midwife.org and www.mothersnaturally.org. Be sure to ask for references and speak to a few mothers who have already given birth with that midwife. Chapter 3 has more questions you can ask midwives before hiring.

Be aware that receiving a recommendation for a midwife from a childbirth educator or friend, or even finding them listed on a website referral list, does not guarantee that she is a legally practicing midwife. Always confirm licensing and certifications, and be aware that hiring a midwife who practices outside the law may put your baby and your health at risk.

You may decide to have a home birth late in your pregnancy, after already receiving care from a medical practitioner who does not attend home births. Midwives are used to couples making the home-birth choice later in the pregnancy, but the one you choose will need to assess your pregnancy to ensure you and your baby are in good health and low risk. Also, many midwives have a cut-off date when they will not accept new clients, usually around week 32 of pregnancy.

Be sure to write a birth plan and discuss your wishes with any midwife or doctor you consider hiring for your home birth. Although home birth medical practitioners are likely to embrace natural childbirth and favor less intervention, you still have plenty of options. In fact, you may find that creating a birth plan is a less stressful and more enjoyable process when you know you are just considering your ideal birth experience and won't have to fight protocol. Possible topics to include in a home birth plan are whether you want a water birth, who gets to "catch" the baby (could be you or your husband!), the kind of mood you'd like at the time of birth, and what family you'd like to include and how.

## Choosing a doula for a home birth

A *doula* is a woman who provides continuous emotional, informational, and physical support throughout labor. You can read more about doulas in general in Chapter 3.

Sometimes, people think doulas are mainly for hospital births because the need for an advocate is much more important in that environment. Also, because home-birth midwives stay with you during much of labor, you may think a doula isn't necessary. In fact, many women find a doula a great addition to their home-birth care team. Some doulas prefer to attend home births, because that setting allows them to focus on what they love most — helping a mother through childbirth — without needing to also fight against protocol. Plus, if your labor isn't well established enough for your midwife to come (or if she's tied up elsewhere), a doula may arrive at your side hours before your midwife to provide support. Later, while your midwife is focused on the baby and the delivery, the doula can be by your side, focused solely on you.

Some midwives include a doula in their care team, so ask your midwife if she does and if you can meet her. If it's not a match, you can always hire an additional doula yourself.

## Paying for your home birth

Usually the cost for a home birth includes the prenatal care provided during pregnancy and postpartum check-ups after birth, and sometimes newborn care for the first few weeks. The fee varies throughout the country, but according to the Midwives Alliance of North America, you can expect to pay between $1,800 and $8,600.

Insurance doesn't usually cover all of a midwife's fees for home-birth care, but some policies do reimburse the fees. You will likely need to pay your midwife up front and then approach the insurance company for reimbursement. Speak to your midwife about how she can help you work with the insurance company.

If your midwife is the only medical practitioner providing home-birth services, you may be able to get your insurance company to extend an in-network exception to get coverage for the fees.

# Getting Your Home Ready for Birthing

Before labor begins, you need to prepare your home and family for the big day! This process includes gathering supplies, including whatever comfort tools you'd like to have, and, if you have older kids, arranging for their care.

# Gathering home-birth supplies

Although your midwife or doctor provides many of the medical supplies for the home birth, she may also give you a list of supplies for you to purchase before Delivery Day. If she doesn't, be sure to ask about it. Here's a checklist of items you may need or want for your home delivery:

❑ **Two sets of fitted and flat sheets for your bed, plus a plastic protective sheet:** After labor begins, you make the bed you'll labor on with one set of sheets, and then on top you place a plastic protective sheet like a shower curtain or drop cloth. On top of this, you put the second set of sheets. This setup allows you to get the top sheets messy during childbirth and then easily strip off the top layers and have a clean, already-made bed for after.

❑ **Six to eight towels and washcloths:** The cloths are for a variety of uses, like creating hot or cold compresses, and, of course, wiping away mess. You need a few more if you're having a water birth.

❑ **Eight cotton receiving blankets:** For gentle swaddling and covering.

❑ **Three cotton newborn hats, two sets of weather-appropriate newborn clothing, and socks:** For keeping the baby dressed and warm.

❑ **Small slow cooker or large pot:** For boiling washcloths and creating warm, moist compresses.

❑ **A disposable 9-x-12 pan or cookie sheet, along with a heating pad:** The cookie sheet can be used as a hard surface for newborn resuscitation, if required. The heating pad, along with receiving blankets, the cookie sheet, and oxygen and resuscitation equipment, may be set up ahead of time, just in case of an emergency.

❑ **A large bowl and a 1-gallon plastic bag:** For the placenta.

❑ **Large overnight maxi pads, bed pads, and adult diapers:** Large adult diapers can be worn instead of regular underwear, to prevent postpartum bleeding leaks on your sheets.

❑ **A peri-bottle, witch hazel, and supplies for sitz bath:** Sitz bath supplies may include a small basin for sitting in, plus sea salts or Epsom salts along with 3 percent hydrogen peroxide. Witch hazel applied to maxi-pads and then placed in the freezer may be helpful for soothing perineal tears. A peri-bottle – used for squirting warm water over the perineum — can be just a water bottle with a squirt top.

❑ **Acetaminophen or ibuprofen:** These painkillers help with postpartum cramps, which may be more intense for mothers who have given birth before.

❑ **A flashlight with batteries:** A flashlight helps the midwife see what's happening, especially if you like the lights dim during labor.

❑ **A large handheld mirror:** You'll use this item if you want to watch the baby being born.

❑ **Robe for you and your partner:** A robe is great if you're getting in and out of a birthing tub. You may want to consider lounging around in a robe for the first several postpartum days, as a way of making clear to your visitors that you're in self-care mode — not hospitality mode!

❑ **At least two large trash bags and two big laundry hampers or boxes:** You'll need to collect dirty laundry and trash someplace.

❑ **Two to three large bottles of hydrogen peroxide:** You may need it to remove blood stains from towels, sheets, or even carpeting.

❑ **At least two small, lined trash cans or buckets:** Trash cans are handy when you need to vomit, which is common during labor.

❑ **Basic baby supplies:** Be sure to have diapers and baby wipes on hand. If you're using cloth diapers, also buy detergent appropriate for laundering the diapers.

❑ **Paper towels and toilet paper:** You certainly don't want to be running out of these the day you're in labor!

❑ **Food and hydration for yourself and your guests:** See Chapter 10 for what to eat and drink during labor. You'll also need food for birth guests, attendants, and your partner, but it doesn't need to be anything fancy! Don't forget about your midwife and her team, who will also need something to eat. Discuss with your midwife ahead of time what she expects or requests.

❑ **Comfort tools:** Get a birth ball, massage tools, essential oils, a personal fan with a mister, or whatever else you need for comfort. See Chapter 8 for more ideas.

❑ **Camera with extra batteries and film:** If you plan to record or take pictures of the birth, have these items ready.

❑ **Your birth plan and an emergency transfer bag:** You may want to write two birth plans, one for your home birth and one in case of transfer. See Chapter 2 for what to pack in a hospital bag.

❑ **An infant car seat:** You'll need a seat in case you need to transfer to the hospital and need it to bring the baby home. You're going to need one eventually anyway.

❑ **Water-birth supplies:** If you intend to labor in water or rent a birthing pool, you'll also need a large plastic drop cloth to protect the floor beneath the birthing pool, bleach to disinfect the bathtub or birthing pool after delivery, and a floating water thermometer. A fish net to catch floating debris and a clean hose (not the one used in your backyard!) for filling the pool is needed as well. You can get more information in the next section.

Be sure to wash all sheets, towels, and baby blankets and clothes at least one month before the birth. Your midwife may suggest you store these items in sealed paper bags (not plastic, which can collect moisture and encourage mold), labeling and placing them in an easy-to-find place.

## Setting up for a water birth at home

If you're considering a water birth, you may be wondering how to do it in your bathtub. Your home's bathtub can be used for labor, but the small space limits movement and it can get icky quickly, with the blood and stool collecting in the tub during delivery. The bathroom also limits the room your midwife has to handle an emergency, which can be a problem if your bathroom isn't particularly large. Someone will also need to clean the tub before and after the birth.

The good news is you can buy or rent a birthing pool. Some women who give birth in hospitals or birth centers without birthing tubs also buy or rent their own (though they need to ask the hospital or center if they will be allowed to set it up). You'll need to clean a birth pool, too, but some pools come with liners, making cleanup easier.

If you want to buy an inflatable birth pool, check out www.waterbirth solutions.com for a variety of pools, including Aquaborn Eco Pools, Eco's Birth Pool in a Box, and La Bassine. After the birth, after you've disinfected the pool, you can use it as a miniature family swimming pool in the backyard (though the pools are not made for frequent use, so it may be a short-term rather than long-term bonus). Expect to pay between $150 and $450 for an inflatable pool, depending on the pool you purchase.

You can also rent or purchase a noninflatable birth pool from www.aqua doula.com. Rentals are $250, and purchases are just over $1,000. Walmart sells Spa-In-A-Box, which can be used as a birthing pool, for about $900. Also be sure to ask your midwife if she knows any local rental options, or she may offer birthing pool rentals herself.

Before labor begins, ensure you have all the nessecary equipment, including a hose long enough to reach a faucet, the correct adapter to connect the clean hose (not your garden hose!) to your kitchen or bathroom faucet, a foot or electronic pump to inflate an inflatable pool, and a large plastic tarp to protect your floor, big enough to contain splashes of water as you get in and out. You may want to set up the pool before labor as a trial run, but if you intend to leave it set up, you'll need to add something to the water to prevent unwanted bacterial growth. Ask your midwife or birthing pool leaser for what you can add to the water. Also, be aware that you may not be able to set it up in your bedroom if it's on the second floor, because of weight limits.

If you have little children around, you must be vigilant that they stay away from the birthing pool before, during, and after labor. The pool should be drained as soon as possible after the birth, and it shouldn't be waiting around too long before. Some pools have locking lids, which is something to consider when choosing a birthing pool. While you're in labor, whoever is watching your children should keep an eye on them if they are in or near the water.

Bowel movements during labor are very common, especially right before and during the actual delivery. If you're laboring in water, this means stool may float to the top as the baby is progressing down the birth canal. Your birth team can use a fish net, the kind they sell in pet stores, to help remove the stool, and hopefully you won't even notice. Be sure the net has never been used in a real aquarium!

## *Taking care of your big kids on the big day*

One benefit to home birth is your kids don't have to be separated from their mama for too long. However, they still need someone to supervise them during labor. Ideally that person won't be your partner, who may want to remain by your side. If your children are young and you think you'll be distracted by their presence or you're concerned the sounds of labor may worry them, consider sending them to a neighbor or family member's home for a sleepover. If this arrangement isn't an option, a babysitter or family member can watch them in your home, though in this case it's a good idea to prepare them for the sounds and busyness of childbirth.

Some families decide to invite their children to the birth. This may mean having them in the room, by your side, or even allowing them to watch the baby's delivery, depending on your comfort level — and theirs. You should still have someone there to support them who can answer their questions or keep them company in another room if they decide not to watch or just get bored. See Chapter 6 for more on including the kids.

If you have any pets, they may need to be cared for during the birth. If your dog doesn't like visitors, you may want to board him elsewhere until after the birth. Also, be sure to have a back-up plan in the event of transfer, so you're not desperately knocking on neighbor's doors in search of a pet sitter when you need to be rushing to the hospital!

# Arranging Support for Your Early Postpartum Days

Most midwives require an adult to stay with you around the clock for the first two to three days after the birth. If your partner can't stay with you 24 hours a day, be sure to get a friend or family member to come instead.

During these early days, you should spend as much time as possible resting in bed with your newborn baby. When you're at home, you may be tempted to run around cleaning and cooking, but all that activity would be a mistake. Resist the urge to play host or hostess to your guests, and let people serve you! To reduce postpartum bleeding and help your body recover, stay in bed and enjoy the bonding time.

Therefore, someone else needs to be in charge of cleaning up and cooking for the family. Organized moms may prepare and freeze enough meals to feed the family for up to a week after the birth. Another option is to stock the house with easily prepared frozen foods and have lots of no-prep meal options. Nuts, bread, cheeses, healthy cold cuts, and spreadable proteins like peanut butter make good snacks for you and your family. Take-out meals are also an option, as well as asking friends and family to take turns delivering home cooked dinners.

If you have young children around, hiring a babysitter can help you rest and allow the kids to continue their daily routines. Even if your young ones decide to curl up in bed next to you most of the day, the babysitter can help them with baths, meals, and trips to the park.

You may also want to consider hiring a postpartum doula. Postpartum doulas specialize in providing support to mothers in the early postpartum days and weeks. They may provide a number of services, including the following:

- ✔ Help with breast-feeding
- ✔ Informational support regarding your recovery from childbirth
- ✔ Newborn care basics, including bathing your baby, dealing with the umbilical cord, and soothing a colicky baby
- ✔ Meal preparation, even running to the store for items and helping cook ahead for a few days
- ✔ Childcare for your older kids, including helping them transition and adapt to the new baby in the house

> ✔ Light housework, like dishwashing and laundry
>
> ✔ Referrals to helpful resources, like lactation consultants for breast-feeding problems or support groups for postpartum depression
>
> ✔ Emotional support and dealing with bossy mothers-in-law and the overwhelming avalanche of advice new moms often face.

Get more information on how to find and hire a postpartum doula at www. dona.org or www.cappa.net.

# Chapter 6

# Including Family and Friends in Your Birth Plan

## In This Chapter

▶ Deciding who (and who not) to invite to the birth

▶ Choosing not to invite any friends or family

▶ Considering family members as childbirth invitees

▶ Evaluating whether someone would make a good birthing buddy

▶ Having your kids with you during labor and delivery

*J*ust a couple hundred years ago, your female relatives surrounded and supported you as you gave birth, while the dad-to-be was left waiting outside. Then, when birth first moved into the hospital, women gave birth surrounded only by hospital staff, essentially alone, and dad stood outside in the hallway. Now, not only dads but also friends and family can attend the birth, and male friends and relatives as well as women may make the guest list! But just because you *can* have more people with you doesn't mean you have to, you'll want to, or even that you should.

In this chapter, we explain your birth guest options and how to decide if someone should or should not be invited, what to do when you want just you and your partner at the birth, whether and how to get your older children involved, and how this all factors into your birth plan.

## Creating Your Guest List

Who to invite to the birth is a personal matter, one that has no right or wrong answers. Maybe you've always imagined giving birth surrounded by your close relatives. Perhaps you just can't imagine laboring without your mother by your side. Or maybe your mother has always imagined being at her grandchildren's birth, but you'd rather she stay down the hallway in the waiting room — or not even in the same building! In this section, we discuss inviting people to be by your side or to wait in the lobby and provide you with some questions to consider before you invite anyone to the birth event.

Deciding who will attend (or not attend) the birth is something that should be done together with your partner. You may be having the baby, but the birth is an important experience for your partner, too! If, for example, your mom makes him extremely uncomfortable, even if you'd really like her to be there, it may be best not to invite her. As you consider guests, make sure to discuss your desires together.

## Assigning guests to front-row seating or the peanut gallery

Inviting friends or family to the birth doesn't necessarily mean they'll be by your side (or in your face, depending on how you feel about them!) the entire birth. You may want some guests to be actively present during labor, whereas you may prefer others to visit your room only after the baby is in your arms. If you want them there right *after* the baby is born, inviting them to wait in the waiting room down the hall is best.

Who may you want to offer front row seating to?

- ✔ **Guests to actively support you:** You believe they can support you, either physically or emotionally.

- ✔ **Guests who you want to experience the big birth moment:** You want them there not necessarily because they'll support you but just to experience the big moment with you. You may ask that these guests only come in the room during the actual delivery, or you may invite them for the entire labor.

- ✔ **Guests you've assigned a job:** You may want a person or two to handle a particular task, like watching over your older children who want to attend the birth but still need supervision.

You should indicate in your birth plan any guests who have an active role in the birth. Include their name, relationship (mother, sister, friend, doula, or whatever), and how you hope they'll be involved. Also be sure to discuss with your guests what you hope or expect from them *before* labor begins! If you hoped your sister could act as your doula but she has no idea that's what you want and plans on waiting outside, it could be awkward or even disappointing for you both.

Check with the hospital or birth center before inviting more than a couple friends or family members. Some facilities have guest limits, and whereas having just your partner, mother, and doula by your side isn't likely to violate the rules, having your partner, your mother, your doula, all your siblings, and all your cousins may be an issue! Facilities usually have no limit to how many people can be in the waiting room. However, most hospital waiting rooms have limited room.

Who may you want to send to the waiting room?

> ✔ **Guests you want with you immediately after the birth but not during:** Maybe you'd love your mother-in-law to see the baby just after the birth, but you're not comfortable with her in the labor and delivery room. The waiting room is best for her.

> ✔ **Guests who will visit you during labor but not stay throughout:** Sometimes seeing a friendly new face for just a moment during labor can refresh and inspire you to keep going or provide some comfort. But that person doesn't need to be there the entire time.

You may be tempted to offer the waiting room to those guests who insist on being at the birth but who you'd rather not attend. The problem with people like this is that they may walk right into the labor room anyway, which can create tension for you and your partner. (And as discussed in Chapter 8, anxiety can intensify labor pains!) If you don't want them in your labor room for even a moment, we recommend that you not invite them to the birth at all, no matter how much they insist. Call them *after* the baby is born!

You (or your guest!) can always decide during the birth that being in the waiting room is better for them than being in your laboring room, or vice versa. Don't feel the need to stick to your original plans after labor begins. You may discover that your cousin, who you expected to wait outside, is a great labor support, while your aunt, who you imagined by your side, would be better off down the hall.

## *Questions to ask yourself about potential guests*

Not everyone belongs in the labor room, even if you want them there or they want to be there. Before you start inviting (or accepting self-invitations), you'll want to carefully consider the following points:

> ✔ **Are you comfortable baring all in front of them?** Both figuratively, as you may moan and cry out during labor, and literally, because childbirth isn't exactly a time of modesty!

✔ **Do they want to be there?** Just because you'd love them to be there doesn't mean they're gung-ho about it. And if they're uncomfortable, you'll sense it, which may negatively affect the birth.

✔ **Do you *really* want them to be there?** Don't allow guilt to affect your choices. Just because your mother or mother-in-law says she'll be heartbroken if she doesn't attend doesn't mean you should say okay. Your comfort level at the birth will affect your labor. If you don't want them there, say no. (Or say yes if the person refuses to listen to your refusals but "forget" to call her when you go into labor! Taking this approach may result in hurt feelings, but if it's the only way to keep someone out of the labor room, your comfort comes before her feelings.)

✔ **Is the guest able to fully support your birth plans?** Can your natural birthing buddy really keep her opinions to herself when you ask for an epidural? Will your epidural-loving sister push you to take some drugs already when the going gets tough? Listen to your gut on this one.

✔ **Is your partner comfortable with this guest?** If your best friend and your partner tend to argue any time they're in the same room, then you probably don't want them in the delivery room together.

✔ **Are they prepared to witness birth?** Especially if you hope for them to be in the room for labor and delivery, the guests best be familiar with childbirth. Childbirth education class or educational birth videos can help.

# Choosing an Intimate Birth: Just You and Dad-To-Be

With all this talk about guests in the labor room, you may get the impression that everyone enjoys lots of company during childbirth. Not so! If the idea of having anyone besides your partner in the room with you makes you cringe, that's fine. You may decide an intimate experience is more for you.

Some people may argue that having an "intimate" birth experience is impossible, especially in a hospital setting, because nurses, maybe a doula, doctors, and even cleaning ladies will be coming in and out of your room all the time. But you can ignore the hubbub and choose to focus on yourselves. Strangers are certainly easier to ignore than meddling relatives.

During labor, if you'd like time alone without hospital staff or your doula, just ask whoever is around if they could leave you and your partner alone for a few minutes or even a couple hours. Depending on what's happening during labor (and if your room doesn't store supplies needed for other patients), they can usually comply.

Don't be surprised if some friends and family ask or assume that you'll include them in the labor room. (After all those years of telling your mom "everyone" is doing something, you may now find yourself on the receiving end, with your mom now claiming "all" her friends are attending their grandchildren's births!) You can be upfront and just tell them you'd like to experience the birth and delivery alone as a couple, promising to call the second the baby is born. Or if being upfront leads to unending confrontation, say you'll call and then conveniently forget to do so until after the baby is born, blaming the excitement and bustle of getting to the hospital or birth center.

If anyone shows up at the hospital before you're ready, you can ask a nurse to help usher him or her out. A nice nurse may be willing to blame the evictions on "hospital policy." Feelings may get hurt, but this is your delivery and you should do everything necessary to feel at ease. After the baby is born, most bad feelings will vanish anyway as the focus turns to the sweet newborn.

# *Inviting the Family (Or Not!)*

Inviting your family to the birth can be a blessing or a huge mistake, depending on your relationship outside the labor room. Keep in mind that family drama not only is likely to come into the labor room but also is likely, with all the hormones and stress in the air, to intensify. On the other hand, sometimes family can support you in ways friends or strangers can't. Witnessing your own grandchild, niece, or nephew enter the world can be quite a miracle.

Following is a rundown of family members you may decide to invite (or *not* invite!):

- ✔ **Your mom:** If you have a wonderful relationship with your mom, and you both want her to be at the birth, then she may be a great support to you. However, if your relationship is tense (like many mother-daughter relationships are), you may want to ask that she wait outside or even arrive after the baby is born.

- ✔ **Your grandmother:** Many women have good relationships with their grandmothers, often with lower tensions than they do with their mothers. However, inviting your grandmother and *not* your mom is bound to create family drama! Proceed with caution if this is your plan.

- ✔ **Your sister(s):** If you're close to your sister, especially if she's already given birth, you may want to have her there.

- ✔ **Your aunt(s):** Aunts are like grandmothers — female relatives that can have motherly relationships with their nieces without the mother-daughter drama. If you have an aunt like this, you may want her at the birth.

- ✔ **Your cousin(s):** It's unusual to invite a cousin to a birth, but in some families, cousins are as close as sisters.

- ✔ **Your dad:** Some women may feel awkward having their father in the labor room, but others can't imagine going through the experience without him. Or you may just like knowing your dad is down the hallway.

- ✔ **Your mother-in-law:** Tension between mothers-in-law and daughters-in-law is extremely common, even if it's normally bubbling just below the surface. Invite your mother-in-law only if you truly feel comfortable with her being there.

- ✔ **Your partner's sister, cousin, or aunt:** With families spread out across different cities and states, it may be that your partner's relatives are nearby while yours are far away. If you've developed a close relationship with your sister-in-law or other female relative of your partner, you may decide to invite her to the birth.

Don't think of this list as the must-invitees to the birth. Consider it only your possible options, inviting just one or a few who you feel close to and who will support your birth plan. Before extending any invitation, be sure to consider the questions in this chapter listed in the sections "Questions to ask yourself about potential guests" and "What makes a good birthing buddy."

# Bringing Your Best Friend

If you and your BFF (best friend forever) are joined at the hip, you may consider it unthinkable to not have her by your side as you make your transition into motherhood. A friend can also make a great labor partner. If the dad-to-be isn't interested or isn't able to offer emotional or physical support during childbirth, your best friend may be the next best thing. Plus, friends are less likely to drudge up drama while you're fighting through contractions, though not every friendship is drama free.

In this section, we explain what makes a good birthing buddy and which friends are better off visiting after the baby's birth.

## What makes a good birthing buddy

Obviously, a birthing buddy should be someone you feel totally at ease with — someone you can be 100 percent yourself around. But to go from being just a good friend to a good birthing buddy, you need someone who also meets the following criteria:

✔ **Experienced with childbirth:** If you have a choice between a friend who has never given birth and one who has, usually it's best to choose the experienced friend. She's more likely to intuit what you need most. On the other hand, some experienced moms may assume you should act and cope the same way they did. There are also some excellent doulas and midwives who have never had a baby. If your closest friend has zero birth experience, consider watching some real birth videos together as preparation, and be sure to take a childbirth education class together.

✔ **Willing to prepare:** A good birth buddy will spend some time before the birth discussing your birth plans and the role you hope she'll play. If your friend will be your main support, taking the role of labor partner, then you should attend a childbirth education class together. See Chapter 7 for more on childbirth education classes.

✔ **Supportive, no matter what choices you make:** If you're planning a natural birth, a supportive friend should also know how to encourage you to keep going when things get tough but also be able to support you fully if you decide mid-labor that an epidural is what you really need. Although you may have little experience with your friend as a labor partner, you likely have experienced her support in other aspects of your life. Go with your gut and be sure whoever you bring into the labor room is someone who will make you feel good, not guilty.

## Friends who don't belong in the labor room

Good friends are not always good birthing buddies. Friends who are best left waiting down the hall or at home include:

✔ **Anyone with an agenda:** If you're hoping for a natural birth and your friend keeps saying you're crazy to even try, or if you're hoping for an epidural and your friend constantly slams you with frightening statistics, make the smart choice and don't invite that friend to your birth. Even if you agree with her, if you suspect your friend will be disappointed if you change your mind, keep her out of the delivery room.

✔ **Squeamish friends:** More likely to be a problem with women who have never given birth, if your friend gags at the very idea of being in the same room as vomit, blood, or poo, she probably won't handle childbirth well. Invite her to visit after the baby's born.

✔ **Friends unwilling to prepare:** If your friend is too busy to talk about your birth plan with you before labor, then she probably shouldn't be invited to the delivery. You don't want to find out too late that her philosophy on childbirth is diametrically opposed to yours. Plus, if she's too busy to prepare for the birth, she may be too busy to come when you're actually in labor (or too busy to stick around during a long labor).

✔ **Friendships full of drama:** Friends usually carry less drama than family, but that's not always true. If your friend tends to be judgmental or has a confrontational relationship with your partner, then you probably don't want her by your side when you're in labor.

# Including Your Older Children at the Birth

With the birth of your first child, you are reborn as a mother. With the birth of subsequent children, your family is reborn: you as a mother of another, and each sibling as an older brother or sister to the new arrival. In recognition of this family change, some mothers and fathers choose to include their older children in the birth. Each family's comfort level with having a family birth experience is different, and of course, each child may react differently to the birth of a new baby. Children attending the birth of a sibling may be as young as toddlers or as old as teenagers.

In this section, we discuss the practical issues of including your children at the birth: dealing with hospital or birth-center policies, preparing your child to attend the birth, and arranging support and supervision for them.

## Dealing with hospital and birth-center policies

If you're giving birth at home, then how and whether to include your kids is your personal choice (though you will still need someone to supervise them in the event of an emergency). However, if you're having your baby at a hospital or birth center, you need to consider the policies of your chosen birth location.

Teenagers are probably not an issue, but the presence of young children, especially toddler to grade-school age, may not be looked upon favorably. Talk to your doctor or midwife first about your children being present. If you're delivering in the hospital, then speak to the hospital's nursing supervisor, labor and delivery floor manager, or risk-management supervisor to find out if the hospital will allow your child to attend. At a birth center, speak to the director before making plans.

If management says no, ask if the facility will allow it if someone besides yourself and your partner supervises the child the entire time. The hospital will want someone to be there designated to care for the children — not your partner, because you wouldn't want him leaving if an issue arose.

You should also discuss your family birth plans with your medical practitioner. Keep in mind that you're not asking if she thinks it's a good idea or not — that's up to you! You're just asking if she'll allow the kids to stay, and under what circumstances they'd need to leave.

If the hospital says no and the doctor says no, you can still take a risk and show up with the kids anyway. You may receive some dirty looks, but they're highly unlikely to refuse their presence completely. Some couples who don't have local family or a babysitter bring along their kids because they have no choice. If your birth plan is to include your child and you've prepared them for the event, you and your child have a great advantage over the ones having a family birth not by choice. On the other hand, if the hospital remains adamant about their policy, your partner may end up in the waiting room with your kids, leaving you alone in the labor room. If you don't have a partner, the staff could end up caring for your children, which could create tension between you and the staff.

## Preparing your kids to attend the birth

Watching your mother give birth can be exciting — you can *really* find out where babies come from! — but also scary, especially if a child isn't prepared. Understanding that it's normal during birth for Mommy to make noises and that babies come out looking kind of gooey and bloody is important. Otherwise, your child may worry that something is wrong. A prepared child, on the other hand, is likely to be curious and highly interested, not fearful.

Of course, helping your teenager prepare and helping your toddler prepare are very different things. That said, here are some ways to get ready:

- ✔ **Talk about where babies come from — at least in part.** For very young kids, you can skip the sex talk and just discuss where in Mommy's body the baby grows and how the baby comes out.

- ✔ **Read books together about birth and babies.** Depending on your kids' age, you may want to read illustrated books written for adults, not just children's books. Seeing birth pictures in a book can help normalize the experience for them.

- ✔ **Watch real birth videos together.** Stick to real births with positive outcomes. See Chapter 8 for birth video ideas.

Prescreen birth videos first, and avoid showing kids birth "reality" television shows.

✔ **Have them attend a sibling birth class.** Some childbirth educators offer classes for children in which they explain what happens during birth. See Chapter 7 for more on finding childbirth education classes.

✔ **Talk, talk, and talk some more about the birth.** Talking with your children before the birth about how excited you are for them to be there and how excited you are about the birth of their new sibling can help them mentally prepare. Talk about where you'll have the baby, what they may see, your birth plans (the aspects that are visual, positive, and understandable to them), and different ways they could help, like by bringing Mommy drinks or puffing up pillows. Also be sure your children know they don't have to be at the birth and can even change their minds in the middle of labor, if they want.

Prepare a birth bag just for your kids. Include things to keep them occupied when they're bored, along with plenty of snacks and drinks. You may also want to bring an illustrated birth book, something you've read together before, so someone can use the book to explain what's happening at the moment with mom and baby.

## Arranging a care provider for your children

Ideally, someone should be assigned to watch over your kids during labor, and that someone should not be your partner (unless you have absolutely no other choice). You and your partner will be focused on the birth, but your children will still need some attention and care, varying with age and maturity. A supervisor can help with breaks, snacks, bathroom visits, and questions. Also, in the event of an emergency, or if you or your kids change your mind about them being at the birth, they will have someone to watch over them.

You can choose a friend or relative, or even hire a babysitter. Your children should be comfortable with whomever you choose, and you should *also* feel comfortable with this person. Take into consideration the information found under "Questions to ask yourself about potential guests."

# Part III

# Planning Childbirth Options for a Normal Birth

## The 5th Wave
By Rich Tennant

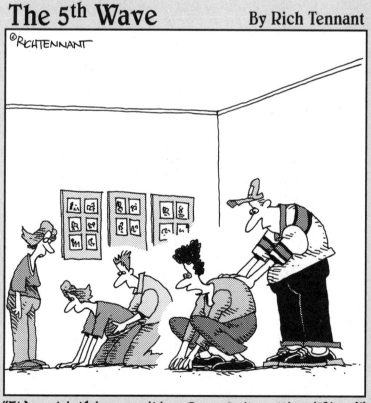

"It's a birthing position, Dan. Quit yelling 'Hike.'"

# In this part . . .

After you decide on the who and where of your birth, you're ready to consider additional options. These chapters get into the nitty-gritty details that will help you truly personalize your birth plan, from ways to stay active in labor to ways to stay calm and keep your cool in an exciting but often tumultuous time.

# Chapter 7

# Getting an Education

. . . . . . . . . . . . . . . . . . . . . . . . . . . . . . . . . . . . . . . . . . . . . . . . . . . . . . . . .

## In This Chapter

▶ Reaping the benefits of childbirth education

▶ Considering what birthing style may be right for you

▶ Selecting a great childbirth class

▶ Benefitting from your previous labor and delivery experiences

. . . . . . . . . . . . . . . . . . . . . . . . . . . . . . . . . . . . . . . . . . . . . . . . . . . . . . . . .

*Y*ou can easily get caught up in getting everything ready for your baby, from painting the nursery to purchasing the car seat, but don't forget about preparing for the most important part — the birth itself! In this chapter, we explain how to get an excellent childbirth education. We give you a primer on what the different childbirth styles have to offer so you can pick the method and classes that are right for you. We also explain how to use your former birthing experiences to shape your next one, if you've been through this before.

## Taking Classes: Childbirth May Be Natural, But It's Not Easy!

Childbirth education classes are a rite of passage for couples expecting their first child, though even experienced moms may benefit from a refresher course. The classes can offer practical insights, inspiration, and information that may improve your birthing experience. If that sounds like a commercial, well, it is. We believe in education!

Some women participate in childbirth education only because their doctors insist, and they drag their unwilling partners to yawn alongside them. Even if you're signing up only to please your doctor, try to approach the classes with an open mind and positive attitude. Childbirth education does *not* have to be boring, especially if you choose a birthing style that fits your personality.

Childbirth education class can benefit you and your partner in a number of ways, some obvious and some not so obvious. Going to classes gives you the following advantages:

- ✔ **Getting the lowdown on labor and delivery in person:** At classes you're able to ask questions (something you can't do with a book). Your instructor may utilize props and video (yes, real birth videos!) to help you understand the birthing process. If you take a class in the hospital, you get to see where you'll be laboring, which can take away the fear of the unknown.

- ✔ **Meeting other couples:** Unless you're lucky enough to be surrounded by friends and family who are at the same stage of impending parenthood as you, getting together with expectant moms and dads can help you feel less isolated and provide future coffee and play dates. Many a mom-to-be has made a new best friend at childbirth class!

- ✔ **Practicing soothing techniques:** You learn new techniques for pain management and get a chance to practice them in a calm, pain-free state. Even if you plan to have an epidural, you won't be able to have one the moment labor begins, so be sure not to doze off during this part of the class!

- ✔ **Gathering options for your birth plan:** A good class helps you understand your options for labor and birth. You can ask your instructor for clarification on issues you don't yet understand, and she may even be willing to look over your birth plan and make suggestions for improvements.

- ✔ **Learning how to be an excellent birth partner:** Labor can be overwhelming for partners as well as for laboring moms (though we wouldn't say it's *as* overwhelming, and you shouldn't either, Dad, if you don't want to sleep on the couch tonight!). Partners benefit from learning about normal labor and delivery, which helps them stay calmer in what can be a nerve-wracking situation. They also learn how to advocate for and support the mom-to-be (not an easy task!).

# Determining Your Birthing Style

Although just about every childbirth education class offers the key benefits listed in the previous section, not every class offers that information in the same way. Finding a class that fits your style best helps you have an enjoyable experience. Childbirth education, like everything else, goes through fads (often determined by the latest celebrity craze), but some methods have proven their staying power despite evolving over the years. The next sections describe some of your options for childbirth education classes.

If a few of the childbirth styles appeal to you but you have limited time and finances or the class you'd love isn't available in your area, you can take a course in one style and just read or listen to materials from others. And in Chapters 8 and 9 you can also find lots of info on natural soothing methods and movement and positions for birth. So read on!

Don't fret too much about choosing the "perfect" method or style for you. Although each method has a unique emphasis, they all pretty much teach the same basic birthing principals: using optimal positions for labor and birth, avoiding unnecessary inventions, making use of comfort measures, and following your instincts during labor. You won't miss "the secret" to childbirth if you take the "wrong" course.

## *Lamaze International*

Once upon a time, Lamaze childbirth classes focused on patterned breathing and strongly coach-led labor. Lamaze was the original inventor of the hee-hee-hoo method of childbirth breathing. Times have changed.

Today, the Lamaze approach emphasizes the normality of birth. Lamaze believes that the role of childbirth education is to empower women to make informed decisions regarding their healthcare, to take responsibility for their health, and to trust their inner wisdom.

Lamaze believes that women have a right to give birth free from medical interventions, and they teach the following "Six Lamaze Healthy Birth Practices" to help mothers have a normal, natural delivery:

- ✔ Allowing labor to begin on its own
- ✔ Moving around throughout labor
- ✔ Bringing along a doula or friend for support
- ✔ Avoiding unnecessary interventions
- ✔ Avoiding lying on your back for pushing
- ✔ Keeping mother and baby together

We cover some of these techniques in Chapter 9 on movement and positions for labor, in Chapter 17 on nourishing your baby (and rooming-in), and in Chapters 3 and 6 on how to hire a doula or bring along a friend for support. Also, in Part IV, you can read up on various interventions used during labor so you know what your options are and how to avoid interventions that aren't necessary during a healthy labor and delivery.

A Lamaze class may be a good fit for you if the following descriptions sound like you:

✔ You'd like to take one of the most well-known and widely available childbirth courses around. (There's a reason people think "Lamaze" when they think childbirth education!)

✔ You're looking for an evidence-based course, which will provide you with birthing tips proven effective in research studies.

✔ When you imagine yourself in labor, you like to see yourself up and active, confidently turning down unnecessary routine interventions, with a doula or friend by your side, and pushing your baby in an upright position, *not* lying on your back!

To learn more or find a Lamaze educator near you, check out www.lamaze.org.

## The Bradley Method

Also known as *husband-coached childbirth,* the Bradley Method puts a strong emphasis on natural childbirth. In fact, their website claims that 90 percent of moms who take their classes have natural (medication-free) childbirth (not accounting for cesarean-section births).

The Bradley Method emphasizes relaxation and normal breathing as the key to reduce labor pains. Instead of using distraction, moms are taught to trust the birth process and their bodies and to turn inward to focused full-body relaxation. You can read about some of these techniques in Chapter 8.

Other unique aspects of the Bradley Method classes are the focus on the labor coach's role, their 12-week-long sessions (the average childbirth course is 6 weeks), detailed discussions on avoiding tears and episiotomies, information on avoiding a cesarean section and how to make the most of one if you need it, and what to do if your baby is born accidently in the car en route to the hospital or birth center.

A Bradley Method course may be right for you if you agree with the following statements:

✔ You're absolutely sure you want a natural childbirth.

✔ You're willing to commit to a 12-week-long course.

✔ Your partner, doula, or birthing buddy is also committed to learning Bradley techniques and taking an active role in supporting you.

✔ When you imagine yourself in intense labor, you see yourself lying on your side or sitting upright, supported by plenty of pillows, and quietly focusing deep within yourself on total relaxation as you breath calmly and normally.

For more on the Bradley Method, or to find a class near you, visit www.
bradleybirth.com.

# *Birthing from Within*

In Birthing from Within classes, you're less likely to focus on medical procedures and more likely to focus on self-discovery. In fact, Birthing from Within
recommends that people who prefer a research-intense class take another
mainstream course alongside Birthing from Within.

Birthing from Within doesn't focus on natural childbirth, and it doesn't promise pain-free labor or any particular outcome. Instead, Birthing from Within
encourages women to see birth as hard work and to remember that positive
actions can't guarantee specific results. Birthing from Within encourages a
"living-in-awareness" approach to labor, including the mindful use of medications and procedures when necessary.

Other unique aspects of Birthing from Within include the use of in-class
experiences (including art projects!) and instruction on self-hypnosis and
visualizations. The classes focus on seeing birth as a rite of passage, and they
address how to "give birth from within" during cesarean section, with pain
medication, or in any other medically assisted birth. (We discuss hypnosis
and visualizations in Chapter 8.)

If you fit the following descriptions, a Birthing from Within course may be
for you:

- You're looking for not only lectures and birthing-technique practices but
  also inner work through art and discussion, preparing you mentally for
  the hard work of labor and emotional transition to parenthood.

- You like the idea of not focusing on the outcome of birth (like having a
  natural birth or not) but instead focusing on what you can control, such
  as birthing awareness, however labor goes.

- When you imagine yourself in labor, you like to see yourself remaining
  active throughout, approaching labor as hard (but doable) work, and
  you imagine yourself as a birthing warrior, claiming your space and
  experience as your rite of passage to motherhood, whether you have a
  natural vaginal birth or cesarean birth.

To learn more or find a class near you, check out www.birthingfrom
within.com.

# HypnoBirthing

HypnoBirthing, also known as the Mongan Method, teaches that the negative stories and myths regarding birth strongly impact mothers. These stories create fear, fear then leads to tension, and tension leads to increased pain. Fear and tension may also prevent the body from birthing normally.

HypnoBirthing is based on the belief that your mind is the most powerful tool in having natural childbirth. Through the use of self-hypnosis and guided imagery, labor doesn't need to be unbearably painful. In fact, some HypnoBirthing mothers report pain-free births. (Coauthor Rachel used HypnoBirthing, and although the delivery wasn't pain free, it was completely tolerable. Her doctor said she never saw anyone "sleep" through labor before!)

A HypnoBirthing course may be for you if these statements sound like you:

- ✔ You're willing to spend time some time each day listening to audio recordings, diligently practicing your self-hypnosis and affirmations.

- ✔ You are hypnotizable. Not everyone is! If you haven't been hypnotized before and aren't sure if it's possible for you, HypnoBirthing may work well for you if you daydream often, you can lose yourself in an activity and not notice people around you, or you can get deeply involved in books or movies.

- ✔ You know that fear may be preventing you from approaching labor and childbirth calmly.

- ✔ When you imagine yourself in labor, you see yourself deeply relaxing your body during contractions while remaining alert and active in between, trusting completely in your body's ability to birth your baby.

If this sounds like you, go to www.hypnobirthing.com to learn more. You can also find more about using the power of your mind in Chapter 8.

# BirthWorks

BirthWorks teaches that women innately know how to labor and give birth and that developing trust in this inner knowing is key to having a healthy, natural childbirth. The program is not a method; it approaches childbirth as a process that should be guided by a woman's instincts.

BirthWorks teaches that emotions can have a strong effect on birth outcomes and so wherever a woman feels most safe is the best place for her to give birth. It also teaches that healing emotional pain caused by a prior negative childbirth experience is an essential part of preparing for the next birth.

In BirthWorks classes, women also learn how to use affirmations to increase positivity toward birth and how to use positions to optimize the pelvic opening for labor and delivery. You can explore some of these techniques in Chapter 8, on the power of the mind, and Chapter 9, on positions for birth.

A BirthWorks course may be for you if these statements are true for you:

- You're working through emotions from a previous negative birth experience and you're looking for more guidance on this issue.
- You're planning a VBAC (vaginal birth after cesarean), something BirthWorks covers especially well.
- You imagine yourself in labor working with both your body and mind to consciously birth your baby, trusting your body's urges, vocalizing when it feels right, and using optimal positions and movements to make way for your baby's passage.

The BirthWorks website, www.birthworks.org, can give you more information.

# ICEA (International Childbirth Education Association)

ICEA, the International Childbirth Education Association, believes that the birth of a baby is also the birth of a new family and many new relationships within the family. ICEA takes a family-centered approach to childbirth, seeing birth as a life-changing event and not just a medical procedure. You can learn more about including your family or kids in birth in Chapter 6.

ICEA educators are pretty much free to create their own unique courses, so classes vary from instructor to instructor. It's an eclectic approach, offering freedom from focusing on just one particular childbirth method. Visit the association's website, www.icea.org, to learn more.

An ICEA childbirth class may be for you if these descriptions fit you:

- You want to include your older children in the birth experience.
- You like the idea of taking an eclectic approach to childbirth preparation rather than learning one technique or style.
- You see yourself making informed decisions throughout labor, using your medical practitioner as a guide — not master — to the birthing experience.

# Choosing a Class

Deciding which class to take goes beyond birthing styles; it also involves finding the right teacher, class size, and price. Two different instructors certified in the same childbirth method may offer very different classroom experiences. Unfortunately, this sort of thing is hard to assess without actually going to the class, but if you try a class and hate it, no rule says you have to continue it. Try a class on another night if it offers a different instructor.

## Comparing private and hospital-sponsored classes

You can find childbirth classes at hospitals and at private centers. Hospital-sponsored classes are partially subsidized and are therefore less expensive than private classes. Lamaze-certified, ICEA-certified, and labor and delivery nurses (who may or may not be certified childbirth instructors) often teach these courses.

Hospital-sponsored classes may provide the inside scoop on the hospital's policies and include an L&D (labor and delivery) floor and postpartum floor tour. They may or may not provide information on all your potential birth-plan options. Some people say hospitals fail to provide this info because they don't want to create "difficult" patients who have their own ideas on how childbirth should go. A hospital-sponsored class typically includes a more eclectic group of parents-to-be than method-focused private classes do, mainly because it's more affordable and not focused on one particular style of childbirth. Private classes also tend to have more couples intent on natural childbirth; hospital-class participants tend to be evenly mixed or slanted more to medicated childbirth.

Private courses are typically more expensive and have smaller class sizes. They're also more likely to focus on a variety of labor and delivery techniques. Although many hospital courses are based on Lamaze, a privately taught Lamaze course may spend more time on natural coping techniques and less on hospital policy. You may decide on a private course because you want to learn a particular style. For example, if you're interested in the Bradley Method, you're unlikely to find it as a hospital-sponsored course.

If you decide to take a private course but still want details on the hospital's policies, take a free tour of the labor and delivery floors and ask the nurses questions after the tour (and before labor begins!).

Private isn't always better. Many good hospital-sponsored childbirth courses and terrible private ones are out there, so be sure to speak to the instructor and ask questions before you enroll, if possible.

## Finding a childbirth class

Call your local hospitals to ask about sponsored classes. Although taking a course offered by the hospital you've chosen for the birth has its advantages, you can take one offered by a different hospital if it seems more appealing.

For private courses, check the websites of the particular birth style you're interested in (some of the different options are given in the earlier section "Determining Your Birthing Style"). Most offer searchable directories or numbers to call for information.

People who know you well may be your best resource. Be sure to ask other moms and dads, your medical practitioner, or your doula about childbirth classes they've taken or heard good things about.

## Asking the instructor some questions

Before you choose a class, get the name and number of the instructor so you can ask some questions. Even within the same birthing style, each instructor offers a unique experience.

Here are some questions you may want to ask the instructor:

- Are you certified? What are your qualifications to teach this course?
- What topics does the class cover? Do the topics lean toward a particular style of labor and birth?
- What is your philosophy on pregnancy and birth?
- What does a typical class session look like?
- Is the class private or offered by a health clinic or hospital? If sponsored, how much freedom do you have over the curriculum and topics covered?
- How many sessions do we meet for? How long are the classes?
- When and where are the classes?
- How much does the class cost? What does that fee include exactly?
- How many couples attend the classes? (Ten or fewer is best.)

✔ How much class time is spent on natural birthing techniques? Does the class include practice opportunities?

✔ Do you offer sibling classes, either to prepare them for the arrival of a new baby or to prepare a child to attend the birth?

✔ Do you talk about birth plans? Are you open to helping me with questions as I write my own plan?

There really are no right or wrong answers to most of these questions. What's most important is if the class and instructor sound like a good fit to you. Go with your gut feeling. However, even if the course sounds wonderful, don't discount practical considerations. For example, if the class is a long drive away or outside of your budget, you need to weigh whether the disadvantages outweigh the benefits.

# Using Your Last Delivery as a Learning Experience

If this isn't your first rodeo and you're an experienced mama, you have some idea of what labor and childbirth is like, and you may even have a better idea of what you want and don't want.

If your last experience went well, you may be more confident than other expectant moms and know how you'd like to labor and deliver. If your birth experience was less than ideal, you can use that knowledge and revisit your options to improve your next birth.

## Changing what didn't work

You're more likely to remember what didn't go well than what went well, and that selective memory has an advantage: It allows you to make changes.

Sit down and make a list of everything you felt went wrong during your last labor, birth, and postpartum period. Don't think too hard about what was preventable and what wasn't — just write, write, write.

Don't forget to ask your partner or doula what they remember from your last birth. They may have insight into how or why things went wrong that can help you have a better birth next time. They may also remember the birth in an entirely different way, and listening to their version of the events can be helpful.

## Diving into books and video about birth

With the hundreds of books and many television shows and documentaries on birth, knowing where to start can be overwhelming. Here are a few birth resources to get you started:

✔ *The Business of Being Born,* **directed by Abby Epstein:** A frank look at what's happening in American hospitals today, this documentary looks at how birth moved out of the home and into hospitals, as well as the move from using midwives to using doctors. The documentary is strongly slanted towards home birth, but even if you're planning a hospital birth, the footage of women laboring without drugs and pushing in a variety of positions is educational and inspiring.

✔ *Birthing from Within: An Extra-Ordinary Guide to Childbirth Preparation,* **by Pam England:** Coauthor Rachel's all-time favorite book about childbirth, *Birthing from Within* takes a unique approach to natural childbirth while acknowledging the time and place for medication or even cesarean delivery. Great for women who have had previous negative birth experiences or who are fearful of the birth process, the book addresses the psychological and emotional side of labor and delivery more so than most books on childbirth.

✔ *The Birth Partner,* **by Penny Simkin:** Considered a classic childbirth preparation book, *The Birth Partner* is especially written for dads, doulas, and anyone else planning to support a laboring woman. If you can't take a childbirth class, this book can help you and your labor partner prepare for childbirth.

After you complete the list, sit back and consider: What can I change? What's out of my control? For the things you can change, make a plan of action. Speak to your medical practitioner, doula, childbirth educator, or partner for advice if you're not sure how to make those changes.

If thinking about your past birth experience causes intense emotions or you find yourself deeply fearful of the upcoming birth, speak to a therapist or a trusted friend. Fear from a traumatic birth can lead to another difficult birth. High stress can interfere with the body's birthing process and your ability to cope with pain. You'll do better if you work through the emotions now *before* contractions begin. See Chapter 20 for more on coping with a negative birth experience.

## *Taking a childbirth education class again*

Childbirth classes aren't only for new moms and dads. Even if you're an experienced birther, you may want to sign up again for the following reasons:

✔ **You felt unprepared last time.** Judging what kind of labor style fits you best can be hard until you've actually been in labor. If the techniques you studied didn't work well last time, maybe a different style or instructor can help you have a better experience.

✔ **You need a refresher.** If you gave birth a couple years ago, maybe it's all fresh in your mind. But if more than a few years have passed, taking a new course can help. Sometimes childbirth instructors offer special refresher courses for experienced couples. Also, if you've given birth before but this is your partner's first birth, you may want to take a class.

✔ **You want to add to your laboring knowledge.** Maybe last time the birth went great but you're eager to learn more tips and tricks. Plus, no two classes are the same, even with the same instructor and same birthing style. You're bound to learn something new.

✔ **You want to meet new moms and dads.** Okay, so maybe you're not supposed to pass notes during class, but you can chat before and after.

The classroom is just one place where you can learn about childbirth techniques and options. There are also hundreds of books on giving birth (like this one!), not to mention films, birthing videos, and websites dedicated to providing inside information. We don't suggest you learn only from books and videos, but we do encourage extra-credit learning outside the classroom.

# Chapter 8

# Natural Methods for Soothing Your Mind and Body

They don't call it "labor" because it's easy and simple. Even moms who rave about their beautiful natural childbirths will admit it required lots of preparation and hard work. Whether you hope for a natural birth or you're determined to get an epidural as quickly as possible, natural coping techniques help you deal with the labor of labor, including all the emotional and physical ups and downs of childbirth and delivery. In this chapter, we explain how to utilize different relaxation tools and choose the techniques that will work best for you.

Although you don't need to list every comfort technique you plan to use in your birth plan, those that require special accommodations — like use of a shower or birthing pool, or the desire to be free from monitoring equipment so you can move freely — should be mentioned clearly in your plan.

## Tapping into the Power of Your Mind

Your most powerful tool when facing labor and delivery is your mind. Just think of the difference between how you feel when talking with a good friend compared to someone who intimidates you. When you're confident and at ease, your body is relaxed, you're able to think straight, and you speak in a clear, articulate manner. When you feel intimidated, your shoulders may tighten, you feel unsure and anxious, thinking on your feet is more difficult, and the ability to speak your mind is noticeably affected.

Women who are fearful of labor and delivery are more likely to feel out of control and less confident advocating for themselves. They may also experience higher levels of pain. Dr. Grantly Dick-Read, in his book *Childbirth Without Fear,* explains that when a woman feels fear during labor, she tenses up and fights the contractions. Fighting against the contractions intensifies the pain. This increased pain leads to even more fear, and when the next contraction comes, she fights the contraction more fiercely, and again, the pain is worse. It's a difficult cycle to break, especially if you don't know it can be any different.

Feeling nervous about birth is normal, especially if this is your first pregnancy or if you've experienced difficult births in the past. The good news is that you can take certain steps to increase your confidence and lower your fear and anxiety. You can train yourself to let go of tension and, instead of fighting the contractions, learn how to ride them like an experienced surfer rides a wave.

## Employing hypnosis and guided imagery

If hypnosis brings to mind a stage magician waving a watch in front of audience volunteers and getting them to perform strange acts, seemingly against their will, forget about that. Therapeutic hypnosis has nothing to do with entertainment hypnosis.

During therapeutic hypnosis, you are put into a trance-like state with the help of a therapist or, with self-hypnosis, an audio recording. Your body feels completely relaxed, and you become more open to suggestion. For birth, these hypnotic suggestions usually aim to reduce your fears, increase the trust you have in your body's birthing process, teach you to deeply relax almost instantly, and decrease your sensations of pain. The reduced fear and ability to deeply relax help break the fear-tension-pain cycle that so often ruins the most dedicated mothers' plans for a natural childbirth.

Guided imagery isn't the same as hypnosis, but the two practices have similarities, and they're often used together. *Guided imagery* involves picturing in vivid detail scenes that induce a state of relaxation. For birth, guided imagery may involve picturing specific outcomes or biological processes, like a breech baby turning head down, effective contractions, and soft, gentle dilation. Or, you may imagine yourself in a safe place, like an empty beach with waves whispering to you in the background. Calming music is often used to increase the effects. Some describe guided imagery as wakeful dreaming or daydreaming with a purpose, and many people actually fall asleep when listening to guided-imagery recordings.

Research has found that hypnosis and guided imagery help women feel more in control, reduce their sensations of pain, decrease the use of interventions (including epidurals), and may even shorten labor. If these results sounds too good to be true, coauthor Rachel can personally vouch for hypnosis: It helped her have an amazing natural childbirth with her second child. With her first child, the fear-tension-pain loop led to the need for an epidural. Hypnosis and guided imagery changed her approach to birth completely!

If you want to try hypnosis for childbirth, you may want to sign up for one of the hypnosis-based childbirth classes. The Mongan Method of HypnoBirthing (www.hypnobirthing.com) has made hypnosis for labor popular, but these classes aren't the only source for hypnotic childbirth preparation. HypnoBabies (www.hypnobabies.com), Leclaire Hypnobirthing (www.leclairemethod.com), and HypBirth (www.hypbirth.com) also offer classes and at-home study packages.

Hypnotherapists, who are usually psychologists or counselors, can also help, and they can personalize the hypnosis to address your specific fears or history. Personal hypnosis can be used along with a hypnosis childbirth method or by itself. For a referral, contact The International Medical and Dental Hypnotherapy Association at 570-869-1021.

Hypnosis isn't for everyone. Some people are not affected at all by hypnosis, while others are highly suggestible. Everyone else falls somewhere in between. If you're a daydreamer, get lost in your thoughts, or tend to get pulled into books or movies, you're more likely to benefit from hypnosis. Guided imagery can help you relax whether or not you're the highly suggestible type.

Healthy Journey's *Healthy Pregnancy & Successful Childbirth* is an excellent guided-imagery audio, created by the queen of guided imagery, Belleruth Naparstek. You can purchase an MP3 or CD from www.healthjourneys.com.

For best results, guided imagery and self-hypnosis recordings require repeated listening. In your rushed everyday life, you may feel like you're "wasting time" listening to relaxation audios every day, but this extra effort is necessary for best results. Making it part of your daily routine, maybe before bed or for a restful lunch break, may help you keep up the habit.

If your hypnosis program includes certain cue words, you may want to include them in your written birth plan. The medical staff probably doesn't need them, but it may be handy for your labor partner or doula. Also, if you need a specific environment — like soft lights or calming music — you should mention this as well. If your hypnosis or guided imagery recording can be used during labor, be sure to bring it along with you on your MP3 player.

## Repeating affirmations and birthing mantras

Affirmations are positive statements meant to bolster confidence. You may be familiar with affirmations from the *Saturday Night Live* skit "Daily Affirmation With Stuart Smalley": "I'm good enough, I'm smart enough, and doggone it, people like me!"

All snickering aside, affirmations can help you prepare for childbirth, and many self-hypnosis and guided-imagery programs include a separate affirmations tract. Birthing affirmations may include lines like, "I trust in my body's ability to birth this baby," or "Each breath leads naturally into the next, soothing and calming me with each exhalation."

You can write your own affirmations or use affirmations from a particular program. To use affirmations, you either read them out loud, if they're written, or if they're an audio, you listen first and then repeat. Ideally, you would say them every day, at least once. You may want to listen while doing household chores or when driving to work. Listening to self-hypnosis or guided-imagery recordings when driving is dangerous, but affirmation tapes are fine to listen to on your daily commute.

Although affirmations are typically used during preparation for labor, birthing mantras are statements or words said during labor itself. A birthing mantra is simply a phrase or word that you repeat to yourself over and over. You may speak the words out loud, whisper them softly with each breath, or simply mentally focus on them in silence.

Birthing mantras can be affirmations, or they can be some other repeated phrase or word that lends you a sense of calm or power. Some women repeat a beloved verse from a religious text, meditation, or prayer. It helps if whatever you choose has a soothing sound or beat and is easy to repeat. Birthing mantras can act as reminders to remain relaxed. For example, you may use the mantra "Let go, let flow," or "Soft eyes, soft cheeks, soft tummy, soft bottom." (Or simply repeat "Soft, soft, soft, soft.")

Think up your own affirmations or birthing mantras — the words should be positive (in other words, not "I am not tense," but "I am relaxed") — or choose one of the examples in this section. Sit in a comfortable position, take a deep breath, and as you exhale, whisper your chosen word or phrase. Try this for a few breaths, in a place you feel safe and at ease, and see if it helps you relax. You may want to practice birthing mantras during Braxton-Hicks contractions, the non-labor contractions that frequently occur during the third trimester. Practicing them when contractions are practically painless will help them be automatic when true labor begins.

## *Educating yourself and trusting in your body's birthing abilities*

Nothing generates fear more than the unknown. One reason the dark can be so frightening, to both children and adults, is because we can't see what's in front of us. We don't know what's coming next!

To reduce tension and fear, having an understanding of birth can be extremely helpful. In fact, many natural childbirth methods emphasize knowledge of the birthing process, down to the nitty-gritty details like how the muscles wrap around the uterus and how contractions work. This information may seem unnecessary, but it can change how you approach and even experience labor.

Trusting in your body's birthing abilities doesn't mean you should ignore the possibility of problems. There is a growing movement to give birth unassisted, without doctors or midwives, as an ultimate way of showing trust in the birthing process. However, balancing trust with caution is important. Ensure that wherever you give birth, you'll have quick access to someone who's trained to aid you or the baby in an emergency.

Besides reading about birth or attending childbirth classes, another way to get familiar with childbirth is watching positive birth videos. A variety of birth videos are on the market, including *Orgasmic Birth, Birth As We Know It, The Business of Being Born,* and *Birth Day* (not the reality show).

You can also watch birth videos online for free. Just search for terms like "natural birth," "hypnobirth," "water birth," and the like. You'll find some home videos uploaded to YouTube.com, but you can also find professionally produced educational birth videos at `www.injoyvideos.com/mothersadvocate`, including footage of women giving birth in a variety of positions.

Not all birth videos are great for childbirth preparation. The recent spate of reality birth shows aren't ideal preparation for birth. The problem with these shows is that they overdramatize the stories to increase tension and keep people watching, and they rarely show natural or low-intervention births. Your friends and family may also feel the need to tell you birth horror stories. You need to hear positive empowering birth stories — not ones that scare you or make you doubt yourself! Don't hesitate to interrupt your friends or shut off the television if a birth story makes you anxious or upset.

A nurse (or friend or family member) may ask you during birth *when* you're going to order an epidural, even if you intend on a drug-free labor. Usually this question is asked out of a genuine concern or belief that natural childbirth isn't really possible or is "crazy." Even if you felt confident before a comment like this, it can plant the seeds of self-doubt, and self-doubt is only a few contractions away from deciding you can't do this after all. Before this situation occurs, you may want to put a sign on the door (and include in your birth plan) a polite request that medication not be offered or suggested, but instead, you will let your wants be known if you decide an epidural is right for you. You should also pass this message to guests attending the birth.

# Breathing in the Calm

When distressed or in pain, people tend to take shallow, quick breaths. This reaction may have been very helpful in the wild when trying to evade the attention of dangerous animals, but it's not so helpful in modern-day life. Rapid breathing upsets the balance of oxygen and carbon dioxide in the bloodstream, which then leads to a number of problems, including heightened anxiety, feelings of panic, heart palpations, and lightheadedness.

The good news is that you have some control over your breathing. Just as shallow breathing leads to a cascade of stress reactions in the body, mimicking deep or relaxed breathing (even if you are secretly freaking out!) leads to a physiological relaxation response: the heart slows, blood pressure regulates, and you get a physical sensation of well-being. You can choose from a number of breathing techniques for labor, each with its own advantages and disadvantages. We describe them in the following sections, so give them a try to see which works best for you.

## Reasons for choosing a drug-free birth

Some people wonder why anyone would choose to go through labor and delivery without drugs. If you don't *have* to feel discomfort, why put yourself through it? Choosing a "natural" childbirth isn't as crazy as it sounds. Here are some common reasons women choose a drug-free birth:

✔ **For the natural-birth high:** Your body serves up a cocktail of hormones as you go through birth and delivery, though some of these hormones are suppressed when you take pain drugs. A "runner's high" has nothing on the high experienced after a drug-free birth.

✔ **To avoid negative side effects of pain drugs:** Epidurals and other pain drugs have their place, and thankfully they are available when needed. They are not, however, completely harmless. (See Chapter 11 for the risks of epidurals and other drugs.)

✔ **To experience an orgasmic birth:** Yes, labor and delivery can produce feelings similar to orgasm, especially if the body is deeply relaxed. The documentary *Orgasmic Birth* takes a close look at the pleasurable side to childbirth.

✔ **Because they can:** There's a myth passed along from some medical practitioners to women, and from woman to woman, that a positive natural childbirth isn't possible. Some women are determined to give birth naturally just to show it is possible and to prove to themselves they can do it.

Breathing practices are meant to help with relaxation. Some people get the wrong idea that breathing alone is the key to natural childbirth, but it's not that simple. Conscious breathing should be used in conjunction with other coping mechanisms.

Although breathing exercises are relaxing to some people, others feel increased anxiety or panic when they think too much about how they are breathing. If thinking about your breath leads to distress, don't do it. Like any natural soothing technique, if it doesn't work for you, try something else.

## Breathing deeply

Deep breathing is a relaxation technique that can be used not only in childbirth but also in any number of high-stress situations — including new parenthood! Deep breathing is often taught as a remedy for insomnia, anxiety, panic, and high blood pressure. It's also thought as a spiritual practice by some world religions. Deep breathing is sometimes referred to as abdominal breathing to differentiate it from shallow chest breathing.

The best way to understand deep breathing is to try it. Get into a comfortable sitting position and sit as tall and straight as you can (deep, abdominal breathing is easier to do if you're not crunched up). Place one hand on your stomach and another on your chest. Just notice your natural breathing first. Pay attention to how your chest and abdomen move along with your breath. Then, when you're ready, take a nice, slow inhalation through your nose, and allow your abdomen to expand as you do. Your chest should only rise along with your abdomen, not on its own. You may want to think of breathing into your tummy instead of your chest. When you've reached the top of the deep breath, let out a gentle, slow exhalation. When you have completely emptied your lungs of breath, start another slow, deep inhalation. You may want to try experimenting exhaling with your mouth closed and with your mouth open to see what feels best.

You can count to yourself as you inhale and exhale, if it helps you breath deeper. First, you may breath in and out to the count of three. If that feels comfortable, you may try counting to four, then five, and even six. During labor, counting can help you slow down your breathing if you're subconsciously breathing quickly. You may also want to pair visualizations with your breathing; for example, you could imagine a blue or white light that starts at your toes and slowly rises up until it reaches your head at the top of your breath, and then, as you exhale, you can imagine the light escaping through your lips, taking along with it any tension in your body.

If you want to practice deep breathing when under stress, try tightly holding an ice cube in your hand. The ice cube will cause some physical discomfort, so you can try comforting techniques while tolerating pain.

## Using yogic breathing

In yoga, breath, also known a *pranayama,* is as important as the famous yoga poses. Yogis believe that yogic breathing increases a person's life energy, or *prana.* You don't have to be a yogi or believe in life energy to benefit from yogic breathing. A number of yoga breathing techniques are taught, but for our purposes, we focus on the two that are most helpful for birth: victorious breath and golden-thread breath.

Victorious breath, also known as *ujjayi,* is slow, deep breathing that involves inhaling and exhaling through the nose while creating a softened Darth Vader–like sound in the throat. Some people compare the sound of victorious breath to waves breaking on a beach or a newborn snoring. Along with the deep breathing, this sound is the key relaxation effect of this breathing technique.

The best way to learn how to create the sound is to take a slow, deep inhalation and then exhale slowly with your mouth open while making a soft *ha* sound. Your throat shouldn't be too tense, but tighten it just enough to make the gentle *ha* sound. After you've tried it with your mouth open, try again with your mouth closed and exhaling through the nose. After you get the hang of making the Darth Vader sound on the exhale, try using the same throat tension to create the sound as you inhale. You may want to close your eyes and picture ocean waves, matching the imagery with your breath.

Breathing with the mouth closed may feel unnatural as labor progresses. Just like when you exercise, strong active labor may trigger you to exhale through your mouth. Golden-thread breath, taught by Uma Dinsmore-Tuli in *Mother's Breath,* is perfect for this. It can be used along with victorious breath (just with open-mouth exhalations) or alone.

To practice golden-thread breath, sit up tall in a comfortable position. Your teeth should be slightly apart, jaw and face relaxed, and your lips just slightly apart, as if a tissue were between them. Take a slow, deep inhalation through the nose, and then gently exhale through your lips while picturing a fine, golden thread spiraling out from between your lips with the breath. Visualize the golden thread spiraling around and around until the exhalation is over and you are ready for your next inhalation. Your lips shouldn't be pursed and you're not really blowing, but just exhaling naturally. You may notice a cooling sensation on your lips and a soft whistling sound as you exhale.

Not all yoga breathing techniques are recommended or are safe for pregnancy and childbirth. If you are part of a yoga class, your instructor should know which techniques are contraindicated. Any breathing practices that involve holding the breath, pulling in the abdomen, or forceful abdominal breathing should not be used during pregnancy or childbirth.

# Practicing patterned breathing

Most people think of patterned breathing when they imagine a laboring woman. When the natural childbirth revolution began with Lamaze in the 1960s, breathing patterns were a key element of comfort. The hee-hee-hoo breathing was meant to help women feel more in control and distract them from contractions, while also giving them an oxygen boost. Although some childbirth educators still teach patterned breathing, the emphasis is lower than it used to be. There are many more ways today to get a sense of control and comfort, and natural or deep breathing is more effective for most women.

However, patterned breathing is helpful for some, so it's worth trying to find out if it works for you. Slow breathing is usually taught along with patterned breathing for early labor. Research has found that using patterned breathing in early labor increases fatigue, so natural breathing is your best option until contractions intensify.

The three patterned breathing styles commonly taught are the cleansing breath, light accelerated breathing, and variable breathing (the hee-hee-hoo).

- ✔ **Cleansing breath:** A cleansing breath is taken at the beginning and end of each contraction. It's meant to provide a good dose of relaxation, while also signaling to your partner and those around you that a contraction has started or finished. To take a cleansing breath, simply take a slow deep inhalation, and then, as you exhale, let out a loud sigh, which can help with releasing any tension. (Read more about vocalizing in this chapter in the section "I Am Birthing, Hear Me Roar!")

- ✔ **Light accelerated breathing:** Light accelerated breathing gives you something to focus on (instead of the discomfort of the contraction) and provides a strong dose of oxygen. After taking a cleansing breath, take in light, shallow inhalations through the nose and exhale through the mouth, at about twice the speed of your regular breathing rhythm. Your breathing should be audible but soft, and your exhalations should be louder than the inhalations. As the contraction peaks, make your breathing lighter and faster, now inhaling and exhaling through the mouth at about one breath to each second. Keep tension out of the shoulders and face as you breath. Then, as the contraction subsides, slow the pace of your breathing, switch back to inhaling through the nose, and take deeper and deeper breaths until the contraction ends. At that time, take another cleansing breath.

  During this breathing pattern, if you should feel dizzy or anxious, switch to slower, deeper breathing.

- ✔ **Variable breathing:** This technique is the famous hee-hee-hoo breathing, and it's usually reserved for intense labor or when you're struggling to relax. Before you begin, take a nice cleansing breath, as described above. Be sure to release all the tension in your body with a sigh as you exhale. Next, inhale and exhale shallow panting-like breaths through the mouth, like a dog on a hot day. (This breathing pattern is sometimes referred to as pant-pant-blow.) Every two or four pants, let out a longer breath with a vocalization like *hoo* or *huh.* Continue this pattern until the contraction ends, when you take a cleansing breath. As with all breathing patterns, if you feel lightheaded or the breathing just doesn't feel right, stop and switch to natural or slow, deep breathing.

Patterned breathing isn't limited to the patterns explained here or elsewhere. Technically, any breathing that is done at varying rates or depths qualifies, and you may develop your own pattern that is soothing to you. The most important thing is to not hyperventilate (which is caused by rapid deep breathing or prolonged shallow breathing) or do anything that causes you to feel uncomfortable or lightheaded.

## *Breathing naturally*

Natural breathing, or instinctual breathing, is gaining popularity as the best way to breathe through birth, and childbirth-education classes today emphasize it (along with deep breathing) more than any other breathing style. You may be wondering why it needs to be mentioned at all. It's natural, right? One reason is because after years of patterned breathing, many women don't realize that natural breathing may be all they need for labor. Also, at one time the role of the labor partner was to coach the woman through breathing patterns. But coaching breathing could interfere with a woman's ability to follow her instincts, and these days people feel very different about childbirth and coaching.

Another reason natural breathing is taught in childbirth classes is because many people don't breath correctly on a day-to-day basis. Young children naturally breath with their abdomens, but as children become adults (and perhaps become more concerned with how their waistlines look), they tend to suck in their stomachs and breathe with their chest and shoulders. When you're pregnant, abdominal breathing is more difficult just because the baby is pressing up into your diaphragm. But even with your baby nestled up under your ribs, you can learn how to breath with the abdomen and not the chest.

Follow these steps to relearn how to breathe:

1. **Get yourself into a comfortable position, sitting up straight or in a semi-reclining position.**

2. **Place one hand on your abdomen and one hand on your chest and just breath naturally.** Notice how your chest and abdomen move with each inhalation and exhalation. Also take note of your shoulders. Are they tense? Do they rise up as you breathe?

3. **After a few breaths, purposely tighten up your shoulders and then release that tension, letting them fall down and away from your ears.**

4. **Take a slow deep breath and visualize your breath filling up your tummy.** Notice how your chest moves slightly but not as much as your abdomen.

5. **Exhale and return to natural breathing. Sit quietly for a few more inhalations and exhalations, allowing your abdomen and not your chest do the hard work of respiration.**

Using natural breathing during childbirth includes following your instincts to sigh, moan, or vocalize in any other way. (More on that in the next section.) Natural breathing means that if you feel like deep breathing, you do that, and if you feel like taking very light short breaths, you do. You may also match your breathing to your movements. For example, if you're standing and swaying your hips gently from side to side through a contraction, you may match your sways to your inhalations and exhalations.

The cleansing breath — that is, a deep inhalation followed by an exhalation with a strong sigh, taken at the start and end of each contraction — can be a nice accompaniment to natural breathing. It lets everyone know a contraction is starting and ending so they can properly support you, and it can also act as an internal reminder to let go of any tension before and after each contraction.

Natural breathing in labor often goes hand in hand with using instinctive pushing for the delivery. Instead of holding your breath and pushing according to the medical caregiver's instructions, you breathe naturally while following your instincts on when to push. If you plan to use instinctive pushing and breathing for the delivery, be sure to write this in your birth plan.

# I Am Birthing, Hear Me Roar!

Take a walk through any labor and delivery floor, and you're bound to hear some brave women birthing loudly. Some women are quieter during delivery — some are naturally quiet birthers, whereas others suppress their urges due to embarrassment or requests from their labor partner or guests. However, vocalizations have a purpose, and there's good reason to let yourself sound off.

## Moaning and groaning

Moaning or groaning during childbirth is normal and natural. This instinctual reaction to contractions and the baby's movements has a soothing effect. The vibrations of your voice reverberate through your body, while the sound fills your ears with a calming tone. During the pushing phase, moaning and groaning can help you push instinctually, almost guiding and encouraging your muscles to bear down in just the right way.

Moaning and groaning also come naturally during bowel movements and during sex. You can use these moments before childbirth to practice your moans and groans. Don't hold back, and just follow your gut (literally!). You may even exaggerate the moaning and groaning just to get a sense for what different intensities feel like. Notice the vibrations in your throat and chest, and see if it doesn't soothe you in some way. Notice if groaning makes your bathroom visits more effective. While your partner will likely be overjoyed at any bedroom moaning action, you may not receive accolades for the bathroom songs. Then again, if you tell your partner the reasoning behind your new bathroom music, maybe he'll join in as a gesture of solidarity.

## Calming yourself with oooms and ahhs

There are so many different ways to vocalize during labor. You may find yourself deeply sighing with each exhale, or using vowels together with sing-song rhythms, like *oh, oo, ah,* or even *i-yi-yi.* These sounds may all come naturally, or they may be something you try out, just to see if it helps. You may intentionally choose vocalizations from meditations or prayers. If you're a yogi, perhaps you'll find a few *oms* escaping your lips. On the other side of the coin, four-letter words may burst out, even if you're not the type who usually swears. Trust us; if you do let an especially colorful word fly, you won't be the first laboring mother to do so!

If your completely normal but lively birthing noises are disturbing other patients or nurses, ask to have your door closed. What if it's offending your guests, like your friends or family? Then remember that this is your birth and your needs come first. If your mother-in-law can't handle it, she should leave. You shouldn't have to silence yourself if it's helping you through labor. See Chapters 6 and 19 for more on handling your birthing support team.

## Easing Physical Tension

In case you haven't already guessed, you should expect some physical tension during labor. (Shocking, we know!) Seriously, though, contractions are just one (very intense) part of the pains of labor. You may also experience backache, headache, shoulder and neck tension, and leg cramps. Some of the tension is directly related to the contractions and position of your baby, but some may unintentionally develop from the movements or positions you use to get through labor. Emotional stress also leads to aches and pains. Although all the techniques mentioned in this chapter and Chapter 9 can help with physical tension, here we give you some tools to attack those aches and pains directly, plus a few preventative techniques.

Many of these techniques require you to move freely or to get into positions that provide comfort but aren't necessarily suitable for fetal-monitoring belts. Your birth plan should make your desire to get out of bed clear, especially if you'll be giving birth in a hospital. If you don't speak up, protocol will likely have you strapped to monitors for the entire labor. See Chapter 9 for more on dealing with obstacles to movement, Chapter 12 for more on the pros and cons of monitoring labor, and Chapter 18 for more on how to work this detail into your written plan.

## Getting comfy

Generally speaking, you should labor in upright and active positions as much as possible, which we speak more about in Chapter 9. However, resting in early labor may help you maintain strength for the long road ahead. As labor progresses, you will naturally tire and need restorative poses that support you completely. Your contractions will continue despite your need for respite, so positions that allow maximum comfort are important.

At the end of pregnancy, lying on your back isn't recommended, because it compresses blood flow to you and the baby. To rest during labor, you'll probably feel best sitting semi-upright; about 40 to 45 degrees allows you to relax but avoid lying flat on your back. If you must lie horizontal, lying on your side works well. You can also try resting on a lounge chair, rocking chair, or even on a bean bag chair, if you have one.

Whichever position you choose, you'll want plenty of pillows for support. Ideally, you don't want tension developing from an unsupportive position. For example, if you're on your side without any support, you'll likely feel tension in your back from your upper leg pulling your body forward and tension in your shoulders, neck, and back from trying to keep from pressing too much on your abdomen while simultaneously trying not to roll onto your back.

Nap time, bedtime, and general relaxation time are great chances to experiment with finding the right amount of support for restful positions. Figuring out how to be comfortable not only helps you later during labor but also may increase the amount of rest you get during your last pregnant weeks. To begin, gather as many pillows as you can. Go ahead and take some couch cushions if you're lacking regular bed pillows. If you want to add to your pillow collection, you can also purchase special pregnancy pillows or just long extended pillows. Pile up a back support to rest sitting semi-upright and be sure to place a pillow below each knee. You may also want pillows to use like arm rests. Be sure your neck is also well supported. When you feel settled, take a few relaxing breaths and scan your body for tension. Is it tension that can be relieved with more support? If yes, tinker with your pillow arrangement. (Don't be surprised if you need a ridiculous number of pillows. Coauthor Rachel slept with seven pillows every night when she was expecting her twins!)

Another time, try a side-lying rest position. Be sure to put pillows behind your back and either between your legs or under your upper leg, if you choose to place it slightly in front of the bottom leg instead of on top. You may need two pillows for the upper leg, or even a pillow to support your abdomen. You may want to hug a pillow as well, using it to support your chest.

During labor, if a particular position feels good and labor is progressing, don't feel like you have to get up. Just rest. However, if labor slows down, then you may need to change positions or become active. You can always return to your comfort position after labor is going strong again.

## Performing progressive muscle relaxation

Progressive muscle relaxation involves tensing and then relaxing muscle groups systematically over the entire body. By feeling muscle tension, you get a better sense of which muscles you need to release to prevent or ease soreness. Progressive muscle relaxation is a good way to learn how to relax, but it can also be used during labor, typically between contractions and not during them.

To try it, get into a comfortable position and close your eyes. Starting at the top of your head, scrunch up your face, including your forehead, your eyes, and your lips. Then release them and take a few relaxing breaths. Tense up your shoulders, arms, and hands, and then release them. Continue tensing and releasing different muscle groups until you get to your toes. See if you feel more relaxed afterward than you did before.

## Experiencing the power of touch

A simple hug, a well-timed hand on the shoulder, or a loving massage: Touch can assure and comfort in so many ways. According to some spiritual beliefs, touch can heal because the hands are seen as a source of powerful energies. Touch can also act as a sort of interference between the pain messages being sent by the contractions and your brain. According to the Gate Control Theory of Pain, you can lessen pain sensations by giving the body and mind something else to process — just like how if you bump your head, you instinctively rub it to lessen the pain. A variety of touch-based comfort measures can be used for labor, and you don't need to be a professional masseuse to perform them effectively. In this section, we give you guidance on using touch to cope during labor.

Everyone reacts to touch differently, and during labor a touchy person may become aversive to massage or a typically non-touchy person may crave it. Your reaction to touch can also change *during* labor, so what works great one hour may be the most irritating thing a few hours later. Staying open to how you feel, expressing your needs to your partner, and taking the time to experiment with soothing touch before childbirth begins can help you and your partner use touch effectively.

### Back massage

When people think of a back massage, they typically picture a kneading of the upper shoulders. Massage also includes any stroking or rubbing of the skin. The labor partner can try circular strokes on the lower back, in time with the mother's inhalations and exhalations (moving slower or faster based on her respirations). Another massage stroke to try is firmly but smoothly running a hand over and down the spine in a smooth motion, starting again at the top with the alternate hand when the other reaches the lower back. You may want back massages between contractions or during them.

The hands are only one way to provide a comforting back massage. You may want to try having someone use a rolling pin, tennis ball, cold soda can, or specialty made massage tools, either directly on your back or over a folded towel. Be sure to also have baby powder, massage oils, or lotion so hands can slide over the skin easily.

### Counterpressure

If you're experiencing back or hip pain during labor, counterpressure may relieve the tension. Unlike massage, counterpressure doesn't involve running the hands over the skin. Instead, the labor partner leans into a particular area with steady and firm pressure. Counterpressure is used most often on the lower back but can also be applied to the hips.

You can try these moves before labor to get a feel for the right area to press. To apply counterpressure to the lower back, the mother may sit on the bed or on an open-backed chair while the labor partner presses with both hands against the sacrum of her back, using either the heel of the hand or the knuckles.

Counterpressure to the lower back can also be applied while the mother is on her hands and knees, with the labor partner standing behind the mother and bending over to press down on the sacrum. The pressure should be aimed down and away so that the hands would slide off the buttocks if the labor partner allowed them to move. Don't direct the pressure toward the spine. See Figure 8-1 for a visual guide.

Another method of applying counterpressure is called the *knee press.* The mother sits in a chair with a rolled-up towel between the small of her back and the back of the chair. Her feet should be hip distance apart and flat on the floor (or on a pillow if they don't reach the floor). The chair should be up against a wall so it can't tip backward. The labor partner kneels in front of the mother and cups the knees, using the heal of the palm to press back, applying pressure directed back toward the hips (see Figure 8-2). This move applies counterpressure through the knees and femur bone, back to the hips, relieving lower back pain.

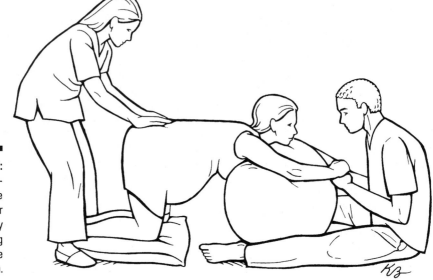

**Figure 8-1:**
Apply coun-
terpressure
to the lower
back by
pressing
firmly on the
sacrum.

*Illustration by Kathryn Born*

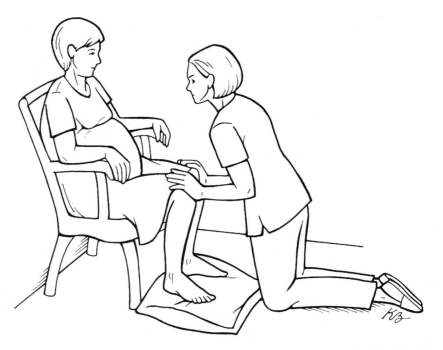

**Figure 8-2:**
Counter-
pressure on
the knees
can relieve
lower back
pain.

*Illustration by Kathryn Born*

To apply counterpressure to the hips, the mother assumes a sitting, kneeling, or hands-and-knees position. The labor partner stands behind the mother and places a hand on the outer side of each hip. Then the labor partner applies pressure to both hips, squeezing the hips together (see Figure 8-3). This technique is sometimes called the *double-hip squeeze*.

### Hand, foot, and head massage

Hand massage during labor can be comforting, especially a circular rubbing of the inner palm with the thumb. A firm or light stroke over the length of the arms, from shoulder to forearm, can also be soothing. The same goes for a foot or head massage. For a foot massage, your labor partner can use the thumbs to apply firm pressure to the bottom of the feet. However, you should try this massage before labor so you and your partner know what feels good and not ticklish. The pads of the fingers can be used for a head massage, rubbing gently the way a hair stylist does when shampooing your hair. The strokes can be firm or light, depending on what feels best in the moment. Also, don't discount the power of a simple hand squeeze, a gentle brushing of the cheek or hair, or a cool cloth rubbed across the forehead.

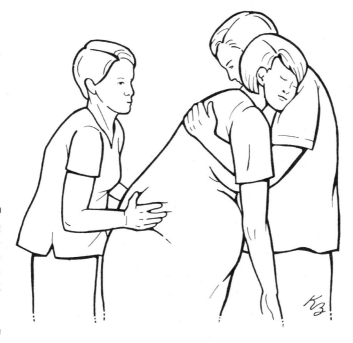

**Figure 8-3:**
The double-hip squeeze can relieve lower back pain during labor.

*Illustration by Kathryn Born*

## Alternative therapies for back pain

Back pain and hip pain during labor can be very difficult to cope with, especially because they're compounded by the contractions! Besides massage and counter pressure, consider these alternative therapies:

✔ **TENS machine:** TENS stands for transcutaneous electrical nerve stimulation. For labor, electrodes are placed on directly on the skin on either side of the spine. The electrodes deliver low-voltage pulsations that some studies have found to provide labor-pain relief. The pulsations are controlled by the mother by a handheld switch, and the intensity of the pulsations can be adjusted on the TENS machine itself. Not all hospitals have TENS machines available, though you may be able to purchase one from a physical therapist with a prescription from your medical practitioner. Ideally, you should try the TENS machine before labor begins and be taught by a physical therapist how to use it.

✔ **Sterile-water papules:** Sterile-water papules are tiny injections of sterile water placed just below the skin. For back labor, the injections are given on the back. Although the injections produce a stinging sensation, they can be helpful in reducing severe back pain during labor. Ask your medical practitioner if she or your birth location offers this therapy.

✔ **Acupressure:** Acupressure works like acupuncture, except instead of using needles you use your finger or thumb to apply pressure to a specific area. Applying finger pressure to the center of the ball of the foot is said to relieve back labor.

✔ **Arnica oil:** Arnica oil used on the back, especially when combined with massage, is said to help with tense or aching muscles, including back pain.

Sometimes when a mother gets an epidural, her birth partner or birthing guests may assume she doesn't need physical support. That's not true! An epidural doesn't always provide complete pain relief; even if it does, the lack of pain doesn't mean that a laboring woman still doesn't experience fear or need support. A hand or head massage can be comforting to many women.

### Effleurage, or light touch massage

Massage doesn't always have to be firm. *Effleurage* is massage that is relatively light, with the hands practically gliding over the skin. Effleurage can be used over many parts of the body, including the back, arms, legs, or hips, but it can also be applied directly to the abdomen. You may find effleurage soothing to provide for yourself. You can run both hands lightly over your lower abdomen to relieve tension during or between contractions.

Some women find this light touch to be extremely annoying as labor progresses, so move on to something else if you feel the need.

### Simple, steady contact

Sometimes the simplest physical contact is all you need. You may want to hold your labor partner's hand or sit together on the bed, leaning against him or her. Your labor partner may sit up against the back of the bed while you lie back against the chest in a semi-sitting position. Steady contact may also include leaning into each other while standing, walking, or gently swaying.

Simple touch may be used as a reminder to release tension from tight areas. Your labor partner may firmly but gently place a hand on your forehead to remind you to release tightness. Firmly touching other commonly tight areas, like your shoulders, chest, hands, or thighs can also help. This relaxation technique is something you can discuss and practice before labor begins.

Your labor partner isn't the only one who can use touch to soothe — you can, too! You may massage your own abdomen, arms, or legs. Or you may want to gently cup your hands and place the heal of your hand over your eyes, with your fingers over the forehead, to calm the mind. Sometimes, people feel embarrassed to self-soothe, especially if they are not alone. If the touch you need is your own, do it and forget about what other people may think.

## Unwinding in wonderful water

Some women can't imagine birth without water therapy. So much about water is soothing — its sounds, its warmth, its ability to lighten your load when submerged, its massage-like touch when directed by a shower head. Here are a few ways to use water to ease physical tension.

### Having a real baby shower

A warm shower can be soothing during labor, especially if you don't want to or can't get into a birthing pool or tub. You can sit on a chair or birth ball (a large physiotherapy exercise ball) so you can rest while enjoying the indoor rain shower. You may stand directly under the water or sit on a chair backward, with your back under the shower and your head resting on a folded towel hung over the chair's back.

A handheld showerhead, especially one with a variety of spray options, can act as a wonderful massage tool. You may enjoy having your partner aim it at your lower back while you sit on a chair or rest on your hands and knees on the shower floor. (Place a few folded towels beneath your knees for comfort.) Your partner can hold the stream steady in one place, or you may prefer that he move it around in circles, trace up and down your spine, or move it back and forth on your lower back.

On a lighter setting, you may aim the shower head yourself at your abdomen, either holding it so it just brushes by your lower abdomen or making circular motions.

### *Enjoying bliss in the birthing pool*

A birthing pool is a personal-size pool used for labor relief and sometimes water birth. Some hospitals and birth centers offer birthing pools or another form of water therapy, like a deep tub or Jacuzzi. If you're having a homebirth, you can rent a birthing pool. (Some birth centers and hospitals also allow you to bring in a rented birthing pool if they have the means to fill and drain them.) See Chapter 5 for more on renting a birthing pool.

Floating in a birthing pool can be tremendously soothing during labor. The buoyancy of the water gives all your joints relief from the weight of your pregnancy, and even contractions are easier to handle when you're fully submerged. Some women dilate quicker when in water, maybe because they are deeply relaxed and the contractions become more effective. This quicker dilation may also be caused by the water's stimulation of the nipples, which causes a release of natural oxytocin. The weightlessness of the pool also allows greater freedom of movement, so you can lunge, squat, sway, or circle your hips in whatever way feels good with less effort. In the water you may have an easier time following your natural instincts for movement, which may help your baby move into the best position for delivery. Being in the water also causes a slight drop in your blood pressure and a slight increase in your pulse, which helps your baby and your uterus get a better supply of oxygen.

If you plan to use a birthing pool, be sure to include it in your birth plan. Hospitals that offer birthing pools don't have enough for every laboring mother, and they may reserve rooms adjacent to a birthing pool for women who specifically request them on admission. So in addition to writing it in your birth plan, speak up and let the hospital staff know right away.

If a birthing pool isn't available, floating in a Jacuzzi or bathtub can also be soothing, although you won't have the freedom of movement and may not be able to fully submerge.

If you're modest, you may want to wear a sports bra or camisole with thin straps in the water as a cover-up. You may also consider wearing a tennis skirt or swim skirt (without the bottom) if you're uncomfortable leaving that area exposed. Another option is to float a few towels in the water, but clothes aren't required. Although the water itself is supportive, a few folded towels placed underneath your knees or a floating pillow or folded towels hung over the side to rest your head on can be helpful. A pool noodle can also be used to lean on in the water. You may also like to add a few drops of essential oils to the water, like lavender or peppermint, to provide a soothing aroma.

Using a birthing pool for labor doesn't necessarily mean you need to give birth in the water. You or your medical practitioner may prefer the birth to be on land, or you both may decide to go ahead and deliver under the water.

However, water birth is contraindicated or controversial in some situations. See Chapter 9 for more on water birth.

You need to take a few precautions when laboring underwater:

✔ Your birthing pool should be clean, though absolute perfection isn't necessary unless vaginal exams will be conducted in the water.

✔ You need to prevent raising your body temperature and causing the baby distress, so the water shouldn't be hotter than 100 degrees Fahrenheit (about 38 degrees Celsius).

✔ Some say you shouldn't enter a birthing pool until a certain dilation, usually 5 centimeters, because the water can slow labor down. However, you can always get out of the water if contractions slow too much and get back in when things pick up again.

✔ Be sure that you (and your partner, if he's in the water with you) drink fluids to stay hydrated. Being in the water throws off the balance of fluids in your body. Sports drinks can help rebalance your electrolytes.

✔ If you're sitting in your bathtub, where the water isn't deep, be sure your bottom remains below the surface of the water. If you bob in and out and your baby's face is born while out of the water, he may begin to breathe and then swallow water if you sit back into the water again. (You can find out more on delivering in water — as opposed to just laboring in water for comfort — in Chapter 9.)

✔ You will need to come out of the tub if you or the baby experience complications or exhibit signs of distress. If you feel lightheaded or unwell when laboring in water, let your medical practitioner know.

# Employing the Art of Distraction

Given that labor can last for hours (and hours and hours), focusing on something *other* than the contractions is an excellent idea — especially during early labor, when you'll likely be chipper, excited, and full of energy. When active labor begins, you may prefer to focus inward, or your preference for distraction may change. For example, you may spend early labor walking around the mall but distract yourself with a focal point during active labor. Distraction can also help if you have an epidural and you're stuck in bed but still anxious about the birth. In this section, we give you some ways to keep your mind focusing on things besides your uterus.

## Going about your day as usual

Early labor is a great time for last-minute nesting. You can decorate the nursery, sort and organize baby clothes, or even go to the mall to purchase more baby supplies (just don't travel alone or too far from your chosen birthing location). If you enjoy puttering around the kitchen, you can bake some treats for serving to your guests after the baby arrives or to bribe the nurses at the hospital. Organized-types may even prepare and freeze a few meals to make your first days at home with baby easier.

Early labor is also a good time to spend with your big kids and to allow the youngest to enjoy his or her last hours being the baby of the family. A trip to the park can help your labor pick up while entertaining the troops. Some women plan on labor projects, even setting aside materials for the big day. Ideas for labor projects include:

- ✔ Baking a birthday cake for your soon-to-be-born baby, complete with decorations

- ✔ Putting together a scrapbook, either digital or on real paper, with pictures documenting the pregnancy, leaving room at the end for birth day pictures

- ✔ Creating fun, messy art with the big kids, making things for themselves or presents for their new brother or sister

- ✔ Getting on your hands and knees to scrub the floors — an Amish tradition during labor! — puts you into the perfection position for optimizing the baby's position in utero.

## Finding focal points

Using focal points may help take your focus away from your body and act as a distraction from the contractions. They may also help you reach a meditative state when used along with breathing techniques. Depending on what you choose to focus on, your focal point may inspire you to keep going. They can be helpful when the contractions are difficult to speak through or when you're trying not to push during transition. Ideas for focal points include your loved ones' eyes, a special photo, or an inspiring painting or poster, perhaps of a place you dream of visiting. If you're the crafty type, you may want to create your own focal point before labor begins, adding words or images that inspire you. A focal point can also be something completely mundane and unplanned, like a thumbtack on a corkboard that just happens to be on the wall of your room, or the intersection of tiles on the floor or ceiling.

You might think focal points are for focusing on, but sometimes the best way to use a focal point is to look *beyond* your chosen focus. If, for example, you're staring at a thumbtack, you look in the direction of the thumbtack but focus your eyes as if you were trying to look at something behind the thumbtack, further away. It can create a meditative state that is calming to some.

## Laughing through labor

Researchers have found that laughter can increase your tolerance for pain, and you probably already know from experience that laughter can lighten up a tense situation, making it easier to cope through. You may spend much of early labor cracking jokes with your partner or even your doctor. You may also want to pull out your favorite comedies or stand-up acts to watch together with your labor partner or birthing guests.

Although the laughs may roll right along during the early hours of labor, at some point, nothing may seem funny. The labor partner and birthing guests should take note of this change and respect it. The laughter is likely to return once the baby's born; likely the teary kind of laughter that comes from pure mama joy.

# Gathering Comfort Tools

When you pack your bag for the big day, don't forget to include comfort tools! Although some of these items may be available for borrowing at your birth center or hospital, you'll need to bring most of them yourself:

- ✔ **A birth ball:** A large physiotherapy or exercise ball can be used to support you in a variety of positions. See Chapter 9 for more details on using a birth ball.

- ✔ **Heat and cold packs:** Gel-based heat packs and cold packs can be purchased from any pharmacy. You may also use a hot-water bottle, a rice-filled sock (put in the microwave to heat up), towels soaked in hot or cold water and then wrung out, or a glove filled with chipped ice.

  For a pleasing, calming scent, add herbs to a rice sock or a few drops of peppermint or lavender essential oil to a wet towel.

- ✔ **Aromatherapy:** Besides adding scent to hot and cold packs, you can bring along scented lotions or massage oils. If you're at home, you can light candles or incense. Herbal teas can offer not only a pleasing smell but also warm hydration. Try out any scented products before labor to make sure you find them pleasurable and not sneeze-worthy.

✔ **MP3 player:** Whether with headphones or with a speaker, an MP3 player can be used to play guided imagery or self-hypnosis recordings, calming music, or even rock music, if you need some inspiration to get active. Nature sounds, drumming music, or other new-age tunes may help set a quiet birthing mood, or you may put together playlists of more mainstream songs relating to birth or babies.

✔ **Lots of pillows:** Hospitals are rarely prepared to give you six pillows. In fact, you're lucky if you can get two! If you need lots of comfy support, bring your own. The nurses may snicker, but hey, at least you'll be comfortable! (Use colorful pillow cases so they don't get mixed up with the hospital linens.)

✔ **Personal fan:** A small handheld fan, especially one with a mister which can be refreshing.

✔ **Massage tools:** Massage tools include things like a rolling pin (for use on the lower back), massage knobs, and massage oils or powders. Stores that sell bath products often sell a variety of massage tools.

# Chapter 9

# Movement and Positions for Labor and Birth

*I*f you imagine yourself laboring on your back in bed for hours, banish that image from your mind. Labor and delivery are usually more effective and easier when you remain active. Of course, labor is also hard work, so you need to rest sometimes! When you do take a break, positions that are upright, comforting, and supportive help childbirth progress. You also have several pushing position options, most of which are significantly more effective than lying on your back with your legs in stirrups.

In this chapter, we explain how to stay upright and active throughout labor, how to move between restful and active positions, what your pushing-position options are, and how to deal with potential obstacles to moving and pushing the way you want. We also stress the importance of addressing these issues in your birth plan and with your practitioner before labor begins.

# You Go, Girl! Staying Active and Upright during Labor

Television shows persist in portraying laboring women on their backs in hospital beds, and with good reason. This position is, unfortunately, how childbirth commonly occurs in hospitals today. However, labor and delivery are less effective when you limit movement and position changes. An empowering and positive childbirth includes walking around, switching between a variety of positions, and pushing upright, perhaps even in a squat — but not on your back! In this section, we discuss the benefits of remaining up and moving, ideal movements for labor, and switching between activity and rest.

## Understanding the benefits of remaining active and upright

When researchers study cultures where childbirth has not yet been institutionalized, they find women naturally move in and out of different positions during labor. Movement and position changes have physiological benefits for the mother and baby, including the following perks:

- **Shortened labor:** Although remaining active doesn't guarantee a short labor, women who move throughout labor tend to have shorter childbirths when compared to women who are restricted to a bed.

- **More effective contractions:** When you're upright (see Figure 9-1a), gravity works with your uterus, and your baby's head presses down against your cervix, making contractions more effective. In contrast, when you're on your back, contractions work against gravity (see Figure 9-1b).

- **Greater tolerance of labor pains:** Effective contractions, along with the distraction of movement, help you cope better. Women who remain upright are less likely to request pain medications for childbirth.

- **More room for baby to maneuver into better birthing position:** You're not the only one moving during labor — your baby is also making tiny position changes. The baby has more wiggle room when the pelvis is active, which is even more important if your baby is posterior, or "sunny-side up." A posterior baby can slow down labor and make it more painful. See Chapter 2 for more on the baby's position during labor.

- **Lower risk of cesarean section birth:** You're less likely to have cesarean section when upright. This reduced chance may be due to the lower likelihood of epidural use (which increases your risk for cesarean section) and the more effectiveness of the contractions.

- **Greater sense of control:** Remaining upright and active improves your sense of well-being, which increases your chances of having a positive childbirth experience, not to mention your chances for having a natural childbirth. See Chapter 8 for more on the power of the mind in labor.

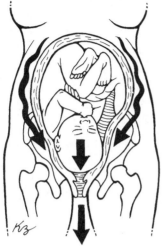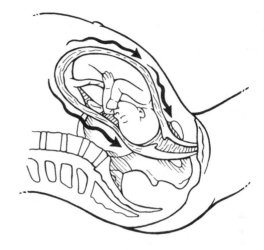

**Figure 9-1:**
Gravity
helps make
the contrac-
tions more
effective.

a. In an upright position, gravity
assists as the uterus contracts.

b. In a reclining position there is very
little gravitational assistance as the
uterus contracts.

# Keeping your body moving

You can keep yourself active and moving in a variety of ways during labor,
but how you move will change as labor intensifies. Follow your instincts for
what feels best and try out new movements if labor stalls. In this section, we
provide you with some movement options for labor.

When you write your birth plan, you may want to include a brief list of movements to try during labor. This list not only shows your caregivers what you
want but can also remind you and your labor partner, because you may forget
after you enter the hospital environment. See the section later in this chapter
"Forgetting that you can move if you want" for more on this phenomena.

## Walking

Walking is great for early labor and sometimes during intense active labor.
Gravity makes contractions more effective, and your pelvic movements help
the baby wiggle toward birth. Walking also provides distraction, which helps
psychologically.

In the early hours of labor, you can walk around your house, getting busy
with labor projects (see Chapter 8 for ideas). You may want to head to a
nearby park with your big kids, or even to the mall for some baby shopping.

When active labor begins, your walks may be confined to a smaller area, because you don't want to deliver in the mall bathroom! You may pace the hallways if you're at the hospital or even walk around the perimeter of your room.

Be sure to have someone with you for your labor walks. If you decide to go away from home, don't be the driver, and remain within easy driving distance of wherever you plan to deliver. Labor also isn't a good time for hiking in the woods or walking on difficult trails, as your coordination won't be great.

In early labor, you may be able to walk during contractions, but as labor intensifies, you'll probably want to stop walking during them. You may stand unsupported, or you may lean onto a wall or your labor partner. The handrails in hospitals make good supports for hallway walking. See the later section "Standing with support" for more ideas.

### Lunging

Lunges are a great way to move during contractions. As you lunge, gravity works with the contractions and the pelvis opens wide to one side, providing extra room for the baby to move. They may also relieve back pain and help a posterior baby turn.

The lunges you do in exercise class are *not* the kind used during labor; labor lunges are easier and more supportive. The two basic kinds of labor lunges are standing with a chair and kneeling on the bed or floor.

To do a standing lunge, follow these steps:

1. **Place a chair in front and slightly to the side of you, on whichever side you want to do the lunge.**

   You can lunge on one side for several contractions or switch back and forth.

   The chair should be sturdy and up against the wall or bed so it doesn't slide. Be sure someone is standing next to you for extra support.

2. **Put your foot closest to the chair up on the seat. Your leg should not be directly in front of you but slightly off to the side.**

3. **During the contraction, lunge by bending at the knee and leaning toward the chair while your leg on the floor remains straight.**

   To prevent injury, your lunging knee shouldn't pass your ankle. You can simply lean into the lunge or you can move slightly in and out of the lunge. Do whatever feels best.

4. **When the contraction is finished, put your leg on the floor to rest.**

Kneeling lunges may be used when you're feeling tired and don't want to stand. These steps walk you through a kneeling lunge:

1. **Kneel on one knee with the other leg out to the side and in front of you, your foot flat and sturdy on the bed or floor.**

   Place some folded towels below the kneeling knee for comfort.

2. **Using a wall, chair, or back of the bed for support, lean into and toward the lunging leg during a contraction (see Figure 9-2).**

Don't wait until labor begins to try these lunges. They will be easier to use and more familiar if you practice during pregnancy. They may also relieve leg cramps, backaches, and tight muscles during pregnancy itself.

### Climbing stairs

Climbing the stairs gives you the benefits of walking and some of the benefits of lunging, because the pelvis gets a wider opening when you take a step up. Also, walking up stairs works against gravity, which may be more effective than just walking. During a contraction, you can just stand still, using the hand railing or labor partner for support, or you can put one foot up on a stair ahead and do a lunge. See the previous section for the correct positioning for labor lunging.

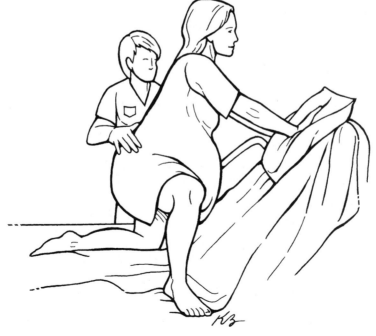

**Figure 9-2:**
In a kneeling lunge, place the foot of the lunging leg flat on the bed or floor, to the front and slightly off to the side.

*Illustration by Kathryn Born*

Be sure to bring someone along with you for climbing stairs, and don't climb up too many flights if you can't come back down via elevator. Climbing stairs can be tiring, so don't overdo it. You want to remain active without exhausting your energy. Take the steps slowly, especially coming back down, and always use the handrail to prevent falls.

### Squatting

Although squatting is used most often for pushing, it can also be used during early labor. Squatting widens the pelvic opening significantly, making room for the baby to descend. It can intensify contractions, which may rev up a stalled labor, and squats may also relieve back pain.

Squatting can be tiring, so unless you're an experienced squatter (lots of yoga perhaps?), don't overdo them. Many women find squats during a contraction too intense to handle, unless they are at the pushing stage. Instead, you can sit in a supported squat between contractions and then stand up or move onto a hands-and-knees position for the actual contraction.

There are a variety of supported squat positions, many of which you can find described later in this chapter under "Positioning Yourself for Pushing." Perhaps one of the best squat positions for labor is an almost-sitting position. Sit on a very low stool, like the kind used for children to reach a sink, or sit on a pile of larger, sturdy books. Place your feet flat on the floor as you would in a squat. You're not supporting your weight in this squat; the stool or books are. If your heels come off the floor, place a folded towel beneath each foot so you are completely supported. You may want to do this supported squat against a wall so you can lean back, or you can lean forward and rest your elbows on your legs.

Although you can squat any time during pregnancy or labor, we don't recommend staying in a deep squat if your baby isn't engaged in the pelvis, or at what is known as the *zero station*. Squatting too much too early can actually hinder the baby's descent. If you're unsure where your baby's at, speak to your medical practitioner.

## Resting when you're feeling tired

With all the benefits of active movement, you may get the impression you should be moving all throughout labor. But constant movement and no rest isn't good either. Labor isn't a sprint; it's a marathon. Pacing is important. You don't want to exhaust yourself during early labor and have no energy left for the end.

How can you know when it's time to move and when it's time to rest?

✔ **Don't overexert yourself.** It may be a bit obvious, but if your body is telling you to slow down, then slow down. Remember that movements, even slow and small ones, are the key. A cardio workout is not required! If you can, try a supported but upright position to reap benefits of gravity while your body rests.

✔ **Take a nap during a slow early labor.** If you've been in labor for hours, try taking a little nap. Your contractions will likely continue, so you may not get the best sleep ever, but even an hour lying down can renew you. See Chapter 8 for how to best rest during labor.

✔ **Get up again after rest periods.** When you stop moving, you may forget to get up and move again. Be sure to go back to movement after a half hour or hour of rest.

✔ **Get up if labor stalls.** If labor has stalled, the best thing you can do is change positions, get up, and move. If your medical practitioner is suggesting induction medications, or even cesarean section, ask if you can try altering your movement and position changes first. (You can even ask your practitioner if you can return home, if labor hasn't truly reached the active stage.) You can also indicate this preference in your birth plan. You may be able to avoid oxytocin (Pitocin) or even surgery with some walking and lunges.

✔ **Get up and move if contractions become overwhelming.** People tend to freeze when they're in pain, and if contractions intensified during your rest, you may not want to move. If staying in one spot is helpful, then stay with it. But you may want to talk about this situation in advance with your labor partner and ask him to gently suggest movement if you come to a point when you feel you can't handle the contractions.

If you're tired of moving around but don't necessarily need to lie down, the supported positions we describe later in "Remaining Upright but Supported" can help you take a load off while still allowing gravity to work with your contractions.

# *Rock-a-Bye Mama: Comforting Moves*

Movement can be comforting, and rocking is one of the most soothing movements. Rocking puts babies to sleep and mamas in the zone. Here are some ways to put rocking moves into your labor repertoire.

# Rocking in a chair

A simple rocking chair can provide an upright but comforting position, along with movement. Rocking chairs are naturally in a semi-reclining position, so you can really sink back into them. You can rock yourself, or you can put your feet up on a rocking ottoman or on the front of the rocking chair while your labor partner rocks you. You can add extra pillows for additional comfort.

Rocking chairs usually allow access to your belly, so you can lightly rub your abdomen. (Turn to Chapter 8 for advice on light massage.) You can also try placing one leg up and to the side on a low stool or chair. As you rock in that position, your pelvis gets the benefits of a lunge, without any strain on your knees or legs.

If your hospital room doesn't have a rocking chair, ask for one. Sometimes they have limited supply or keep them in the "natural" laboring rooms. Don't assume it's not available if you don't see it.

# Dancing slowly

Slow dancing is a romantic way to get comfort and movement working together. You may slow dance while facing your partner, placing your arms up around his neck, your elbows resting up by his shoulders. Or try dancing with your back to your partner, which provides access to your belly for light massage.

You don't need any fancy "dance" moves. Simple swaying is great. Turn down the lights, put on some romantic or calming music, and, if you're not at a hospital, light some candles. The combination of movement and mood can be extremely soothing and memorable.

# Rocking on a birth ball

A birth ball is a large physiotherapy ball, which you may have seen used in exercise videos. If you hire a doula or midwife, she may have a birth ball to lend, and some birth centers and hospitals have them too (but check before you assume!). In any case, a birth ball is well worth purchasing, because you can use it during pregnancy for back pain relief and exercise and later in the postpartum period for active sitting to strengthen your core muscles. After birth, you can lull to sleep a fussy baby by sitting on the ball and gently bouncing. Look for a ball that is strong enough to carry your pregnant weight (a rating up to 300 lbs is best) and won't slip.

The size of the ball also matters, as you want your feet to be flat on the floor but have enough height to sit comfortably, with your knees at about a 90 degree angle. This size turns out to be approximately 65 cm in diameter for women up to 5 feet, 5 inches and slightly bigger for taller women.

You can use a birth ball in a variety of positions, including hands and knees, standing (not *on* the ball, obviously!), and sitting. Sitting on a birth ball offers an almost squatting pose of the pelvis, because of the way your bottom rests on the ball. One of the greatest benefits of sitting on a birth ball, as opposed to sitting on a chair or bed, is that you get ease of movement. You can gently rock from side to side, back and forth, or even a little of both. Your labor partner can kneel or stand behind you, placing a hand on your back, holding your hips, or applying the double hip squeeze for back labor, described in Chapter 8. See sections "Standing with support" and "Getting on your knees" for more birth ball ideas.

Sitting on a birth ball with confidence takes practice, so try it during pregnancy if you can. Have something to steady yourself with, like a table top or the back of a chair, and during labor, have a labor support person nearby, just in case you lose your balance or need extra support.

# Remaining Upright but Supported

You can't keep moving all through labor, and in fact, you shouldn't. You need to rest, too! Whenever you rest, take advantage of gravity by remaining upright. Staying upright will also boost your mood and make contractions more effective and less painful than lying down. In this section, you find a variety of upright but supported positions to try.

Just as we suggest you write in your birth plan the movements you'd like to use during labor, you can also list the positions you want to try. This list acts as a quick reminder to you and your labor partner and lets your caregivers know what you want.

## Standing with support

Standing isn't the most restful position, but it's one that can be supported. Some women tolerate contractions better standing up. You may also use a supported standing position during a contraction in the midst of walking or stair climbing.

Supported standing can be very simple, like leaning into a labor-support partner. You may stand side by side, with your labor partner's arm around your shoulder, or you may stand facing each other, with your arms around your labor partner's neck and shoulders. You can lean back against your labor partner as well, though he should be against a wall so he doesn't fall himself.

Supported standing can also be done by bending over a tall table or bed. You can place a birth ball on a bed or table to get better height and so you can really relax into the position, as shown in Figure 9-3.

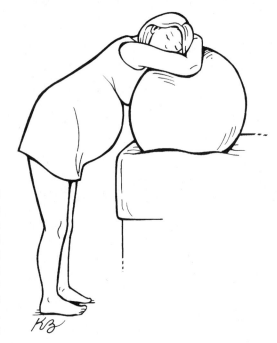

**Figure 9-3:**
Placing the birth ball on the bed gives you something to rest on while standing.

*Illustration by Kathryn Born*

## Sitting upright

Sitting upright means you're either sitting straight up or leaning slightly forward. You may sit on the edge of a bed, resting your head on your labor partner's shoulder. If you sit backward on a chair, you can lean forward, resting your arms or head on the back of the chair. This is a good position for back massage or for in the shower so the spray hits your back.

## Sitting semi-upright

Sometimes you need or want to lie back, but lying flat on your back can cause dizziness and restrict blood flow. Instead, try sitting semi-upright, at about a 45-degree angle. Pile up pillows behind you (see Chapter 8 for guidance) and tuck a pillow beneath one hip so you're almost on your side, to help with blood flow. This position allows good fetal monitoring. Be sure the bed is adjusted to this degree before the belts are strapped on, to avoid having to reposition the belts after things are set.

Don't sit this way too long, however, because your baby may rotate into a posterior position, which can make labor more painful. (See Chapter 2 for more on posterior babies.)

You may also try leaning back onto your partner. He sits on the bed, and you sit in front of him, leaning back onto his chest for support. He can lightly massage your abdomen in this position, too.

Most hospital beds can be adjusted into a variety of positions. Just because the bed is in one position when you get to the room doesn't mean it should stay like that! Ask your nurse to explain your options so you can use it to your advantage.

## Sitting on the toilet

Sitting on the toilet may seem like an awkward place to have your baby, but the position is actually good for labor. The toilet seat, especially if it's low to the ground, allows you to sit in a somewhat squatting position without straining to support yourself. Also, you may be able to relax and release tension in your abdomen and bottom more easily, making contractions more effective and less painful. You can lean back or lean forward, supporting yourself with the back of a chair or a birth ball on top of a chair. Leaning forward while on the toilet also encourages your baby to rotate into an anterior position for labor.

Whether or not you decide to sit in the bathroom long, you should be sure to urinate frequently throughout labor. A full bladder irritates the uterus and may make contractions more painful.

If while sitting on the toilet you start to feel a lot of pressure or the urge to push, let a nurse or your medical practitioner know. Even if you think you're having a bowel movement, it may actually be the baby!

# Getting on your knees

Although many positions speed up labor, sometimes you need things to slow down. Resting on your hands and knees can relieve back pain and help slow down rapid labor. Getting into a chest-and-knees position (see Figure 9-4a), with your head resting on the bed and your bottom in the air, can really help with overwhelming contractions. This position may also help a posterior baby turn.

You can choose from a variety of hands-and-knees positions. You can lean against the back of the hospital bed or hug a birth ball (see Figure 9-4b). You can pile pillows up and lean into those while kneeling. You can also lean on a chair while kneeling on the floor. If you're in a birthing pool, you can lean over onto the edge. Be sure to cushion your knees with some folded towels or a folded blanket.

The hands-and-knees position can be used for a variety of comfort techniques, like applying counterpressure to the lower back, which we explain in Chapter 8. You can also do pelvic tilts, either between contractions or during them.

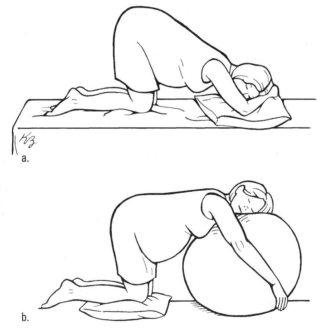

**Figure 9-4:**
The chest-knees position can help turn a posterior baby (a). A birth ball can give you support while in a hands-and-knees position (b).

a.

b.

*Illustration by Kathryn Born*

# *Handling Possible Obstacles to Movement in a Hospital*

Remaining upright and active is rarely an issue for women delivering at a birth center or at home, because medical practitioners attending deliveries in these locations encourage movement. If you enter a hospital, however, remaining active gets complicated.

## *Working with a continuous fetal monitor*

When you arrive at labor and delivery, you'll likely have initial monitoring of your contractions and the baby's heart tones. Two straps will be placed around your belly, one checking on the baby and the other measuring the frequency and intensity of your contractions. Fetal monitoring has a variety of advantages and disadvantages, which we discuss more thoroughly in Chapter 12.

As long as you aren't lying flat on your back, this initial monitoring isn't usually a big issue. Monitoring does become a problem, however, when the belts are on continuously. You can't get up, walk, or change positions as long as the belts are strapped on. Some hospitals have a policy that if you're in bed, you have to be monitored (like airplanes insisting you wear your seatbelt if you're sitting down!). Also, continuous monitoring may be required during inductions or if you take any pain medications, especially an epidural.

You can indicate in your birth plan and to the nurses that you want to remain active as much as possible during labor and therefore want minimal monitoring. Even if you tell them when you're admitted, you'll probably have to call for them to remove the belts. If monitoring is necessary for medical reasons, you may be able to use a telemetry monitoring device that uses radio signals to send your baby's heart tones to a recording device. It's also possible to intermittently check on the baby with a handheld Doppler device, which is often used during prenatal checkups, but not all nurses and medical practitioners are familiar with monitoring labor with a Doppler.

Speak with your medical practitioner about these issues *before* labor begins. You should also check on your chosen hospital's policies, inquiring about the availability of telemetry monitoring or handheld Doppler devices for active childbirth.

## Dragging along an IV pole

Many hospitals require or strongly insist that you receive intravenous (IV) fluids, regardless of whether or not you need them. This requirement usually goes along with policies about no food or drink. An IV may also be needed if you're having an induction, receiving antibiotics for Strep B, or getting pain medications. An IV is essential if you have an epidural, which often causes a severe drop in blood pressure when first injected. (We discuss advantages and disadvantages of IV fluids in Chapter 10.)

If you don't actually "need" the IV, you can turn it down. This choice is something to indicate in your birth plan. Some hospitals are not willing to completely forgo an IV, in which case you can request a *saline lock*. It's basically the IV set up in your hand or arm without the actual tubing and fluids, so you can move around as you like, but if medications are needed quickly, an IV needle doesn't need to be placed.

Even if you do require an IV, it shouldn't stop you from moving around. Most IV poles have wheels. Carefully navigate the tubes so you don't get tangled, and ask your nurse to help you get moving.

## Changing positions with an epidural

An epidural severely limits your movements. If possible, ask the nurse if you can sit as upright as possible in bed so you at least have gravity on your side. You may, however, be required to lie flat on your side. Ask the nurse if she can help you change sides or positions every so often. Nurses usually do this anyway, but if they're especially busy, a reminder won't hurt.

A *walking epidural* may enable you to have more movement, but you'll still be quite limited. Not all hospitals offer walking epidurals, so be sure to ask when considering where to deliver. Speak to the anesthesiologist about your options. A nurse may need to help you change positions and move even with a walking epidural. Get more details on epidurals in Chapter 12.

## Forgetting that you can move if you want

When you enter the hospital, you're surrounded by protocol and authority. Someone tells you wait here, stay still for this, move over for that. You change out of your dignified clothing and put on a gown that hardly closes properly. Continuous monitoring belts may be placed without any suggestion that they can be removed after an initial screening. Machines are beeping and blinking, and quite frankly, you may feel intimidated and overwhelmed.

You may come to a hospital ready to be active during labor, but if your nurse isn't also pro-movement, those plans may be quickly forgotten. If you think your nurse will read your birth plans carefully and help you implement them, you're sadly mistaken. Nurses are busy, protocol is not easy to go against, and the only advocate for your birth plan is you.

Knowing this possibility may happen, however, prepares you to tackle the situation. A doula can be a big help, because she is less likely to be swayed by the hospital environment. Your partner can also be your advocate, if he knows how. See Chapter 19 for more on advocating for your birth plan.

# Positioning Yourself for Pushing: Beyond the Bed and Stirrups

Just like you have position options for the first stage of labor, you also have plenty of options for the pushing stage. The most commonly known delivery position — lying on your back with your legs in stirrups — isn't the most effective. In this section, we explain the benefits of pushing upright, the pros and cons of various delivery positions, and how to handle potential obstacles to pushing the way you want.

The pushing stage can be short or take up to a couple hours, especially for first-time mothers. As you review your pushing options, don't think you need to choose just one position and stay there. Switching between positions is not only possible but preferable, both for your sake and the baby's. When you write your birth plan, you can indicate that you want the freedom to switch between a variety of positions, instead of listing just one or two preferred poses.

Ideally, you should follow your instincts and your medical practitioner's guidance to find positions that feel right and offer the most advantages. Determining the right positions may require trial and error, trying one pose for a few contractions and another for the next. However, don't wait until labor to try out these poses! Some positions, like squatting, take practice. Not only will you develop strength with practice, but you'll also learn the poses in a kinesthetic way and figure out how to best support yourself (or be supported) in the poses. Just don't actually push during your practice sessions.

## *Understanding the benefits to upright pushing*

Although lying on your back to push may be the best pose for certain situations, pushing in an upright position is typically preferred. Here are some benefits of upright pushing:

- ✔ **Shorter pushing stage:** Pushing upright may reduce the time you need to push, which will be easier on you and your baby. It's especially important if the baby needs to be born quickly due to signs of fetal distress.

- ✔ **Less pain:** Contractions are more effective, and pushing may be less painful when you're upright.

- ✔ **Better fetal heart tones:** When compared to lying on the back, fetal heart tones are better in upright pushing positions. Blood flow is better in upright positions, which can be compromised on your back.

- ✔ **Fewer episiotomies:** Pushing upright lowers your chances of having an episiotomy. Studies have found varying rates on vaginal tears in upright positions, some finding them less frequent and others finding them to be more common. However, natural tearing may be preferred to an episiotomy. See Chapter 13 for more on episiotomy.

- ✔ **Greater sense of control:** Pushing from an upright position increases your sense of control and power, which can help you have a more positive birth experience.

- ✔ **Lower rates of cesarean delivery, forceps delivery, and vacuum delivery:** Researchers have found that women who had an epidural but who used an upright pushing position had lower rates of cesarean section, forceps delivery, and vacuum delivery than women pushing on their backs with an epidural.

With all these great benefits, you may wonder why the most commonly used pushing position is lying on the back. Upright pushing is great for the mom and baby, but it isn't convenient for the medical practitioner, who will have to work harder to assist in the delivery. Many medical practitioners, especially older obstetricians, don't feel comfortable with upright pushing positions at all simply because they aren't used to them.

You should speak to your doctor or midwife about their willingness to allow you to push in an upright position *before* you go into labor. Find out what they're cool with and what's out of the question. Can you squat on the floor? What about on the bed? Are they okay with hands and knees or kneeling? You don't want to have a confrontation on this when you're about to push!

## Squatting

Squatting is, in most situations, the ideal pushing position. When you squat, you get all the benefits of an upright position. Your baby, uterus, and birth canal are aligned perfectly for delivery, and your pelvic outlet is up to 30 percent wider than when lying on your back. Squatting is the fastest way to push out your baby, so not only does it lead to a shorter pushing stage, but it's also good if the baby must be delivered quickly.

A possible disadvantage includes a higher potential for vaginal tears, though this risk is debatable, with some studies showing more tearing and others showing less. Some people believe tearing can be prevented by better support, placing a folded towel or blanket beneath your heels so you're not balancing on the balls of your feet, which creates tension in the perineum.

Squatting can also be physically tiring. For that reason, supported squats like the three shown in Figure 9-5 are most often used during labor, many requiring help from your labor partner or a nurse. You can do a standing squat with the help of your partner (see Figure 9-5a). You can squat on the bed, with a person on either side of you (see Figure 9-5b). A squat bar, which is a metal bar that can be attached to most labor and delivery beds, can help you support yourself in a squat (see Figure 9-5c).

A squat bar can also be used in an alternative way by looping a towel or sheet around the center horizontal bar and placing your feet on the vertical part of the bar by the bed. Then you push downward while pulling back on the towel or sheet. If you want to try a squat bar, be sure to include that in your birth plan and let your nurse know early on so someone can track it down and set things up for you.

## Using a birthing stool

Birthing stools, shown in Figure 9-6, provide many of the benefits of squatting but with less effort and more support. A birthing stool or cushion is a stool that's low to the ground, with a cutout in the center to make room for delivery. Pushing on a birthing stool is similar to the way you use a toilet, which may be a more familiar experience than pushing a baby out!

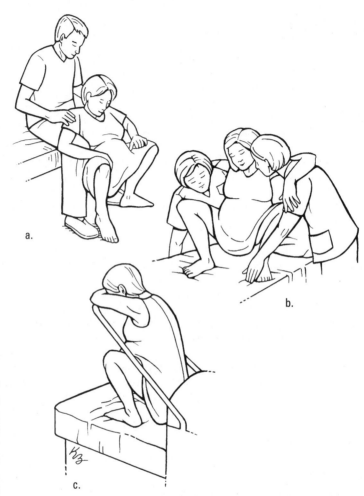

**Figure 9-5:**
Squatting
to push is
much easier
with
support.

a.

b.

c.

*Illustration by Kathryn Born*

Birthing stools aren't widely available. Your hospital or birthing center may have them, but you'll need to ask. Your doula, doctor, or midwife may have one to lend, so be sure to ask before you go into labor. If a birthing stool is not available, you may get somewhat similar results by pushing sitting up straight on the edge of the bed or on a very low stool, though this position may not feel as sturdy or comfortable. You can also try sitting on a pile of pillows, a sort of makeshift birthing cushion.

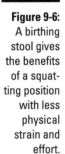

**Figure 9-6:**
A birthing stool gives the benefits of a squatting position with less physical strain and effort.

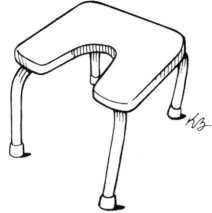

*Illustration by Kathryn Born*

## Resting on your hands and knees

A hands-and-knees position, especially if you're more kneeling than bent over, is a good pushing position for the start of the pushing stage. You may also use the back of the bed, a birth ball, or a chair to support yourself. This position is less tiring, making it a good one if you're exhausted. See the section on "Getting on your knees" earlier in this chapter for illustrations of this position.

Hands and knees can also be helpful if you need to slow down delivery. Rapid delivery may cause severe tearing, and allowing the perineum to stretch at a slower rate can prevent this. This position may also relieve back pain or help a posterior baby turn. You may use the hands-and-knees position in the beginning of the pushing stage and then switch to a supported squatting position for the last few pushes.

## Sitting partially upright

Semi-upright sitting is an upright position best used if you have an epidural, because it doesn't require you to support yourself with your legs. Semi-upright sitting can also accommodate fetal monitoring belts, if they are necessary. In a sitting position, you may hold your own legs back or a nurse and your labor partner can help hold them up. This position is the most common for upright pushing because it's convenient for the medical practitioner.

Although partially upright sitting may seem to have the same pelvic advantages as a squat, it doesn't. The baby and birth canal aren't lined up as well, the pelvic outlet is not as wide as it is in a squat, and the perineum is more at risk for tearing. That said, it is still a better position than flat on your back.

## Lying on your side

Lying on your side is good if you need to rest or you need to slow down a rapid delivery. This position can also be used if you have an epidural. You don't get the benefits of an upright position, but it's better than lying on your back, which compromises blood flow and may cause you to feel lightheaded or cause fetal distress. This position may also be the least likely to cause vaginal tearing. In a side-lying position, someone will help you hold up your upper leg, as you curl up and push, almost like squatting sideways. See Figure 9-7 for a visual guide.

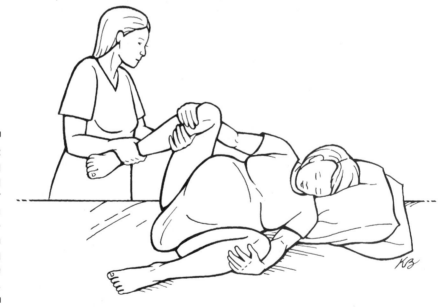

**Figure 9-7:** Pushing while lying on your side, with a labor support person helping support the upper leg.

*Illustration by Kathryn Born*

# Lying on your back

Lying on your back is the worst possible position for pushing your baby. When you're on your back, you're likely to feel lightheaded and your baby is more likely to experience fetal distress. You're pushing your baby up, going against gravity. You're also more at risk for needing a vaginally assisted delivery, which may require forceps, vacuum, or episiotomy. This position also increases the risk for a cesarean section.

If your medical practitioner is insisting on delivery on your back, ask if you can try semi-upright pushing, with the bed as upright as possible, or try a side lying position. Remember, hospital beds are adjustable; you should be able to raise the back for delivery and have the stirrups adjusted to a more angled or lower position, if your practitioner insists on using them. These positions are still fairly easy for your medical practitioner to use but are better for you and your baby. Better yet, if your doctor won't allow you to use a different pushing position, switch doctors before delivery time!

# Getting submerged for water birth

Water births are all the rave, and with some good reason. Mothers who experience water birth report that they feel more relaxed and experience less pain. The water's buoyancy makes squatting and other upright positions easier. Some say being born into water is more peaceful for the baby, and babies born via water are said to be calmer and cry less. However, no primitive society is known to have practiced water birth, so whether or not human babies are meant to be born via water is questionable.

Water birth is generally considered safe with an experienced medical practitioner and no other labor complications, but some risks exist, including the following:

- ✔ While taking the baby out from the water, the umbilical cord may snap, causing maternal or fetal blood loss.

- ✔ The baby may breathe under water if not brought quickly but gently to the surface, which can cause drowning, though this tragedy occurs rarely. If the mother is kneeling in a shallow bathtub and her bottom comes out of the water during the pushing phase, the baby may be exposed to air and begin breathing. If the mother sits back down into the water, the baby can drown.

- ✔ If the baby breathes underwater and lives, she may still experience respiratory problems (also rare).

Although deaths have been reported, the majority of water-birth studies have concluded that birth via water for low-risk women is safe. This type of delivery is not a do-it-yourself project, however; try water birth only with an experienced attendant present.

Some water-birth advocates recommend allowing the baby to float up slowly to the surface instead of gently but immediately bringing the baby up after the birth. However, this delay seriously increases the risk of anoxia (lack of oxygen) and death for the baby.

You may not be able to have a water birth if your pregnancy or delivery has complications. If your baby is breech or you're carrying multiples, water birth may not be safe. Other reasons you may not be able to have a water birth include abnormal bleeding, meconium in the amniotic fluid, or receiving an epidural. Even if you can't give birth in the water, you may still be able to labor in water and switch to land for the birth. Speak to your medical practitioner for guidance.

Not all medical practitioners are experienced or comfortable with water birth. If you think you'd like a water birth, be sure not only to note this in your birth plans but also to discuss it with your medical practitioner way before labor begins. You'll also need to find out if the hospital or birth center has birthing pools available. If you're having a home birth, you'll need to rent one. See Chapter 12 for information on renting a birthing pool.

# Preparing for Potential Obstacles to Pushing the Way You Want

Epidural anesthesia will limit your options for pushing. Partially upright sitting or sitting on the edge of the bed with a lot of support are probably your only upright pushing positions available with an epidural. You can push while lying on your side, which has advantages, or on your back, which is not recommended. A walking epidural may allow you more pushing options, but not all hospitals offer them. See Chapter 11 for more information.

Epidurals can also interfere with your physical ability to push by dulling the pressure sensations that trigger the pushing urge. Some practitioners let an epidural "wear off" or turn down the amount of medication running through a continuous epidural infusion to help you feel the contractions. If you have an epidural that interferes with the pushing sensation, your doctor may let you *labor down,* which means letting the force of the contractions alone move the baby down through the birth canal.

Continuous monitoring can also interfere with pushing the way you want. An epidural requires continuous monitoring because of potential risks to you and your baby from the medication. Other situations may also require monitoring, in which case you'll be limited to the positions available to someone with an epidural. A radio telemetry monitoring device may help, but not all hospitals have them available.

One of the biggest obstacles to conquer is your medical practitioner's willingness to attend a delivery in a nontraditional position. Although research shows upright positions are best and some practitioners and hospitals encourage them, plenty of doctors are still uncomfortable or unwilling to use them. Hospital policies may also limit your pushing options, like requiring you to only push on the bed. Squatting and hands-and-knees positions can be done on a bed, but other poses, like a supported standing squat, are not possible unless your hospital has a squatting bar positioned on the end of the bed.

Be sure to speak to your medical practitioner early in your pregnancy about pushing positions, and also ask hospitals about their delivery rules. This preparation is a vital part of your birth plan, and although writing down your preferences will help you advocate for yourself, it won't change the mind of a stubborn doctor or override difficult hospital policies.

# Chapter 10

# Nourishing Your Laboring Body

*In This Chapter*

▶ Understanding the pros and cons of eating during labor

▶ Choosing the best foods and fluids

▶ Consuming food and drinks during intense labor or before a scheduled cesarean section

▶ Allowing or rejecting IV fluids during labor

*I*f you were to go for a long, long walk, one that involved lots of hill climbs, exertion, and plenty of sweating, you'd be prepared to hydrate and nourish your body. During childbirth, your body is also working hard! You also burn extra calories from staying active during labor, whether from just walking the hallways in the hospital or from changing positions frequently and pushing at the end of labor. Because you need hydration and energy during labor, you need fluids. But taking in adequate fluid by mouth is a challenge during labor. Many doctors and hospitals have policies forbidding fluids or foods by mouth, and even if your doctor approves, not all foods and drinks are good for labor.

In this chapter, we explain the benefits to eating and drinking during labor, the possible pitfalls, the best foods and drinks to choose, and how to deal with anti-food policies. We also discuss the pros and cons of routine intravenous (IV) fluids — an intervention introduced to counteract the negative effect of policies against eating and drinking — and explain your IV options for labor.

As with all labor decisions, talk with your medical practitioner before labor starts to determine how best to include your choices in your birth plan.

## *To Eat or Not to Eat during Labor*

For the past 20 years, women have been advised to not eat or drink during labor. The only item on the menu? Ice chips. "Nothing by mouth" restrictions started in the 1940s, prompted by a study stating that aspiration, a complication of general anesthesia where vomiting causes particles to get into the lungs, could be prevented if foods and fluids were avoided during labor. At that time, general anesthesia was frequently used for cesarean sections.

Today, however, general anesthesia is rarely used for C-sections, and anesthesia techniques have greatly improved.

Researchers have taken a new look at food and drink restrictions, and guidelines of many major health organizations have also changed their stance on fluids and food during labor. In this section, we explain the benefits to eating and drinking during labor, the possible risks, what your options are, and how to decide what you want to include in your birth plan (because the issue isn't black and white!). We also help you deal with policies against food and drink if you feel it's right for you.

## *Reaping the benefits of eating and drinking during labor*

Although most women don't want to eat much during intense labor, during the early hours of labor eating and drinking may instinctively feel like the right thing to do. Here are some of the benefits to nourishing your body naturally during labor:

- **Providing fuel for your laboring body:** Childbirth isn't called labor for nothing! It's hard work, and hard work requires fuel and fluids.

- **Preventing ketosis and dehydration:** Ketosis is what happens when the body isn't getting enough carbohydrates or hydration to function properly. Without a source of fuel, the body taps into the fat stores. Ketosis can lead to feelings of weakness, fever, and inefficient muscle function, including the uterus. IV fluids are often used to prevent and treat ketosis during labor, but the latest research shows that, in low-risk women, preventing ketosis with real fluids (and sometimes food) by mouth is better.

- **Offering comfort:** We're not talking about "comfort foods" per se, like macaroni and cheese (which you should *not* be eating during labor!) but just the soothing feeling of drinking a warm beverage or eating something light, like toast, can help you feel grounded and reenergized.

- **Increasing a sense of well-being and health:** Being told you can't eat or drink may make you feel like something is wrong with you, which can raise anxiety levels. On the other hand, knowing you can drink or even eat some light foods may help reinforce the idea that childbirth is not an illness, but a normal (albeit somewhat risky) function of life.

- **Shortening labor (maybe):** Some, but not all, studies have found that eating and drinking during labor may shorten labor by anywhere from 45 to 90 minutes.

These benefits apply to women with low-risk pregnancies. It's important to discuss your risk level with your medical practitioner. If she doesn't want you to ingest anything, find out if the restriction is because of routine or because you have risk factors that may make eating and drinking during labor potentially dangerous.

## Understanding potential problems with eating and drinking during labor

The main reason food and drink are restricted during labor is to reduce the risk of aspiration during general anesthesia. Also known as *Mendelson's syndrome,* aspiration during surgery occurs when the contents of the stomach get into the lungs. It can lead to irritation or infection, and in some cases can be deadly. Not eating and drinking before surgery under general anesthesia reduces your risk of aspiration.

Aspiration is extremely uncommon today because anesthesiology techniques have greatly improved over the years. Despite more and more women drinking and eating lightly during labor, deaths from aspiration remain very low. To give you an idea, in Britain between 2003 and 2004, among 2,113,831 deliveries, six deaths were directly related to anesthesia, and none of them were due to aspiration.

General anesthesia is also rarely used today for cesarean section. Most C-sections are done under an epidural or spinal, which does not carry risks of aspiration. However, if you have a C-section scheduled, you will be asked to avoid food and drink beforehand as a precaution, in case the anesthesiologist has difficulty placing the catheter that delivers the numbing agent to the epidural or spinal space. In a true obstetrical emergency, general anesthesia may be used because it's faster to administer and works more quickly than a spinal or epidural. See the later section "Eating and Drinking before Scheduled Cesarean Section" for more on what to expect.

Formerly, people thought that eating and drinking during labor caused increased vomiting (which is common during labor) or slowing down of labor, but the vast majority of the research has not found this to be the case. Many women vomit during labor whether they've eaten or not.

## Exploring your options: Not a black-and-white issue

When deciding whether and what to eat and drink during labor, you have many options. Of course, you need to discuss your best options with your medical practitioner. You also need to take into consideration the policies of your childbirth location and your medical practitioner's allowances.

That said, following are your potential options:

- ✔ **Ice chips only:** This choice may be your only or best one if your doctor considers you high risk. It may also be what you prefer, if you decide you'd rather not take any risks, which is understandable. Just be sure to not restrict yourself too early, like when labor hasn't been well established yet. In most low-risk cases, you don't need to avoid all food and drink before you're ready to go to the hospital.

- ✔ **Nourishing fluids:** More and more doctors and hospitals are allowing fluids during labor. Specifically, research has found that isotonic sports drinks can reduce dehydration and ketosis during labor without increasing gastric volume (that is, the amount of stuff in your tummy). For more on what to drink, see the later section "Hydrating healthfully in early labor."

- ✔ **Fluids plus liquid-like foods:** You may want to try nourishing fluids plus very gentle foods that are practically liquids, like gelatin, clear soup broth, or very thin applesauce.

- ✔ **Light foods plus fluids:** Some women do well on fluids plus breakfast-like foods: toast, biscuits, low-fat yogurt, simple egg preparations (no fancy omelets!), and easily digestible fruits, like bananas. For more on what to eat during labor, see subsection "Serving up smart options for eating during early labor."

- ✔ **Slightly heavier foods:** This option includes foods like chicken, sandwiches, and other heartier options. Your doctor is unlikely to go for this one, but some midwives may approve of this kind of fare, especially in very early labor.

Besides deciding what to eat and drink, you can also choose when to do so. For example, you may eat and drink as you please before you come to the hospital, but when there, follow whatever policy they have or whatever you have worked out with your medical practitioner.

## Dealing with hospital policies against food and drink

Old habits die hard. Even though the current research supports low-risk women drinking during labor and some studies support women eating light foods, most hospitals haven't changed their policies accordingly. Your doctor may also be unwilling to take a risk and allow you to eat or drink during labor, especially if the hospital forbids it.

When discussing the issue with your medical practitioner, it may help to mention that the American Congress of Obstetricians and Gynecologists, the Society of Obstetricians and Gynecologists of Canada, and the American Society of Anesthesiologists have guidelines allowing liquid diets during labor for low-risk women. Also, the World Health Organization recommends that low-risk women not be restricted from light food or oral fluids during labor. If you have a great doctor, this information may help sway him to approve of your birth plans, but don't be surprised if this discussion bumps up against the ego of some docs.

You must discuss with your medical practitioner your birth plans regarding fluids and foods before labor, especially if you're giving birth at a hospital. Just because your doctor agrees to allow you to eat or drink doesn't mean the nurses will be okay with it without written or verbal approval from your doc. If your medical practitioner approves fluids or food during labor but the hospital doesn't, be sure to have your doctor give the nurses an order that allows you to eat. Otherwise, you will have difficulty getting your nurse to allow you to eat.

Unless your doctor has restricted fluids and food during labor for a specific medical reason, or you have a scheduled C-section, you can always just eat and drink as you like while laboring at home. Unless you must rush to the hospital or you have very quick labors, staying at home as long as you feel comfortable may help avoid these conflicts.

# Eating and Drinking during Early and Intense Labor

If eating and drinking is part of your birth plan, the next thing to decide on is *what* and *how* to eat and drink — and it shouldn't be Chinese takeout with a few brewskies on the side! In this section, we explain your safest options for eating and drinking.

## Serving up smart options for eating during early labor

When considering what to eat during labor, keep in mind that your goals are to nourish your body, remain energized, and stay hydrated. The foods you choose should be healthy but not too taxing on your digestive system. A big pasta meal, for example, is not only way too heavy for your laboring stomach but also may make you feel tired and bloated, things you don't need during labor.

Keep in mind the following guidelines when considering what to eat:

- ✔ **Low fat:** Fatty foods are difficult to digest and may make you feel run down.

- ✔ **Low fiber:** Although high fiber is usually best for you, during labor, you want the opposite. For example, toast made from white bread is a much better choice than whole-grain toast, and plain yogurt is preferred over yogurt with fruit pieces.

- ✔ **Energizing but healthy:** High-sugar treats may give you a boost, but they also lead to a crash. Instead, if you're craving something sweet, choose healthier options, like a banana or applesauce.

Breakfast foods or the diet you'd keep while recovering from a stomach virus are best for early labor. Try toast made from white bread, biscuits, white rice, instant oatmeal, dry cereal, well-cooked vegetables, bananas, cooked fruits (like applesauce), low-fat plain yogurt, soup, or plain eggs. Cantaloupe has natural pain-relieving properties, making it an especially juicy choice. You may even eat very well-cooked tender chicken, but no steaks!

How often and how much you eat should also be slightly different than your regular eating habits. Avoid eating big meals, and instead, nibble on things as you feel hungry. You don't want your tummy to be too full — it's unnecessary and may make you feel uncomfortable.

Listen to your body. You may plan on eating during labor but find you actually feel nauseated and don't want to eat. That's okay. If you want to eat, eat, but if you don't, don't!

## Hydrating healthfully in early labor

The majority of medical practitioners today still discourage solid foods during labor, but an increasing amount of doctors are allowing fluids. Not all fluids, however, are ideal for labor.

Most research on labor has looked at the effect of isotonic sports drinks, like Gatorade and Powerade. These drinks are high in carbohydrates, so they not only rehydrate you but also give you a boost of energy. Some women, however, feel nauseated by the high sugar content in these drinks, and they may prefer to drink an oral electrolyte solution meant for children, like Pedialyte.

Following are some other liquids recommended by the American Congress of Obstetricians and Gynecologists for low-risk women:

- ✔ **Water**
- ✔ **Fruit juice** (without pulp)
- ✔ **Carbonated beverages**
- ✔ **Plain tea** (without added milk or cream, though you could add sugar or honey)
- ✔ **Black coffee** (just be aware that too much caffeine may affect your baby's fetal heart tones)
- ✔ **Soup broth** (without any solid particles)

How often you drink is up to you, though frequent sipping is much preferred over downing a lot of liquid at once. Drink when thirsty, as opposed to drinking just to drink. You may want to use a water bottle and straws so you can sip easily from a variety of positions.

## Eating and drinking during intense labor

Early labor lasts for hours (and hours), and if eating or drinking is part of your birth plan, that stage is when you're most likely to do so. However, a time will come when even if you could eat, you won't want to. This may occur during transition (the very end of active labor, from about 7 centimeters dilation and on), or even slightly before. Not only will you not want to eat, you're also likely to vomit occasionally.

During intense labor, you'll likely only want fluids (if that), and ceasing to eat is probably what's best for you. Your labor partner may bring out the ice chips at this time, even if you had been eating and drinking earlier, just to help with dry mouth and lips.

# Eating and Drinking before Scheduled Cesarean Section

If you have a scheduled cesarean section, your doctor will likely tell you to not eat for at least eight hours before the scheduled surgery. Hopefully, your surgery will be scheduled in the morning, so you won't notice the fast much. However, with more docs doing scheduled C-sections, your scheduled time may run into the late morning, so ask your doctor — or the anesthesiologist, if she calls to go over your history ahead of time — when to stop eating or drinking in this case.

The American Society of Anesthesiologists says that low-risk patients who have scheduled cesarean sections with an epidural or spinal may have a moderate amount of clear liquid up to two hours before surgery. Clear liquids are completely devoid of particles, so no juice with pulp or tea with cream.

However, this recommendation is not appropriate for all women, like those who are very obese, suffer from diabetes, have airway complications, or are otherwise at risk for general anesthesia. Be sure to discuss with your doctor what she suggests before surgery day, and let the staff know when you arrive for surgery what you ate or drank, if anything.

# Deciding Whether to Accept IV Fluids

Intravenous fluids, or IV fluids, may seem like the best option for nourishment during labor because they come without any risks of aspiration during surgery. However, IV fluids are not completely risk free. Sometimes IV fluids are essential, and sometimes regular food and drink are best. In this section, we explain the pros and cons to IV fluids and what your IV options are for your birth plan.

## Pros and cons of IV fluids during labor

Routine administration of intravenous (IV) fluids began mainly to counteract the negative effects of restricting food and drink to laboring women by providing them with hydration and nourishment. Additionally, some procedures specifically require IV fluids, like if you get an epidural, require oxytocin to induce or speed along labor, or require antibiotics. However, if you hope to give birth without drugs, IV fluids aren't necessarily the best choice.

Following are some of the benefits to IV fluids:

- **Hydration without risk of aspiration:** If you're getting all your nourishment from an IV, you don't need to eat or drink during labor, and the risk of aspiration during surgery is lower.

- **Easier to give medication:** Some medications require IV fluids. And having an IV in place makes administering medication simpler in an emergency. A saline lock can also provide this convenience, which is discussed in the section "Considering your IV options."

- **Rehydration in the event of excess vomiting:** Some vomiting is common during labor, but if you experience excessive vomiting, IV fluids can be a lifesaver for easy rehydration.

Here are the possible disadvantages to IV fluids:

- ✓ **Restricted movements:** You can move around with an IV, but it's cumbersome. Most IVs are on poles with wheels, allowing you to walk around, but you'll need to be careful not to get tangled in the tubes.

- ✓ **Over hydration:** IV fluids don't necessarily provide you with the most balanced nourishment. If you get overhydrated, you may experience excess swelling, and in severe cases, difficulties breathing. Some studies have found that newborns can also become overhydrated from their mothers' IVs, which may lead to steeper drops in weight after birth. This weight reduction may be misinterpreted as the baby not getting enough breast milk, when actually the baby is just losing the excess fluids from its mother's IV during labor.

- ✓ **Low blood sugar in newborns (possibly):** The excess glucose in IV fluids can lead to hypoglycemia in the baby. To prevent an overload of glucose, many hospitals use lactated ringer solution during labor, which doesn't contain any glucose. If you receive IV fluids containing glucose and your baby develops hypoglycemia, frequent breast-feeding should help, but in some cases, the low blood sugar causes the baby to feel lethargic and unwilling to suck. This problem may lead to the need for supplementation with expressed breast milk, donor milk, or formula. In severe cases, your baby may require intravenous glucose.

- ✓ **Physical and possibly emotional discomfort:** Having the IV feeds into the idea that you are sick, which can have a negative effect on your confidence during labor. IVs are also uncomfortable, which is fine if you really need one, but can be frustrating if you don't.

## Considering your IV options

Your IV options are partially dependent on the rest of your birth plans. For example, if you're certain you want an epidural, you really have no reason to turn down IV fluids, because you'll need them. If you hope to give birth without drugs, however, you may want to exercise some of your other options. Those options include:

- ✓ **No IV fluids; getting hydration from oral intake:** The World Health Organization recommends this approach for low-risk women, and if your medical practitioner has given you advance approval of oral liquids during labor, you may turn down the IV altogether.

- ✓ **Saline lock with no IV fluids:** A saline lock is basically the IV setup in the arm without the attached tubing and fluids. You'll still need to get hydration from other sources, but in the event of an emergency, the IV is partially set up and ready to go. Some hospitals require it for women attempting a VBAC (vaginal birth after cesarean). If your doctor or nurse is hesitant to forgo the IV altogether, she may be willing to try this option.

✔ **Accept IV fluids:** If you don't want to eat or drink during labor, or you're feeling weak and dehydrated from a prolonged labor, IV fluids may be right for you.

In the following situations, you're required to have an IV:

✔ **If you get an epidural:** IV fluids are required due to the drop in blood pressure you may experience.

✔ **If you need labor augmentation:** If you are induced with oxytocin, or your labor needs speeding along, you'll need an IV.

✔ **If you require antibiotics:** If your Strep B culture was positive, you'll require intravenous antibiotics during labor.

✔ **If you become dehydrated:** If you have not had enough fluids or you vomit excessively, the best thing for dehydration is IV fluids.

✔ **If you're diabetic:** Your practitioner will often administer IV insulin and fluids to keep your glucose levels in balance during labor.

✔ **If you have severe pregnancy-induced hypertension:** You may need magnesium sulfate, a drug to reduce your risk of having seizures.

As with all aspects of your birth plan, you should discuss with your doctor your preferences for IV fluids before labor. If you're giving birth at home or at a birth center, your medical practitioner is unlikely to require IV fluids. But if you're giving birth in a hospital, your doctor or midwife must take into consideration not only her own preferences but also the hospital's policies. Some medical practitioners have no problem going against norms, whereas others are hesitant to take risks.

Your place of birth and your chosen birth attendant have a strong influence on how much flexibility you have with turning down routine IV fluids. As with many other issues affecting natural childbirth, asking your medical practitioner about her philosophy on childbirth early on will help you avoid problems on delivery day.

# Part IV
# Knowing Your Options for Interventions and Medications

## The 5th Wave
By Rich Tennant

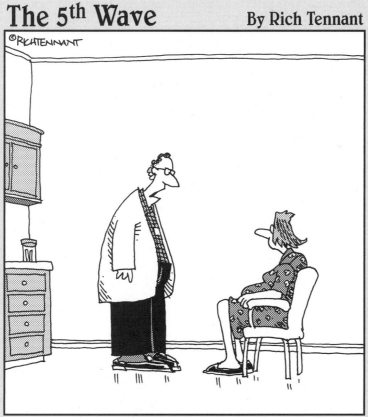

"There's a new pain medication available to expecting mothers that will keep you numb through labor, delivery, and the next 18 years of your life."

## In this part . . .

No two births are ever alike, and very few follow precisely what you read in a book. In this part, we describe the types of medications available in labor as well as the most common interventions during birth, including cesarean section. We also help you make your way through the maze of hospital regulations so that you can write a birth plan describing the type of birth you want.

# Chapter 11

# Ouch! It Hurts! Medications for Pain

*P*opular culture portrays labor pains in one of two ways: A pregnant woman gently moans, puts her hand on her stomach, and has a baby several minutes later, or she screams in agony for hours on end and then passes out and has the baby. As you may suspect, neither portrayal comes close to the truth. Labor is painful, but it rarely causes you to pass out. One contraction normally doesn't result in a newborn baby, either.

When creating your birth plan, pain medication options may play a prominent part. Whether you want nothing or want everything, creating your birth plan is easier if you know the pros and cons of different medications. In this chapter, we give you the knowledge you need to make informed decisions.

## Preparing for Some Pain

Does labor always hurt? Perhaps somewhere, at some time, some woman has given birth to a baby without any pain whatsoever. But unless you have a very high pain threshold, expect to have some discomfort during labor. How you deal with the discomfort is completely up to you.

Writing in your birth plan that you absolutely do not want any pain medication doesn't mean you can't change your mind during labor.

The medications used in labor must be given carefully. If you choose to have it, you need enough to decrease your discomfort but not so much that it affects your baby. Timing is everything when giving pain medication in labor. Giving sedating medication within a few hours before the time of delivery can make your baby very sleepy and slow to breathe.

Research has found that epidural anesthesia also affects your baby, even though it's injected directly into the epidural space. Epidurals can affect your baby in indirect ways as well, by lengthening your labor or by causing your blood pressure to drop, reducing blood flow to your baby. (Refer to the section "Opting for an Epidural" later in this chapter for more on the benefits and risks of epidurals.) Some studies also indicate that epidural anesthesia may interfere with breast-feeding success.

In this section, we preview your options for pain medications and highlight some reasons why you may want to forego painkillers for a natural delivery.

## Putting in your order

Your birth plan should address your wishes concerning pain medication. Unfortunately, knowing just what type of medication you may need is difficult in advance. You may experience more discomfort in labor than you expect — or less! Leave your options open on whether or not you want an epidural or intravenous sedation.

Just writing your wishes for pain management in your birth plan doesn't necessarily make them happen when you want them to. Most doctors prefer not to give epidural anesthesia or intravenous sedation until a certain point in labor because the medications may slow your labor. Sedatives can't be given too close to the time of birth, or the baby may not breathe properly.

Even if you don't put in your order for pain medication in advance in your birth plan, you have options. If your baby is posterior (see Chapter 2 for more about posterior babies) and your labor drags on and on, with increasing back pain, you may change your mind about not taking anything. No one is going to chastise you for this about-face, especially if you deliver in the hospital. If anything, most labor and delivery nurses don't like to see their patients suffer and may offer pain medications more than you'd like.

Only one person can determine what you need in labor — and that's you. Particularly if this delivery is your first baby, you almost always have time to get an epidural if you decide you want one.

## Considering going natural

Why would anyone consider natural childbirth when there are so many other options for pain management during labor? Natural childbirth goes in and out of fashion, but you may not want to take pain medication in labor for one of the following reasons:

- ✔ **You want the empowering experience of giving birth naturally.** This idea isn't just hippie-speak left over from the '60s. Many women want to fully experience childbirth without artificial aids.

- ✔ **Your baby may be more alert and better able to breast-feed right after birth if you don't take any medication.** Intravenous sedation can cause sleepy babies; epidural anesthesia can cause a temporary decrease in muscle tone in newborns.

- ✔ **You want to be able to move during labor.** You generally can't walk around after taking IV sedation or an epidural because of the risk of falls, and lack of movement may slow labor.

- ✔ **You want to deliver in water.** You can't have a water birth if you have an epidural, because of decreased control of your legs and also the risk of infection.

- ✔ **You may have a history of unusual reactions to many medications and don't want to take the risk.**

- ✔ **You want a short labor.** Epidural anesthesia reduces the urge to push and can lengthen your labor. (However, you can let the epidural wear down when you're ready to push in order to reduce this effect.)

- ✔ **You want to avoid interventions.** Epidurals can increase the risk of interventions such as forceps or cesarean delivery, although not all studies have shown this.

Most hospital labor and delivery nurses are more used to patients demanding pain medication than refusing it. Expect your nurse to ask more than once if you're sure you don't want something for the pain. Encourage her to glance through your birth plan so she can see what types of interventions you plan to use to help with the discomfort. (See Chapters 8 and 9 for suggestions on ways to get through labor with or without medication.)

Give your partner, doula, or other support person permission to speak on your behalf if you're getting frequent and unwanted offers of pain medication. Don't take offers of pain medication as an indication that you're not handling labor well; hospital personnel are generally just trying to help. If you want a natural delivery, make that clear. Also make sure your support people understand that it's your prerogative — and no one else's — to change your mind if you decide to take something.

# Opting for an Epidural

More than half of all laboring women in the United States receive epidural anesthesia for their deliveries; in some parts of the country and in some hospitals, the percentage is much higher. An *epidural* refers to the placement of local anesthesia or narcotics into the epidural space near the spine. An anesthesiologist or anesthetist places the catheter, which usually remains in place for future injection as needed, through your back and tapes the catheter in place. In some hospitals, a continuous epidural infusion runs via a pump; in others, you can give yourself a bolus of anesthesia when you need it, within certain parameters set by the anesthesiologist. In some cases, the anesthesiologist will inject more medication when needed.

Drugs injected into the epidural space outside the spinal cord numb the nerves that cause pain in your abdomen and lower extremities. Drugs used in epidural anesthesia include anesthetics such as lidocaine as well as narcotics such as sublimaze (brand name Fentanyl). Complete pain relief can take up to 20 minutes.

Epidural placement differs from that of spinal anesthesia; spinals cause more complete numbing and inability to move from the mid-chest down to your feet and are more often used for cesarean sections than for labor, although some anesthesiologists also use epidural anesthesia for cesareans. In some hospitals, anesthesiologists use a spinal-epidural combination, first injecting the spinal dose and then pulling the catheter back into the epidural space and leaving it there for future epidural injections. The spinal injection is done only once.

Even if you decide in advance to have an epidural during labor, you still should include your wishes about the administration of the epidural in your birth plan. We discuss your options for epidural anesthesia a bit later in this section, under "Deciding between epidural options."

## Enjoying the benefits

Epidurals offer the most complete pain relief of the common pain medication options in the United States. Although *hot spots* — areas where the epidural doesn't deliver complete pain relief — are possible, in most cases, having an epidural greatly reduces the discomfort of childbirth.

An epidural also comes with the following benefits:

- ✔ It allows you to doze off and get enough rest so that you're not exhausted when the time comes to push.
- ✔ It makes labor a more pleasant experience for you and probably for your birth attendants as well.

✔ The amount of medication can be increased or decreased; changing your position can also help the medication reach areas that aren't well numbed.

✔ Less of the anesthesia reaches your baby than if you received intravenous sedation, so you can have epidural anesthesia right up until the time your baby is born. Unlike narcotics, which can make breathing difficult for your baby, epidural anesthesia doesn't depress breathing.

## *Uncovering the potential risks*

Epidurals are not as benign a choice for labor as you may think. Epidural anesthesia does reach the baby and can have effects on her even after birth. Some of the side effects of epidural anesthesia include:

✔ **An increased risk of interventions such as forceps, vacuum extraction, labor augmentation with oxytocin (Pitocin), or cesarean delivery:** Having an epidural can weaken contractions and interfere with your baby's ability to navigate the birth canal without assistance, which increases the need for assisted delivery and/or oxytocin to strengthen contractions.

✔ **A drop in blood pressure:** The fluid you receive through the IV before the epidural is placed helps keep your blood pressure up. A drop in your blood pressure means your baby gets less oxygen, which can lead to fetal distress and the need for an emergency cesarean delivery. However, even with the IV, a drop in blood pressure can still occur.

✔ **A rise in temperature:** The cause of the rise in temperature after epidural anesthesia isn't completely clear. But because your doctor can't tell whether infection or the epidural is the cause of your temperature going up, you will be given intravenous antibiotics so that you or your baby don't suffer any ill effects from infection. A fever can also make your baby's heart beat faster, which can cause concern and may lead your practitioner to do a C-section. If your baby has a fever at birth, she may be admitted to the NICU to be watched for signs of infection or to receive IV antibiotics.

✔ **Difficulty breast-feeding:** Some studies have shown that babies whose moms had epidural anesthesia have more difficulty latching on during breast-feeding for the first few days after delivery. (See Chapter 17 for how to deal with breast-feeding challenges.)

✔ **Difficulty urinating:** Because your bottom gets numb with an epidural, you may not be able to tell when your bladder is full. A full bladder can keep the baby's head from coming down properly and slow the pushing stage of labor. In some hospitals, placement of a Foley catheter is routine if you have an epidural. If you don't want this procedure, talk to your doctor about alternatives such as using a bedpan, although many women can't feel their bladder well enough to do this. Another possible option is intermittent catheterization instead of an in-dwelling catheter.

✔ **Headache:** Headache can occur and may be severe if the anesthesiologist inadvertently enters the spinal space. Leakage of a small amount of spinal fluid can cause severe headache, although this type of pain develops in less than 1 percent of people having epidurals.

✔ **Hot spots:** Epidural anesthesia may not spread to all areas of your body equally, resulting in areas where you still feel pain. Changing position helps the anesthesia flow to a different area, which numbs the nerves that haven't been numbed well. If a large area doesn't get numb, even if you shift position, you may need to have the epidural redone.

✔ **Itching:** The medications used in the epidural can cause annoying itching.

✔ **Inability to move during labor:** Some epidurals can make your legs feel so heavy that you need help even to turn from side to side. You may be tempted to just stay in one position rather than make the effort to move, but inactivity can slow labor.

✔ **Nausea and/or vomiting:** Feeling ill and throwing up are common side effects in labor, whether or not you have an epidural, but in some cases, the anesthesia seems to cause them.

✔ **Shivering:** The required intravenous fluid infusion may cause this effect, or the medications themselves may cause it.

Rare complications of epidural anesthesia include maternal seizures, infection at the injection site, or temporary or permanent nerve damage.

## Deciding between epidural options

Not all hospitals or anesthesiologists offer all epidural options, so ask your doctor what options you'll have before you go into labor. Don't bother including an option in your birth plan if you can't have it! If your hospital does offer several options, ask your doctor which he prefers and why. If he gives you carte blanche on which option to choose, state your preference clearly in your birth plan as well as discussing it with the anesthesiologist.

In every type of epidural, the anesthesiologist leaves the catheter in the epidural space so you can be given more medication without have to sit up and have the catheter placed all over again. Some hospitals offer a continuous epidural, where medication flows constantly into the epidural space via a pump that is managed by the nursing staff. In some cases, you can control the medication flow yourself via a PCA pump. Continuous epidurals have two benefits:

> ✔ The pain relief is more steady and doesn't wear down when the dose wears off.
>
> ✔ The anesthesiologist doesn't have to come back to reinject the catheter at regular intervals.

If the hospital doesn't offer continuous epidurals, you will need to let your nurse know when your pain starts to increase so she can call the anesthesiologist.

When an epidural starts to wear off, your pain level can increase quickly; because you're going from no discomfort to the full discomfort of contractions, you can feel even more uncomfortable than you did before the epidural. Let your nurse know as soon as you notice an increase in discomfort. It can take some time to get the anesthesiologist to your room, especially if it's at night and the hospital has only one anesthesiologist, who may be busy doing a surgery or another epidural.

### Walking epidurals

Walking epidurals sound like a really good idea, but they generally don't work as well as planned. A *walking epidural* is simply an epidural with less medication used and positioning so that your legs don't get as numb as with a traditional epidural.

If your epidural doesn't make your legs too numb to walk well, you may also not get good pain relief. And even though the term *walking epidural* is used, most women still don't have enough strength in their legs to actually walk around.

### Turning down the epidural for pushing

Epidurals often interfere with the pushing reflex because you can't feel the muscles needed to push. If you have a single-dose epidural, you can just stop getting reinjections; as the anesthesia wears off, you can feel the contractions well enough to push. If you have a continuous epidural, your anesthesiologist can adjust the dosage to help you feel the contractions.

If you have an epidural, some doctors prefer to let you *labor down,* which means letting the force of the contractions rather than your pushing efforts bring the baby down. This approach is great if it works that way, but if your baby is in an unusual position or if your contractions aren't forceful enough, this technique can lengthen this stage of labor and increases the risk that you'll need a cesarean delivery. Your birth plan can include an option for letting the epidural wear down to give you a chance to push and see if it helps if this occurs.

## *Receiving the epidural*

An epidural can be given at any stage of labor, but it usually isn't given in very early labor because it can slow progress. When epidural anesthesia is given in early labor, some doctors start oxytocin (Pitocin), a drug to induce labor, to offset the slowing in labor or decrease in the force of the contractions.

Here's what you can expect when the anesthesiologist places your epidural catheter:

1. You're infused with a large amount of IV fluid, approximately one bag, to offset the drop in blood pressure that may occur with epidural anesthesia.

   This infusion can be uncomfortable because the fluid is at room temperature and feels cold.

2. You either sit on the side of the bed, with assistance from your nurse or your birth attendants, or lie curled up on your side.

   You need to remain still and in this position through several contractions.

3. The nurse places a blood-pressure cuff around your arm.

   After the solution is injected, your blood pressure must be taken very frequently.

4. Your back is cleaned with a cold sterilizing solution, and the anesthesiologist palpates your back, looking for the landmarks for proper placement.

5. The epidural catheter is placed into the epidural space on the mid back (see Figure 11-1). You will feel the injection, much like a bee sting, to numb the skin. After the skin becomes numb, you will feel only pressure as the anesthesiologist places the catheter. Some people feel something like an electric shock when the catheter is placed.

   You may feel some uncomfortable poking and prodding at this point. Sometimes the doctor has difficultly placing the catheter due to your anatomy, and more than one needle stick may be necessary. This problem isn't anyone's fault, and getting the catheter correctly placed is important for good pain relief.

6. After the catheter is in place, a test dose is given and blood pressure is carefully assessed to make sure the catheter is in the right place and to make sure blood pressure doesn't fall too low to maintain blood flow to the baby.

   At this point, the automatic cuff is set to register your blood pressure every minute or so for a short period. Some women find this repeated tightening very uncomfortable. Keeping your arm as still as possible allows the machine to work quickly, so try to hold still.

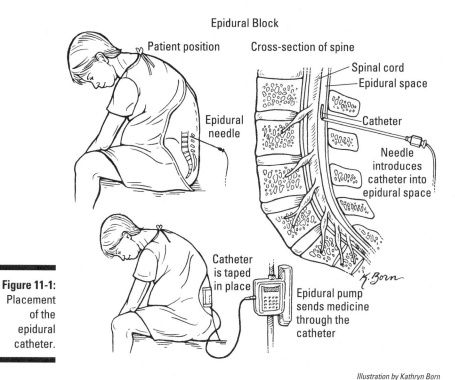

Epidural Block

Patient position      Cross-section of spine

Spinal cord
Epidural space

Epidural
needle

Catheter

Needle
introduces
catheter into
epidural space

**Figure 11-1:**
Placement
of the
epidural
catheter.

Catheter
is taped
in place

Epidural pump
sends medicine
through the
catheter

*Illustration by Kathryn Born*

# Reducing Pain with Narcotics and Other Drugs

Some doctors would rather not give an epidural until your labor is well established, because they feel that epidurals can slow labor if given too soon. In the
interim, your doctor may suggest intravenous or intramuscular sedation with
narcotics. And in some cases, you may prefer to manage labor with narcotics
rather than an epidural. Narcotics, like any other type of drug, come with
pros and cons during labor.

## Benefitting from non-epidural medications

Unlike an epidural, narcotic or narcotic-like medications do not make you
numb or relieve all the pain, but that doesn't mean they don't have a place in
childbirth. Consider some of the ways narcotics can help in labor:

✔ **They can take the edge off contractions so you can get through them more easily.** During active labor, narcotics have less of an effect but may make you slightly more comfortable and able to get through labor.

✔ **In early labor, narcotics can help you rest so that you're not exhausted when active labor starts.** The prodromal stage of labor can last up to 24 hours. If you're too uncomfortable to sleep during that time, you'll be worn out when active labor starts.

## Realizing the potential risks

Narcotics have potent side effects. One problem with taking narcotics in labor is that they affect the baby directly. Narcotics cross the placenta, so if you get sleepy, so will your baby. Before putting narcotics on your birth-plan wish list, be aware that:

✔ **Narcotics can stop labor if given in the very early stages.** If you're having irregular or nonproductive contractions, pausing labor can be a benefit if it allows you to get some sleep before active labor starts. However, it can also delay the start of active labor.

✔ **If you take narcotics four hours or less before you have your baby, your baby may be very sleepy at birth.** Babies under the effects of narcotics may suffer from respiratory depression, which means that they don't breathe properly after birth. Your baby could need resuscitation or careful observation in the nursery until the narcotics wear off.

✔ **You can have a reaction to narcotics.** Everyone has different reactions and tolerances to medications such as narcotics. You could develop itchy skin, feel anxious, or have allergy symptoms such as hives or breathing difficulties. Some women feel dizzy and nauseated after taking narcotics.

✔ **Your baby's heart rate may slow or show other changes before birth from the effects of the narcotic, causing concern for her well-being.** If your doctor doesn't like the changes he sees on the fetal heart monitor, he may suggest a cesarean section.

## Perusing the drug menu

Most doctors have certain narcotic medications that they like — or don't like — to use during labor. Most choose medications that are more easily reversible if you or your baby has an adverse reaction to the medication. Although you probably won't be able to dictate to your doctor which drug you'd like to have, it's good to know what your options may be and the side effects of each.

## Fetal heartbeat facts

When you're listening to the fetal monitor, you may wonder exactly what your baby's heart rate should sound like. Normally, the fetal heart rate

✔ Beats between 110 and 160 beats per minute, although variations do occur in healthy babies

✔ Speeds up, or accelerates, (called, logically enough, an *acceleration*) when your baby moves around and often slows down during a contraction (called a *deceleration*)

A slow heart is called *bradycardia,* and the term *tachycardia* describes an abnormally fast heart

rate. Fetal distress can cause either bradycardia or tachycardia; fever in you or your baby can also cause tachycardia.

A drop in your baby's heart rate that starts around the middle of the contraction and doesn't return to baseline until after the end of the contraction is called a *late deceleration.* This is considered a more serious sign of fetal distress than a deceleration that occurs during a contraction but recovers by the end of the contraction. This type of deceleration is called an *early deceleration.*

If you receive IV narcotics, you probably will have to stay in bed due to the risk of falls from getting dizzy or lightheaded.

Ask your doctor ahead of time which medications he normally suggests during labor and why so that you can do your homework and read up on your choices before putting them into your birth plan. The following medications are commonly used during labor in the United States:

✔ **Meperidine (Demerol):** Meperidine is a narcotic with a long history of use for pain management, although it's used less frequently in labor today than previously. It can be given either through an IV or in an intramuscular injection. The effects last between two and six hours. Because meperidine is a narcotic, your doctor can reverse its effects by giving naloxone (brand name Narcan), a drug that negates the effects of narcotics. This reversal can be helpful if you have an adverse reaction or if your baby is very sleepy when born. Intramuscular meperidine and other pain medications wear off more slowly than IV medications.

✔ **Nalbuphine (Nubain):** Nalbuphine is a synthetic narcotic agonist-antagonist, meaning it has some properties similar to narcotics and some that are the opposite of narcotic effects. It causes little nausea compared to meperidine, but it does cause sedation and feelings of dysphoria, a state of feeling unwell and unhappy, in some people. Narcan cannot reverse the effects of nalbuphine.

✔ **Promethazine (Phenergan):** Promethazine helps reduce nausea and vomiting, which often occur with meperidine. Your doctor may combine the two in an injection.

✔ **Butorphanol:** Like nalbuphine, this drug is a narcotic agonist-antagonist. You may have had this drug in a previous labor under the brand name Stadol, but the drug is now sold only in generic form. Butorphanol, like nalbuphine, can also cause both sedation and dysphoria.

✔ **Nitrous oxide:** A frequently used anesthetic in other countries, nitrous oxide, often called " laughing gas," is being used in more American hospitals. You can self-administer small amounts of the anesthetic, which could help you get over a tough spot in labor. However, nitrous oxide can cause drowsiness or decreased memory of birth. Nitrous oxide doesn't appear to effect newborn alertness.

## Numbing pain with local anesthetics

If you receive an *episiotomy,* a cut made into the skin that enlarges the vaginal opening, or have a tear during delivery that needs suturing, your doctor may inject a local anesthetic into the area either before cutting the episiotomy or afterward, before he stitches. Your vagina is often fairly numb from stretching, so you don't feel the actual episiotomy cut or tear. Local anesthetics can hurt when injected and can make the injected tissues swell. Talk to your doctor about the pros and cons of local anesthesia and include your choice for or against local anesthesia in your birth plan.

# Taking Pain Medications after Delivery

The discomfort of labor doesn't end the minute your baby comes out. Depending on the birth interventions you had, you may suffer longer from the uncomfortable aftereffects of birth than you did with your entire labor. As unfair as this postdelivery pain may seem, we recommend that you plan ahead for the possibly painful aftereffects of labor and decide ahead of time how you want to handle them so you can put your choices in your birth plan.

## Treating pain from the episiotomy

Although some women go through a vaginal birth with no tears or without an episiotomy, most first-time moms experience some tearing if they don't have an episiotomy. Unless you have the most minute of tears, you can expect your doctor to put you back together again with a few stitches.

As you may expect, stitches in your vagina can hurt. They hurt when you sit, they hurt when you walk, and they can hurt for a week or more. While soaking in warm water, shining a heat lamp on the area, or using a donut-shaped ring to sit on can all help with the discomfort, your practitioner may also order oral pain medication to help you cope. The medications he orders may be simply over-the-counter analgesics or narcotics, depending on how sore you are and whether or not you're breast-feeding. (Medications do pass through the breast milk to your baby but are not generally contraindicated for moms who are breast-feeding.)

## Managing pain from the uterine contractions

You would think your uterus would be tired from all that labor contracting and would take a break after you give birth, but that's not the case. Uterine contractions help shrink your uterus back down to its previous size, and your uterus wants to get right to it, so it starts contracting — and keeps contracting — right after you deliver. Afterbirth pains, as uterine cramping after delivery is often called, also help prevent excessive bleeding by clamping down on the blood vessels that were connected to the placenta. So these pains, although often quite unpleasant, have a valuable purpose.

Afterbirth pains are most noticeable in the first three days or so after delivery. First-time moms often have less discomfort than moms who have had several children. A bag of flour or heavy bag of rice on your abdomen may help with the pain. Lying face down on your abdomen can also help.

Afterbirth pains often intensify when you breast-feed. Any medication your doctor orders for discomfort after delivery will help with afterpains as well. Ibuprofen, an anti-inflammatory medication, inhibits prostaglandin release, a key hormone that leads to cramping. Taking ibuprofen on a schedule, instead of waiting until the pain starts, can help reduce the cramping pains.

## Dealing with painful breasts

You can have sore breasts after your give birth whether you breast-feed or not, but the type of pain you experience can differ depending on whether you're trying to produce milk or dry it up. The following factors can contribute to breast soreness after delivery:

✔ **Engorgement:** If you're breast-feeding, you can relieve the pain of engorgement, the experience of having your breasts go overnight from triple A to triple D, by nursing frequently. If you're not breast-feeding, getting through the engorgement stage can be quite uncomfortable. Placing ice packs under your armpits and wearing a supportive bra can help. Cool cabbage leaves placed inside your bra can also help with engorgement. Taking over-the-counter ibuprofen, which reduces inflammation, can also provide comfort.

✔ **Nipple soreness:** Sore nipples are usually a specialty of breast-feeding. Although some lactation consultants swear that breast-feeding should never cause sore nipples, many women do have sore nipples for the first few days of nursing. (See Chapter 17 for more on establishing breast-feeding.) Medications used to treat sore nipples generally don't have side effects for you or your baby, but if you worry about their effects, you can put breast milk on the nipple after a feeding to help it heal.

## Taking pain medications after cesarean delivery

Obviously, popping a few over-the-counter analgesics isn't going to combat the incisional pain you experience after cesarean section. If you had epidural anesthesia for your cesarean, your anesthesiologist may leave the catheter in place and inject longer-acting medication to help with the pain after delivery for 24 hours or so. Your doctor may also order narcotic pain medications to take by mouth or via injection. (See Chapter 14 for more about having your baby by C-section.)

Some doctors utilize a small pump containing pain mediation and tubing that inserts directly into the cesarean incision for pain relief. Called an On-Q, this type of anesthesia is not available from all practitioners.

If you're breast-feeding, the effects of narcotic medications on your baby may concern you. Although a small amount of medication will pass through the breast milk to your baby, the risk is negligible compared to the benefits of breast-feeding.

Try to take your pain medication right after breast-feeding to give the medication more time to leave your system before your baby's next feeding.

Even oral narcotics can make you dizzy and unsteady on your feet, especially when you're recovering from major surgery such as a cesarean. Don't carry your baby around the room if you're feeling woozy, and don't have the baby in bed with you if your partner or other birth attendant isn't with you.

# Chapter 12

# Tuning In: Monitoring Labor and the Baby

**D**uring your labor, your medical practitioner uses several methods — some invasive, some not — to keep track of your labor progress and to measure how well your baby is tolerating labor. In this chapter, we look at the different ways of monitoring and show you how they may fit into your birth plan.

## Monitoring the Fetal Heartbeat

Few sounds are as reassuring during labor as the beep-beep-beep of the fetal monitor recording your baby's heart rate. But fetal monitoring can come at a price and can also increase your anxiety level during labor if you're too focused on every single change in fetal heart tones.

Fetal monitoring is one area where hospital policy can impact your birth plan. If you give birth in the hospital, hospital policy will probably dictate a period of fetal monitoring, around 20 to 30 minutes, when you first arrive at the hospital.

In some cases, your medical practitioner may want you to have continuous fetal monitoring, meaning you're tethered to the monitor for your entire labor. You should discuss this possibility well before labor starts, because obstetricians in particular have strong fears of lawsuits if something goes wrong and they didn't monitor you frequently. On the other hand, if you're having a midwife attend your birth, she may just listen to fetal heart tones with a type of monitoring device called a fetoscope or a hand-held fetal

Doppler. If you're delivering at home, you have much more say, in most cases, over the type of monitoring you have and how often you're monitored, although your provider should have some say in what she considers a safe amount of monitoring. Also, you don't want your practitioner to use technology or methods she isn't familiar with.

The method your practitioner uses to monitor can impact your mobility in labor, so ask ahead of time and find out how much leeway you have with the usual monitoring methods. Incorporate any changes from routine into your birth plan.

## Getting familiar with the equipment

The fetal monitor used in most hospitals looks like a plastic box with a confusing array of plugs and screens. It normally sits inside or on a rolling cabinet. The monitor connects to you via two belts that fit around your abdomen (see Figure 12-1). Following is a list of the parts of the fetal monitor that you'll want to know about:

- ✔ **A round disc that transmits ultrasound signals, which are translated into your baby's heart rate:** Conducting gel is smeared on the disc to transmit the sound waves. It's attached to a wire that plugs into the machine and is attached to you by a stretchy belt.

- ✔ **A rectangular plastic piece called a *tocodynamometer:*** This piece of equipment records contractions by picking up the tightening of the uterus through the abdominal wall. The staff may refer to it — understandably — by the much shorter nickname of *toco.* It's also plugged in to the machine and attached to you by a belt.

- ✔ **A screen that shows your baby's heart rate as a squiggly line and, below that, hills (or mountains!) that represent your contractions.**

- ✔ **Specially printed paper with tiny squares:** The paper is similar to the paper used for an EKG, which feeds out continuously underneath the digital screen. The squares represent a certain period of time. Hospital staff may refer to the paper simply as "the strip."

Some systems allow women to walk around more easily in labor while still transmitting the baby's heart rate via radio signals. Unfortunately, they aren't in widespread use in hospitals, although they're certainly easier to work with if you want to be up and around during labor — and you should be; it's good for you!

Don't ask for a piece of the strip to take home for your baby book. The fetal monitoring strip is part of the legal medical record and often plays a crucial role in court cases. The last thing a hospital or doctor wants if something should happen and you go to court is for part of the strip to be missing.

Losing the signal is easy if you change position, so don't be alarmed if your baby's heart rate suddenly disappears. If the baby is in distress, his heart won't suddenly stop beating. Warning signs such as slowing of the heart rate or an increase will occur first. The monitor will alarm if your baby's heart rate falls outside normal parameters. In many hospitals, a bank of monitors at the nurse's station allows the staff to monitor your baby even when they're not in the room.

In some cases, if you shift position, the monitor may start recording your heart rate rather than your baby's. Because your heart rate is slower than your baby's, it could set off the alarm. If this happens, your nurse repositions the round disc to pick up the baby's heart rate. The staff can change the volume on the monitor so you can't hear it if you want to try to sleep.

You can remove the belts or simply unplug them to walk or to get up to use the bathroom, unless your doctor wants continuous monitoring. In most cases, you don't need continuous monitoring in the early part of labor, although the staff might want to "run a strip" for 20 minutes out of every hour. Hospital policies and doctor preferences vary.

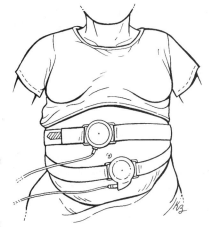

**Figure 12-1:**
Fetal moni-
toring belts.

*Illustration by Kathryn Born*

## Comparing continuous and intermittent monitoring

If you give birth in a hospital, you can assume that you will need some degree of fetal monitoring. The fact that obstetrics is the field of medicine most prone to lawsuits makes this practice inevitable, because no doctor wants to stand up in court and explain why she ignored fetal monitoring as a way to check your baby's well-being during labor. You are also likely to want some degree of monitoring to reassure you that your baby is doing well.

Monitoring gets a bad rap in natural childbirth circles, and while continuous monitoring can create problems during a normal, low-risk labor, intermittent monitoring can allow you freedom to move while also ensuring your baby's well-being. Before you create a birth plan refusing fetal monitoring altogether, keep in mind that monitoring isn't all bad. Plus, few practitioners — neither midwives nor OBs — will agree to zero monitoring. Don't bother frustrating yourself with a request that won't be met.

### Continuous monitoring

Many hospitals place monitoring devices that plug into the large, nonportable monitor as soon as you set foot in labor and delivery and take them off only when you get up to go to the bathroom — if then. Continuous monitoring has advantages for the staff but is less advantageous for you. Here are some benefits of continuous fetal monitoring:

- ✔ **Staff convenience:** Many hospitals have central monitoring banks at the nurse's station so that doctors and nurses can see your baby's heart rate and your contraction patterns without coming into the room.

- ✔ **Quick response to a drop in your baby's heart rate:** A sudden drop in your baby's heart rate will bring several staff members on the run to your room. If your baby experiences true fetal distress, the faster the staff responds, the less likely your baby is to experience any complications from lack of oxygen.

- ✔ **Reassurance for you:** Hearing the constant beat of your baby's heart may help calm you during labor and help you focus on why you're there — to have a baby!

Continuous monitoring also comes with these downsides:

- ✔ **Feeling like you're tied to the bed:** Not being able to move around in labor can increase your discomfort. You may feel especially tied-down if your baby's heart rate is hard to monitor and you need to remain in one position for the heartbeat to record.

- ✔ **Slowing down your labor:** Especially in the early stages of labor, immobility can slow contractions.

- ✔ **Making you uncomfortable:** The belts and monitoring devices can feel heavy, itchy, and cumbersome, especially during contractions.

- ✔ **Increasing the number of medical interventions you have during birth, including forceps, vacuum delivery, and C-section:** Continuous monitoring is more likely to pick up drops in the fetal heart tones that aren't significant but that can panic your doctor and the staff.

### *Intermittent monitoring*

You may find the need for fetal monitoring frustrating if you're planning on a natural birth in the hospital. The best way to circumvent hospital rules is to find a doctor who agrees that intermittent fetal monitoring is best in a low-risk pregnancy. Your best chance of finding a like-minded practitioner is to ask childbirth educators who teach natural childbirth methods.

Although continuous monitoring is the routine in most hospitals, your doctor may well agree to intermittent monitoring, in which you are monitored for 20 minutes out of every hour, leaving you free to move for the majority of each hour as long as things are progressing normally. However, just putting these requests into your birth plan is not enough. Your doctor will need to give the staff an order to monitor less frequently than hospital policy likely dictates.

The nurses aren't trying to give you a hard time; they just can't go against hospital policy without a doctor's order. Getting them on your side by explaining to them why you want to keep moving — perhaps because you're determined to give birth naturally or you hope to avoid a C-section — can help overcome the reticence some nurses have to encourage women to move around during labor. See Chapter 9 for more on the benefits of staying active throughout labor.

If you give birth with a midwife, you have a much higher chance of having your wishes met, especially if you give birth at home, where contraction monitors aren't available. Midwives are trained in intermittent monitoring using a Doppler (see the later section "Using a fetoscope or hand-held Doppler") and palpation.

If your doctor agrees that you don't need continuous fetal monitoring, include this point in your birth plan and remind your nurse to check with your doctor about it when calling to update her on your condition. Keep in mind, however, that this area of your birth plan can easily go out the window for a variety of reasons, including:

- ✔ **Changes in your baby's heart rate that concern the staff:** If your nurse or doctor sees any indication of fetal distress on your monitor strip, you can resign yourself to wearing the belt for your entire labor — and in this case, you probably won't object, because it's for your baby's safety.

- ✔ **Needing oxytocin (Pitocin) to strengthen your labor:** Oxytocin increases the strength and sometimes the length of contractions. Stronger, longer contraction can affect your baby's oxygenation, so continuous monitoring for fetal distress is necessary. Stronger, longer contractions can also cause uterine rupture in rare cases.

- ✔ **Getting an epidural or other pain medication:** Epidural anesthesia can cause a drop in your blood pressure, decreasing oxygenation to your baby, which fetal monitoring can detect.

✓ **If your nurse gets busy:** If your nurse doesn't get back to you right after your 20-minute strip finishes because she's in with another delivery, you could end up waiting a bit for someone else to remove your monitor so you can get out of bed.

## Deciding on internal fetal monitoring

Most doctors don't routinely do internal fetal monitoring. They can't place the internal fetal monitor unless your membranes have ruptured (your water has broken), and the monitoring is invasive because a small electrode must be attached to your baby's scalp by screwing a tiny wire into the scalp (see Figure 12-2).

Internal monitoring has both advantages and disadvantages. Here's the upside:

✓ **One less belt around your abdomen during labor:** The belts are often uncomfortable, so this can be a relief.

✓ **A more accurate depiction of your baby's heart rate:** This information is important if your doctor is concerned about fetal distress. An internal monitor ensures that the baby's heart rate, not yours, is recorded. It also gives a more accurate picture of variability, the difference in the baby's heartbeat over time. A healthy heart doesn't beat at the exact rate all the time; it varies with activity, stress, and fever, among other things. A "flat" heartbeat, one that changes very little from beat to beat, can indicate fetal distress.

✓ **More freedom to move around:** Because the monitor is directly attached to your baby, the signal won't be lost if you shift position.

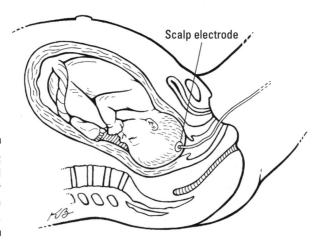

Scalp electrode

**Figure 12-2:**
The internal
fetal monitor
attaches to
baby's head.

*Illustration by Kathryn Born*

On the other hand, the disadvantages of internal fetal monitoring include:

- **Skin infections:** Infection can occur from the wire placement.

- **Improper placement:** Because your medical practitioner can't actually see your baby's scalp, she could place the lead in the wrong place. If your baby isn't in the normal birth position (see Chapter 2 for more on the way babies can "present"), the lead could end up in his butt or, in rare cases, somewhere on his face. In rare cases, this misplacement can lead to permanent scarring or damage.

## Using a fetoscope or hand-held Doppler

If your birth attendant is a midwife, she may use a fetoscope, a low-tech but time-honored method of listening to your baby's heart rate. If your labor and your baby are both perfectly normal, a fetoscope is an adequate way to listen to the baby's heart rate. Your midwife may listen to the heart rate before, during, and after contractions for signs of a drop during or after contractions.

Shown in Figure 12-3, a fetoscope looks like a stethoscope with a bell-shaped piece to press against your abdomen to better magnify the fetal heart rate. Hospital staff rarely if ever use fetoscopes; most don't even have one on the premises.

A hand-held Doppler is a small ultrasonic device that amplifies the baby's heart rate so you can hear it, but it doesn't record it. The Doppler is rarely used in hospitals because it doesn't provide a readout that documents fetal heart tones, but most midwives use Dopplers for intermittent auscultation of the baby's heartbeat.

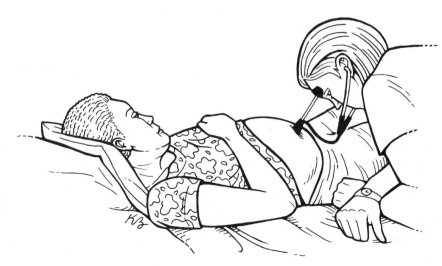

**Figure 12-3:**
A fetoscope
works
much like
a stetho-
scope.

*Illustration by Kathryn Born*

# Checking Your Contractions

External fetal monitoring generally comes as a package deal: Hospital staff check both your baby's heart rate and your contractions at the same time, with two different devices strapped to your abdomen. As with the fetal-monitoring system, your doctor can decide to place an internal catheter to get a more accurate reading of your contractions if your labor isn't progressing as expected or if any question of fetal distress arises.

Both internal and external contraction monitoring systems have pros and cons. Most hospitals start out with the external monitor and later may switch to the internal contraction monitor, which is a soft catheter placed inside the uterus. Like the internal fetal monitor, you must have ruptured membranes to place this monitor.

External contraction monitoring has the following disadvantages:

- **The belt and toco are uncomfortable.** They're especially uncomfortable during a contraction, when your abdomen tightens.

- **You may not get an accurate reading of your contractions.** This problem is more common if the mother is overweight. The amount of body fat between the uterus and monitor and the nurse's skill at placing the toco can affect the reading. Contractions on an external monitor may appear huge when they're really very mild or vice versa.

- **You can't move around much.** Movement can shift the toco and affect the readout.

Internal monitoring, on the other hand, has the following advantages:

- **An exact measurement of the strength of your contractions:** If you're thin, you may be extremely disappointed to see your mountainous contractions dwindle down to little hills after the placement of an internal monitor.

- **A more accurate picture of how your baby is responding to the contractions:** If you have both types of internal monitors, you'll get an especially accurate view. If your baby is having trouble tolerating labor, his heart rate may start to drop at the middle of a contraction and not return to baseline until after the end of the contraction (called a *late deceleration*). This change is easier to see with internal monitoring. Your practitioner will want to try measures such as turning you on your left side and starting oxygen to improve your baby's oxygenation.

- **A more accurate adjustment of medications used to strengthen labor contractions:** Hyperstimulation of the uterus can cause problems for you and your baby.

- **The ability to move around and change positions without disrupting the monitor:** You still can't get up and walk around, but you can shift in bed and change positions without disturbing the monitor.

The disadvantages of internal monitoring include:

✔ **The risk of infection:** The risk increases any time you introduce a foreign object into the normally sterile environment of the uterus.

✔ **Your doctor needs to artificially rupture your membranes:** Your doctor has to break your water to place the catheter that records the pressure inside the uterus. You may prefer to have your membranes break naturally on their own.

✔ **The risk of fetal injury:** Improper placement can cause injuries to the baby.

# Undergoing Ultrasounds Before or During Labor

Ultrasounds during labor are only done if the medical team spots a problem. For instance, your nurse does a vaginal exam when you come into the hospital. She gets a funny look on her face and then says she needs to call your doctor. If this happens, you can bet that what she felt wasn't the baby's head. Your baby may have turned into a breech position or other atypical presentation. If this situation happens, your doctor will likely do an ultrasound to check on the baby's position.

In today's world, where ultrasounds have become routine in pregnancy, it's not often that twins are missed before you get to the delivery room, but if you haven't had an ultrasound during your pregnancy, it's possible. If your doctor thinks you might have an extra passenger onboard, she may do an ultrasound to confirm her suspicions.

# Examining the Cervix during Labor

Vaginal exams are nobody's favorite part of the labor process. Having someone poking and prodding at your cervix is uncomfortable, especially if an exam occurs during a contraction. Some practitioners and nurses also have a much gentler touch than others. You can certainly include preferences about vaginal exams in your birth plan, including who can do them and how often.

## What exactly are they doing down there?

Cervical checks evaluate several factors that can indicate your labor progression. Before labor begins, your cervix is generally located at the back of the vagina. It's around 3 centimeters (1.2 inches) thick and tightly closed. The interior is filled with mucus that seals off the opening between uterus and vagina.

As labor begins, or even a few weeks before, your cervix moves forward in the vagina, which makes it easier to feel. As labor starts and progresses, the following changes occur:

- **The cervix becomes thinner, a process known as *effacement*.** Medical personnel refer to effacement in percentages; a cervix that's 50 percent effaced is half as thick as it was before labor started. Many women start to efface before they go into labor. A cervix that's 100 percent effaced feels as thin as a piece of paper.

- **The os, or opening of the cervix, begins to dilate.** Your practitioner generally uses two gloved fingers to assess the opening, or dilation, of the cervix. Dilation can range from closed to 10 centimeters. At 10 centimeters, your doctor may say you're "complete," which means completely dilated.

- **The baby begins to descend into the pelvis.** Medical practitioners measure this descent by comparing the location of the baby's head to the ischial spines, found on either side of pelvis. When the baby's head is at the same level, he's said to be at 0 station. When the head is above this level, it's described as floating if it isn't settled in the pelvis. At –3 station, the head is three fingerbreadths above the ischial spines. As the baby moves into the pelvis past the ischial spines, descent is described as +1 through +3, until the baby's head is on the perineum.

Your medical practitioner may refer to your progress as 3 (centimeters dilated), 70 (percent effaced), and –1 (station). Now you can decipher the code!

## Understanding the frequency of checks

Every time someone sticks her hand into your vagina, the risk of infection increases, especially after your water breaks. But a vaginal exam is the best way to obtain precise and often essential information about how your labor is progressing. You can't expect not to have any exams at all if you're in the hospital, but you can refuse to allow the entire student nursing class to have a go at figuring out how dilated you are.

On the other hand, you're probably as curious as Nurse Sticky Fingers about how your labor is progressing, and it's hard to turn down a chance to find out what's happening, even at the price of some discomfort.

Unfortunately, when things really start cooking, you may need pain medication, which usually necessitates an exam to make sure you're not too close to delivery for narcotics or that you're far enough along for an epidural. And after you have an epidural and can't really feel the contractions or the urge to push, vaginal exams are the only way to make sure the medication hasn't slowed your labor too much.

Medical practitioners differ considerably when it comes to vaginal exams. For whatever reason, some like to check more frequently than others. You can ask not to be checked during a contraction unless there's a good reason to do so. Your nurse will need to check you when you first enter the hospital so she can call your doctor with the information (unless she's already in the hospital). After that, the main reason to do a vaginal exam is to see if you're progressing well. Your doctor will undoubtedly do a vaginal exam when she comes in, even if the nurse just did one, because she wants to find out for herself what's going on.

If you really want to minimize vaginal exams, talk to your doctor before you go into labor about how to incorporate this request into your birth plan. Keep in mind that some exams may be necessary, because if you're not making any progress in labor other alternative, such as labor augmentation or cesarean, may need to be considered.

## *Evaluating labor's progression without repeated checks*

The progress of labor can be monitored without a vaginal exam. If you're laboring at home with a CNM or lay midwife, who may be less likely to do frequent vaginal exams, or if you have a doctor who agrees to doing them only when necessary, she may look for the following clues that labor is moving along:

- ✔ **A change in your conversation:** Early in labor, you can generally walk and talk through your contractions. When you can't walk or talk through them, labor is intensifying.

- ✔ **A change in the amount of bloody show:** As your cervix opens, small blood vessels break and bleed — not a lot, but enough to stain the mucus that comes out as the cervix thins and dilates. Commonly known as *bloody show,* this blood-stained mucus increases as your cervix dilates, letting more of the protective mucus fall out.

- ✔ **Feeling like you've lost control:** This feeling often shows up during transition, the period of labor when you're not quite ready to push but starting to feel urges, around 8 to 10 centimeters. Irrationality is your overwhelming characteristic during transition. Many women start demanding an epidural, even if they've been adamant about not having one. Swearing at partners is also common, so warn yours!

✔ **The urge to push along with poop production:** This occurrence embarrasses many women, but bowel movements are a natural part of giving birth. The rectum is flattened as the baby moves through, so whatever was in will now come out. It's a good thing in the eyes of your practitioners: It means the baby's coming!

✔ **Bulging of the vagina:** Before the baby's head becomes visible, your birthing attendants may notice the vagina beginning to bulge as you push.

✔ **A protruding rectum, flattened upper buttock crevice, and dimples in the lower back:** All these physical signs indicate the baby is moving down and out!

# Chapter 13

# Helping the Baby Out: Interventions for Vaginal Birth

. . . . . . . . . . . . . . . . . . . . . . . . . . . . . . . . . . . . . . . . . . .

## In This Chapter

▶ Getting labor started with different induction techniques

▶ Increasing labor effectiveness

▶ Considering the pros and cons of an episiotomy

▶ Helping the baby out with forceps or suction

▶ Delivering the placenta

. . . . . . . . . . . . . . . . . . . . . . . . . . . . . . . . . . . . . . . . . . .

*W*omen who can't wait to get pregnant often can't wait for pregnancy to end by the ninth month. Whether you just can't wait to meet your baby or you can't wait to see your feet again, being ready (and maybe a little anxious!) for labor to start at the end of pregnancy is perfectly normal. If you have questions about labor induction or interventions to help your baby out, this chapter is for you.

Doctors often have sound medical reasons for artificially inducing labor. However, inducing labor can increase your risk of complications, including an increased risk of cesarean birth. After you're in labor, they may have reasons for suggesting interventions that facilitate your labor or delivery in one way or another, such as using instruments to deliver the baby or giving you medications to help you deliver the placenta. In this chapter, we look at the interventions your doctor may offer for vaginal birth, and we consider how those options may impact your birth plan.

# Deciding to Induce

Although the end of pregnancy may seem endless, asking to be induced generally isn't a good idea unless you and your doctor have identified sound medical reasons for doing so. After all, if induction fails, you're committed to delivery if your doctor has already ruptured your membranes.

If you do need to be induced, talk to your doctor about all the options and possible risks, and make sure you note in your birth plan any forms of induction that you don't want unless absolutely necessary.

## Considering reasons for induction

Inducing labor early should never be done strictly for patient or physician convenience. Although you may be tempted to determine the exact date of your baby's birth and end pregnancy a little early, inducing labor does have risks (see the next section for details).

But sometimes induction is necessary for your safety or your baby's. Following are some of the reasons why your doctor may suggest inducing:

- **Maternal medical conditions pose a risk to you.** These conditions include high blood pressure, pregnancy-induced hypertension, severe diabetes, systemic lupus, or other heart disease.

- **Fetal medical conditions need prompt evaluation and treatment to keep your baby safe.** These conditions include intrauterine growth retardation, infection, or problems with major organs, such as the heart, lungs, or brain.

- **You're nearing 42 weeks gestation, which is 2 weeks past the normal 40 weeks of pregnancy.** If you haven't delivered by 42 weeks, the placenta starts to age, reducing the flow of oxygen to your baby. Your medical practitioner can do simple monitoring tests that show that the baby is still doing well; if he sees signs of stress, he may recommend induction.

Your personal life situations may or may not be a reason to consider induction. For example, your partner's leaving for military service in a foreign country a week after your due date is possibly a reason to consider induction, if you have a favorable cervix. But your partner's big business meeting out of town the week before your due date generally shouldn't be. However, when deciding to induce for nonmedical reasons, you should also take into consideration the potential risks of induction (more on this topic in the next section).

Most of the time, life isn't neatly wrapped into black-and-white choices, but consider carefully whether your social calendar is more important than your health or that of your baby.

## *Respecting reasons not to induce*

Reasons not to induce labor include your doctor's standing appointment at the golf course or his desire not to come in during the middle of the night. If you don't want an induction scheduled for "physician convenience," make this very clear to your doctor beforehand.

Induction brings its own set of risks, including an increased risk of cesarean delivery. According to a study of more than 7,800 women that published in the medical journal *Obstetrics and Gynecology,* first-time moms who had their labors induced had a C-section rate twice that of moms who weren't induced. Other risks associated with induction include

- ✔ **Fetal distress:** Induction can cause stronger contractions that are closer together, which can reduce oxygen flow to the baby. Poor oxygenation causes a drop in fetal heart rate, which often leads doctors to do C-sections for fetal distress.

- ✔ **Failure to progress:** If your cervix isn't ready at the time of induction and it doesn't have enough time to efface and dilate during induction, your medical practitioner may decide to do a C-section for failure to progress.

- ✔ **Uterine rupture:** Induction with medications may cause uterine rupture, so some medical practitioners won't use drugs to induce women with previous uterine surgery, including a C-section delivery.

- ✔ **Marginally premature delivery:** If your baby isn't as mature as the dates indicate, she may be born slightly premature. Even slightly premature babies can have breathing and feeding problems, plus they have a higher risk of complications such as jaundice.

- ✔ **Postpartum hemorrhage:** Induction increases the chance that your uterus won't contract forcefully enough after delivery to prevent heavy bleeding.

- ✔ **A more painful labor:** Induction often increases contraction strength and frequency very quickly before your body has time to adjust. Contractions may also be harder than natural contractions.

- ✔ **Less freedom in labor:** Induction requires close monitoring, which may leave you stuck in bed (unless your hospital is equipped with telemetry monitoring units). You also won't be able to eat or drink during labor, and you'll be required to have an IV through which the medications will be given. Laboring in water will also be out of the question.

# Evaluating options for induction

If you're considering induction, you need to be familiar with all your options. Besides using medication, you can use natural ways to try to get labor started, although these methods may not be safe in all instances. Talk to your doctor or medical provider before trying home remedies for stimulating labor. Some may just give you a whopping case of diarrhea, while others could be dangerous. In the following sections, we go over some of the most well-known options for labor induction, including both natural remedies and medications.

Just because something is "natural" doesn't mean it's necessarily a safe way to try to start your labor.

### Drinking castor oil

Castor oil, a traditional method for bringing on labor, will certainly give you stomach cramps and probably diarrhea to match. But those stomach cramps may or may not start uterine contractions that will produce cervical changes. Don't try castor oil without your medical practitioner's approval.

### Eating herbs

Many herbs act as mild uterine stimulants, meaning they tone the uterus to ready it for labor. In doing so, some of the herbs can cause uterine contractions. Commonly used herbs for labor induction or uterine toning include evening primrose oil, black haw, black and blue cohosh, and red raspberry leaves.

Although many of these herbs are easily available from natural food stores and pharmacies, talk to your medical practitioner before taking any herbs to stimulate labor, and never take them before 37 weeks of pregnancy.

### Stimulating nipples

Your doctor may suggest nipple stimulation — exactly what it sounds like — to start contractions. Nipple stimulation releases *oxytocin,* a hormone that can cause uterine contractions. However, nipple stimulation will start labor only if your cervix is *inducible,* meaning that you've already started to dilate and the cervix is soft and thinned out. And it's more likely to augment labor that's already begun than to start labor on its own.

### Having sex

Another time-honored home remedy for getting labor going if you're ready to go into labor anyway is sex. Semen contains prostaglandins that can soften the cervix, while oxytocin released from orgasm and nipple stimulation stimulates uterine contractions. The main issue with this induction method is that you may not find it appealing when you're nine months pregnant.

Don't have sex if your bag or water has ruptured, due to the increased risk of infection.

### Walking around the block

Some women swear that increasing their physical activity helps induce labor. Taking a walk around the block is perfectly fine, but don't run up and down staircases or do other vigorous exercise in hopes of starting labor. You may just fall and injure yourself, ending up in the hospital for reasons less pleasant than giving birth.

Normal physical activity as fine, as long as you don't push yourself to the point of exhaustion.

### Stripping your membranes

Stripping your membranes isn't a home remedy, but your medical practitioner may use it during your appointment if he wants to get things moving. In fact, your practitioner may not even tell you he's using this technique. During a vaginal exam at the end of pregnancy, if your cervix is *ripe* (or softened and thinning), he may gently separate the bag of waters from the uterine wall. Doing so doesn't rupture the membranes, but it does release prostaglandins, hormones that cause uterine contractions. It's not always effective for getting labor going, though. If stripping the membranes does unintentionally break your water, then you may end up requiring further induction interventions if labor doesn't begin on its own. (After your water breaks, most medical practitioners want you to deliver within a certain time frame due to the risk of infection.)

### Using prostaglandin gels

Sometimes medical professionals choose to use gels that contain prostaglandins to help ripen the cervix. For example, if you haven't started to dilate and your cervix is still thick and closed but your doctor has identified compelling medical reasons to get your labor started, he may insert prostaglandin gels or suppositories to jump-start the process.

Getting your cervix ripe gives you a better chance of successful induction with oxytocin (Pitocin) the next day or the day after that (see the next section for details on oxytocin). Prostaglandins are difficult to control. For instance, if they cause very strong contractions, gel forms that melt aren't easy to remove from the vagina. For this reason, some forms of prostaglandin are time-released in a container that can be removed by pulling an attached string, and others can be given by mouth. Side effects of prostaglandins can include diarrhea as well as maternal fever, which can raise your baby's heart rate. In rare cases, prostaglandins can cause uterine hyperstimulation and increase your risk of cesarean section for fetal distress.

### Taking oxytocin (Pitocin)

Doctors use oxytocin (Pitocin), a synthetic hormone, both to induce labor and to enhance contractions in a slow labor. Usually doctors give oxytocin intravenously, but a form that absorbs through the cheek is also available.

Your doctor can regulate the effect of oxytocin by administering more or less of the drug via a pump that calibrates precise amounts of the medication. Medical practitioners carefully control the amount of oxytocin being administered, starting at a lower dose and gradually turning up the dose until your contractions become stronger or more regular. Oxytocin should be given only in the hospital, where continuous monitoring is possible.

In some cases, your practitioner may also use an intrauterine catheter to measure exactly how strong your contractions are to more accurately adjust oxytocin doses. (See Chapter 12 for more about internal monitoring and its pros and cons.)

### Rupturing your membranes

Breaking the bag of water that surrounds your baby can sometimes start labor if your cervix is ripe, but this induction method also puts a time limit on your labor, because some practitioners want you to do deliver within a certain time period after your water breaks in order to decrease the risk of infection. Some practitioners rupture membranes when they start oxytocin.

## Choosing the date

If you or your baby has health issues that aren't emergent but that necessitate early induction or you have very pressing and legitimate reasons for wanting to have your baby by a certain date, your doctor may try to wait until you reach 37 weeks of pregnancy, which is the conventional definition of *full-term*. Waiting until 39 weeks is better if possible, unless you have pressing reasons for earlier induction.

Most practitioners won't induce until you get closer to the full 40-plus weeks, unless they have a compelling reason for induction. Even with an ultrasound, pinpointing exactly how many weeks along your baby is can be difficult, and no practitioner wants to induce a baby he thought was 38 weeks but who turns out to be slightly premature.

# Pressing on the Gas: Speeding Up Labor

After labor starts, your practitioner may want to try measures to strengthen your contractions and move your labor along more quickly. Like induction, speeding along labor has risks and should only be done for sound medical reasons. The same medication used to start labor, oxytocin, can be used to augment labor. Some doctors may suggest breaking your water to get contractions moving, although their reason for this step may also be to place an intrauterine catheter to better monitor the contraction strength. (See Chapter 12 for more on monitoring in labor.)

As with any other intervention, feel free to question the decision to speed along your labor, and clarify with your doctor exactly why he thinks it's necessary and what the possible side effects may be.

## Relying on meds: Oxytocin (Pitocin)

Many practitioners use oxytocin (Pitocin) to nudge a sluggish labor into productivity as well as to start labor. You receive oxytocin intravenously with a pump to carefully regulate the amount you get. Fortunately, you generally don't need another IV line for this; the oxytocin line usually plugs into the IV line you already have for hydration.

Here are a few of the most common reasons your practitioner may want to augment labor with oxytocin:

✔ You haven't had any cervical change despite several hours of regular contractions.

✔ Your practitioner inserts an internal contraction monitor and finds that the contractions aren't as strong as they looked on the external monitor. (See Chapter 12 for more on external and internal monitors and their benefits and drawbacks.)

✔ Your contractions and labor progress slow after receiving epidural anesthesia or other forms of pain medication.

✔ Your water has broken and you aren't having many contractions yet. Your doctor may not want labor to last much beyond 24 hours if your water breaks because of the risk of infection, although this preference varies from practitioner to practitioner and is not a rule set in stone.

 If you really don't want oxytocin and prefer to let your body take a little more time to get your contractions going, note this in your birth plan and mention it to your practitioner when he or your nurse comes into the room with the pump and extension tubing to start an oxytocin drip. Another way to avoid having a discussion about labor augmentation when you're not ready is to stay home during early labor, and only come into the hospital when your contractions are strong enough that you can't talk through them.

The risks of oxytocin for labor augmentation are the same as for labor induction — an increased risk of fetal distress and cesarean delivery.

## Breaking the water

Artificial rupture of your membranes can sometimes get labor moving more quickly because your baby's head puts more direct pressure on the cervix, which can help with dilation. However, it also brings several risks for you and your baby, including the following:

- ✔ **Infection:** The bag of water protects your baby from bacteria that can now move up the vaginal tract and into the uterus. If your labor continues to move very slowly, especially if you start running a fever, you may end up in the operating room for your delivery. Frequent vaginal exams after your water breaks can increase your risk for infection.

- ✔ **Cord prolapse:** Most medical practitioners won't rupture your membranes unless your baby's head is low and well applied to the cervix, because rupturing the membranes could cause the umbilical cord to *prolapse,* or fall in front of the baby's head. As the baby's head descends, the cord can be compressed, reducing oxygen flow to your baby. Cord prolapse is a medical emergency that usually necessitates a C-section. Cord *compression,* where part of the cord is compressed between the baby and uterine wall, can also cause fetal distress. Infusing fluid into the uterus can often remove the pressure on the cord.

# You Want to Cut Me Where?! Receiving an Episiotomy

About 30 years ago, nearly every woman delivering in an American hospital got an *episiotomy,* a cut in the vaginal tissue that enlarges the vaginal opening and makes it easier to get the baby out (see Figure 13-1). Statistics haven't changed all that much; about 25 percent of moms still leave the hospital with an episiotomy after birth today. Many — but not all — women who don't have an episiotomy do tear during delivery, but they may tear much less than the doctor cuts; around 70 percent who deliver vaginally will need stitches.

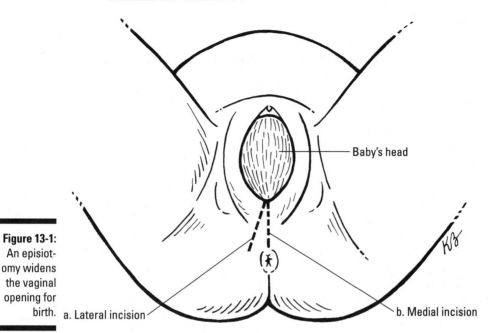

Baby's head

**Figure 13-1:**
An episiot-
omy widens
the vaginal
opening for
birth. a. Lateral incision

b. Medial incision

*Illustration by Kathryn Born*

Few issues in modern obstetrics have been as hotly debated as the routine use of episiotomies. You may already have strong feelings about whether or not you want an episiotomy. If you don't have a strong preference, keep reading to find a helpful list of pros and cons as well as a quick look at some other low-tech but effective interventions you and your birth attendants can do during labor to reduce your risk of tearing. Talk to your doctor about this issue well before delivery and make note of your preferences in your birth plan.

## Pros and cons of episiotomy

Like most medical procedures, episiotomies have both pros and cons. For one, an episiotomy can shorten a delivery if your practitioner wants to deliver your baby quickly. An episiotomy also allows the use of forceps, which can help facilitate a delivery and keep you from having to have a C-section.

# How to do perineal massage

Perineal massage may decrease your risk of tearing during vaginal birth, and you can start using it several months before your due date. To do perineal massage before you ever get near the delivery suite, follow these steps:

1. **Wash your hands to prevent infection and cut your nails short so you don't scratch yourself.**

2. **Get into a comfortable semi-reclining position with your knees bent and legs slightly apart. Position a large mirror to help you see what you're doing.**

3. **Have oil at hand to use for the massage.**

   You can use vitamin E squeezed from vitamin E capsules, vaginal lubricant, or vegetable oil. Don't use baby oil, mineral oil, or petroleum jelly for perineal massage.

4. **Gently massage the perineal tissue, stretching it gently down at the back of the vagina and to the side in the front and side portions.**

   This step shouldn't hurt; if it does, you're pulling too hard or stretching too much. You can insert several fingers and press gently down and out in a *U*-shaped motion or put your finger and thumb on either side of the tissue and gently stretch. You may feel a slight burning sensation when you stretch.

   *Note:* Avoid the urethra, the opening that leads to the bladder. Massaging around this area can lead to bruising or an infection.

   Your birth attendants can do the same stretching during labor and when you're pushing, although some practitioners feel that it increases the risk of trauma when done during labor and delivery.

---

Here are the two main pros for letting natural tearing take its course (and avoiding an episiotomy):

- ✔ **You may tear so little that you don't even need stitches.** As a result, you'll heal naturally, which is less painful than having to deal with the pull of stitches.

- ✔ **Nature decides how much you tear, so you won't tear any more than you need to in order to get the baby out.** Some women have very minor tears, much smaller than the typical episiotomy.

On the minus side for allowing natural tearing:

- ✔ **Natural tears can be jagged and difficult to stitch back together.** In contrast, an episiotomy cut is straight and easier to suture.

- ✔ **A natural tear, like an episiotomy, can extend into the rectum.** Medically termed a *fourth-degree tear,* a tear that extends to your rectum often heals poorly and has a higher risk of infection. An episiotomy cut that isn't large enough to accommodate your baby may extend and become a fourth-degree tear as well, so an episiotomy won't protect you from this complication.

## Alternative options

Some birth practitioners prefer to let their patients tear naturally because they'll tear only as much as they need. These practitioners often use alternative methods, such as the following, to stretch the perineum naturally and avoid tearing:

- ✔ **Perineal massage:** You can start doing perineal massage several months before labor. However, not every woman is comfortable with perineal massage. For directions on how to use this technique, see the nearby sidebar "How to do perineal massage."

- ✔ **Warm compresses:** Applying warm compresses to the perineum makes the skin more stretchy and pliable. Just be sure to make them warm, not hot. Warm compresses can also feel good during labor, even without the stretching benefit.

- ✔ **Favorable positioning:** The *dorsal lithotomy position* (the medical term for the legs-in-stirrups, typical U.S.-hospital delivery position) puts maximum stress on the perineum. The position stretches the skin tightly, making it more likely to tear. Lying on your side or going on your hands and knees for delivery reduces your risk of tearing. Also, having your legs out of stirrups puts less pressure on the perineum and decreases the risk of tearing. (See Chapter 9 for more on pushing positions.)

- ✔ **Soft pushing:** A few years ago, most deliveries in the United States sounded more like a football game than the birth of a baby. Nurses, family members, and staff urged a laboring women to push harder and harder, holding her breath and bearing down as hard as she could. Today, more practitioners use *soft pushing,* or pushing only when you have the urge and not holding your breath. It's also sometimes called *instinctive pushing.*

- ✔ **Laboring down:** This technique is when you let the baby descend naturally with the force of contractions. Many practitioners use laboring down particularly when you've had an epidural and can't feel the urge to push well.

# Assisting the Delivery

Sometimes your baby gets so far and just can't seem to navigate the last few inches of the vaginal canal. If this happens to you, your doctor may suggest using forceps or vacuum suction to get the baby out. Forceps, which look like large salad spoons, have gone in and out of favor over the years; today many practitioners prefer to use vacuum suction. Both have risks, but they can prevent cesarean delivery in some, though not all, cases.

If your baby isn't experiencing fetal distress, consider putting a request in your birth plan that asks your practitioner to try position changes to help the baby navigate the various twists and turns of the vaginal canal before he tries using an instrument for delivery. Sometimes just changing positions gives the baby a more favorable path through the birth canal.

## Forceps versus suction

Doctors have been using forceps to help with delivery for hundreds of years. Made out of metal, forceps have two metal pieces that resemble salad tongs that lock together and fit around the sides of the baby's head. When your practitioner applies the blades to the baby's head, he can slowly guide the baby down, usually pulling during the force of the contractions (see Figure 13-2a).

Forceps come in many different styles, including one type designed for use with breech deliveries, where the baby's buttocks comes out first. (See Chapter 14 for more on breech deliveries.) Practitioners often have preferences on which type of forceps they prefer.

Vacuum suction is a newer option. Many younger practitioners may have trained almost exclusively with using vacuum suction rather than forceps. With vacuum suction, your practitioner puts a soft suction cup on your baby's head and then applies suction to keep it on. He monitors the pressure to make sure it doesn't go too high. He pulls during contractions to move the baby down (see Figure 13-2b).

**Figure 13-2:**
Forceps and vacuum suction can help deliver a baby who's hung up in the birth canal.

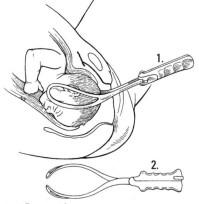

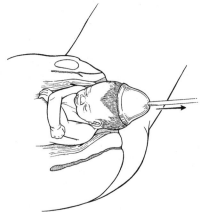

a. 1. Forceps in use
   2. Top view of forceps

b. Vacuum extractor

*Illustration by Kathryn Born*

If the suction cup pops off more than one or two times because the pressure isn't high enough to keep it on, most practitioners will stop vacuum attempts because of the risk of turning the pressure up too high. The same holds true of a forceps delivery; if your practitioner doesn't feel the baby making significant movement in three pulls, he may abandon the effort. At this point, he may schedule you for C-section delivery.

# Pros and cons of assistance methods

Forceps and vacuums can negate the need for cesarean birth, but they work only if the baby is low enough in the pelvis and moves easily with each pull. Doctors no longer use *high forceps,* forceps designed for use when the baby's head isn't engaged in the pelvis, because of the risk of damage to you or your baby.

Disadvantages of forceps and vacuum suction range from minor to severe and include the following:

- ✓ **A cone head created by vacuum suction:** Many babies have a cone head at the time of delivery even without suction. But babies who have a vacuum delivery often have a little cone that's slightly off-center to one side of the head, depending on the cup placement. This is generally harmless — although not very pretty and probably not very comfortable for the baby — and fixes itself within two to three days.

- ✓ **Lacerations:** About 10 percent of babies delivered with either vacuum suction or forceps have scalp abrasions, or small cuts. If your baby's head isn't in the exact position your practitioner thinks it is, the forceps or suction cup may pull on areas of the face rather than on the stronger top or sides of the head. Forceps have caused lacerations on the face or eyes.

- ✓ **Cephalohematoma:** Cephalohematomas form when blood pools under the baby's scalp. This type of bleeding doesn't affect the brain, but it can take a week or two to resolve.

- ✓ **Hemorrhage:** The most serious complication of vacuum delivery is intracranial hemorrhage, or hemorrhage into the baby's brain. This complication is extremely rare, occurring in just 0.35 percent of vacuum deliveries.

- ✓ **Neonatal jaundice:** The large amount of blood pooling under the scalp in cephalohematomas can increase the chance that your baby will be jaundiced. Jaundice occurs when red blood cells break down and bilirubin accumulates faster than the body can eliminate it. More broken red blood cells from trauma increases bilirubin levels.

- ✓ **More painful delivery and/or recovery for you:** You need an episiotomy to make room for the forceps to be inserted into the vagina. You may also experience lacerations or damage to the pelvis floor or perineum.

# Helping the Placenta Out

After your baby's out, you probably won't give a second thought to the placenta, the amazing organ that has nourished your baby for the last nine months. Your practitioner does, though; it's one of the main reasons he's still sitting on the little stool between your legs after you've delivered your baby. Most placentas don't need much help being delivered. After your baby's out and you no longer need the placenta, it usually detaches from the uterine wall on its own.

Your practitioner may notice the cut umbilical cord moving slightly, which is often his signal to gently remove the placenta by carefully pulling on the cord, often wrapping the cord around a pair of ring forceps or other tool to prevent putting too much traction on the placenta. You may feel some uterine cramping when the placenta detaches.

You can put a note in your birth plan stating that you don't want your practitioner to pull on the cord, an action that can present several risks if the placenta hasn't completely detached:

- ✔ **Uterine inversion:** This rare complication occurs when the placenta is still attached to the uterine wall; the top of the uterus inverts and comes through the open cervix. Uterine inversion can cause severe shock and even death.

- ✔ **Cord rupture:** If the umbilical cord ruptures, you can hemorrhage, losing dangerous amounts of blood through the torn cord.

Whether or not your medical practitioner pulls on the cord, if your placenta doesn't detach on its own, he may need to bring in some bigger guns to remove it, such as medication or surgical intervention.

In most American hospitals, doctors routinely give new moms oxytocin (Pitocin) as soon as the baby delivers to help the uterine blood vessel clamp down, reducing blood loss and helping the placenta release from the uterine wall. If you're having a home or midwife-assisted delivery, you may or may not get oxytocin, depending on your individual situation. You can discuss (and put in your birth plan) whether your medical practitioner routinely uses oxytocin or whether he may consider using it only if medically necessary.

According to the March of Dimes, in about 1 out of every 530 deliveries, the placenta decides it's really happy right where it is and doesn't detach from the uterine wall without medical persuasion. Different hospitals have different criteria for defining a *retained placenta,* but most define it as a placenta that doesn't deliver within 30 to 60 minutes after birth. Possible causes of retained placenta include

✔ **Uterine atony:** The uterine wall doesn't contract well enough to expel the placenta.

✔ **Trapped placenta:** The placenta has released from the uterine wall but is stuck behind the closed cervix.

✔ **Placenta accreta:** The placenta has attached too deeply into the uterine wall.

If you have a retained placenta, your doctor may prescribe oxytocin or methylergonovine maleate (Methergine), another drug that causes the uterus to contract, to increase uterine tone enough to expel the placenta. In some cases, your practitioner may give you nitroglycerin to get the placenta out. Rest assured that he won't give you this drug in blast doses and that the placenta won't fly out of you after you take it!

Another option sometimes used by midwives is repositioning — either by putting one leg up on a chair or going into a squat — which allows the placenta to fall out.

Both massage and drugs can cause painful contractions — just when you thought you were done with those! However, not getting the placenta out isn't an option.

Removing a placenta accreta isn't as easy as removing a retained placenta from other causes. No amount of pulling will remove a placenta that's grown too far into the uterine wall or muscle without doing serious damage. If the placenta hasn't implanted too deeply, a dilatation and curettage can remove it.

# Chapter 14

# Cesarean Section: Yes, You Have Options

The C-section rate in the United States and other developed countries has skyrocketed in the last 25 years. In fact, nearly one in three pregnant women in the U.S. now have a cesarean delivery, with rates much higher in some hospitals and parts of the country and among first-time moms.

Whether you have a scheduled cesarean delivery or you face an unexpected one during labor, knowing what to expect and what you can and can't negotiate is an essential part of putting together your birth plan. In this chapter, we give you the tools you need to have a successful cesarean delivery.

# Understanding What Cesarean Delivery Involves

To know what your options are with cesarean birth, you first need to understand what the surgery involves. In cesarean delivery — which probably has nothing to do with Julius Caesar, despite the name and legends — your doctor makes an incision through your abdomen into the uterus.

Although cesarean birth has become commonplace in hospitals today, remember that it's still a major abdominal surgery, and as such, it comes with risks for both you and your baby.

## Reviewing the process

Most scheduled C-sections follow a routine course. If you're scheduled to have a cesarean, here's what to expect:

1. Your doctor tells you a time to come to the hospital the morning before your surgery. At the hospital, you may have to sign consent forms.

   Don't eat or drink anything, including sips of water, for eight hours before your surgery. This requirement is to ensure that you don't vomit and aspirate if you have to use general anesthesia, a rare but possible scenario. (See the section "Receiving Pain Medications for a C-Section" for more about anesthesia.)

2. You receive intravenous infusion to replace fluid and blood loss and to administer medications.

3. You have a Foley catheter placed into your bladder to keep it empty during surgery; a full bladder is more likely to be injured during surgery. Your doctor can place the catheter after you receive anesthesia, although some practitioners prefer to do so while you're still able to move and cooperate. Talk to your doctor about adding a note to your birth plan about putting the catheter in after you're numb.

4. The nurses may give you a mini-prep to shave the area where the incision will go, if you haven't done this yourself.

5. You likely receive regional anesthesia, either with an epidural or a spinal, in the operating room (see the later section "Receiving Pain Medications for a C-Section"). If regional anesthesia doesn't work or can't be done for some reason, you may be put to sleep with general anesthesia, but this practice is rare.

6. The anesthesiologist places electrodes on your chest to connect to an EKG that monitors your heart during the surgery.

7. After you're numb, you doctor begins the surgery. Your partner normally gets to sit somewhere near your head.

   The incision made for a C-section is usually made low and is called a *low transverse incision;* it's called a *bikini cut* because it follows where the top of your bikini line would be, if you still felt like wearing one! See Figure 14-1a for a visual of this type of incision. The incision on the skin and the incision on the uterus may not go in the same direction. A low transverse incision lets you try a vaginal birth after cesarean.

If your baby is in an unusual position and is difficult to "extract" with a low incision, you may need an up-and-down incision made in the upper part of the uterus, called a *classical incision*. (See Figure 14-1b for an example.)

Doctors use a vertical incision on the uterus only if your baby or the placenta is in an unusual position. A *low vertical incision* is a type of vertical incision done in the lower portion of the uterus (see Figure 14-1c).

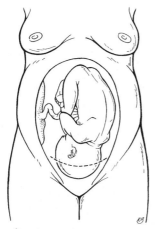

a. Low transverse

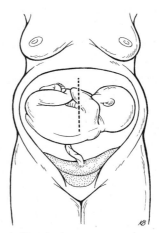

b. Classical

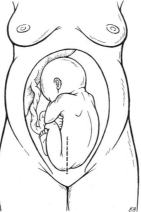

c. Low vertical

**Figure 14-1:**
Three types
of cesarean
incisions.

*Illustration by Kathryn Born*

8. After making the first incision, your doctor generally takes less than 10 minutes to get your baby out. You may feel some tugging sensations as the doctor removes your baby from the uterus.

   The doctor or nurse may give you your baby immediately or take him to a warmer for weighing and cleanup. At this point, you can incorporate many of your desires into your birth plan, such as having your partner cut the cord, not weighing the baby right away, or letting the baby nurse immediately. Hospitals are often less likely to grant exceptions to the rules during a C-section, so discuss your wishes with your doctor before your surgery, if possible.

9. Your practitioner repairs the uterus and the layers of the abdominal wall with stitches. Don't panic! You're still numb during these procedures.

10. After everything is back together, you go to recovery for about an hour. In many hospitals, you need to be able to move your legs before you can go to your room. You won't be able to walk at this point, so you go to your room by gurney. In many hospitals today, your baby will go to recovery with you, unless he's having medical issues.

An unscheduled cesarean birth follows the same steps, although the scene may be somewhat more chaotic, depending on the circumstances. You may already have an IV and a Foley catheter if you've been in labor and have had an epidural. If time allows, the anesthesiologist may use your current epidural, beefing up the dosage to make you more numb for surgery. She will administer general anesthesia if there isn't time for an epidural, one of the few times general anesthesia is used in obstetrics.

## Explaining the risks

Even routine surgeries have risks. Having a C-section increases the following risks:

- **Longer hospital stay:** Most moms come home within one to two days after vaginal delivery and three to five days after cesarean.

- **Nausea and vomiting:** Manipulation of the abdominal organs during a C-section increases your risk of nausea and vomiting afterward, but this complication is short-lived.

- **Bowel problems:** Manipulation of the intestines, bed rest, and the use of pain medications that slow bowel motility often cause constipation after any type of abdominal surgery, including C-sections.

- **Headache:** About 10 percent of women who have spinal anesthesia during a C-section develop a post-surgical headache. Headache can develop if a small amount of spinal fluid leaks out of the spinal space. If the headache is severe, a *blood patch* (which puts a small amount of blood into the space to restore the pressure within the spinal fluid) can help relieve the headache.

✔ **Infection:** As many as 5 to 10 percent of women who have a C-section develop an infection after the fact. This rate is five times more than those women who have a vaginal delivery. Fortunately, most infections are easily treated with antibiotics.

✔ **Blood loss:** Every birth results in some blood loss, but having a C-section increases your risk of hemorrhage to approximately 6 percent, compared to up to 4 percent for a vaginal delivery. Most women lose about 500 cubic centimeters (cc) of blood during vaginal birth, compared to 1,000 cc during C-section birth. Because your blood volume increases during pregnancy, this amount of blood loss normally doesn't cause any problems, but severe bleeding can cause anemia.

✔ **Increased chance of future C-sections:** Because most American doctors prefer repeat cesarean delivery to trying a vaginal birth after a mom has had a cesarean, all your deliveries in the future may be surgical births. The risk of complications increases with each cesarean. For example, your risk of placental problems and adhesions in the uterus increases with every C-section you have; these problems could interfere with your ability to get pregnant in the future and could also lead to future surgeries.

✔ **Higher incidence of respiratory distress for your baby:** Although you may think being lifted out of the uterus is less stressful than squeezing through the birth canal, labor helps remove fluid from the baby's lungs that can cause respiratory difficulties after birth.

✔ **Injury to the baby during delivery:** These risks can include cuts from the scalpel or other injuries that result when the baby's position makes him difficult to extract through the incision.

✔ **Injury to your bowel or bladder during surgery:** These problems can lead to future difficulties with bowel or bladder control or require surgeries to repair the damage.

✔ **Blood clots:** Your risk of deep vein thrombosis increases five- to tenfold during pregnancy. Any type of surgery, including cesarean delivery, further increases your risk.

✔ **Maternal death:** The maternal death rate after vaginal delivery is 0.2 per 100,000 births compared to 2.2 in 100,000 after a cesarean delivery. General anesthesia (normally done only with emergency cesarean delivery) increases the rate of maternal deaths because of the risk of aspiration.

# Addressing a Scheduled C-Section in Your Birth Plan

In some cases, cesarean delivery is a given. If your baby has decided to enter the world upside down or sideways, for example, your doctor will probably schedule a C-section, though some medical practitioners may allow a trial of labor for certain breech positions. Similarly, if you have certain disorders, such as genital herpes, that make vaginal delivery dangerous for your baby, your doctor may go ahead and schedule a cesarean ahead of time.

If you're having a scheduled C-section, you still have plenty of choices to make that can impact your birth plan, including when to schedule the birth, who will be present in the operating room, when you want to hold your baby, and how and when you want to breast-feed. This section covers your options for turning an upside-down or sideways baby, dealing with herpes, having an elective C-section, and choosing a date and time for your delivery. We talk about the other decisions you need to make concerning your time in the operating room later in this chapter.

## Sorting out upside-down and sideways babies

Having a breech baby is one of the most common reasons doctors use planned C-sections. Thirty years ago, doctors delivered breech babies vaginally, and a few still may do so today. But because breech deliveries are more complex and have a higher potential for complications and lawsuits, most doctors have decided that scheduling a C-section is the safest option. The fact that few younger doctors have even been trained how to deliver breech babies vaginally has also contributed to the decrease in vaginal breech deliveries.

Breech babies have three times more risk of complications when delivered vaginally compared to when delivered via C-section. And babies who are *transverse,* or sideways in the uterus, will never come out vaginally. So in many breech situations, C-section is a good option. But before you sign up for a C-section, consider trying the techniques that we describe in the following sections to try to turn your baby into a more favorable position for vaginal delivery.

### Trying a version

Trying to turn a breech baby manually from the outside — a procedure called a *version* — may help you avoid a cesarean if you really don't want one. Versions are normally done under ultrasound guidance, and they can be uncomfortable. You may be given a drug to relax you and another one to relax your uterus to reduce the risk of starting labor. In some cases, the baby may turn right back where he was comfortable before, but this readjustment is less likely in the last few weeks of pregnancy, usually around 37 weeks. Versions have about a 58 percent success rate.

Most of the time, versions are tried in the last few weeks of pregnancy, but your practitioner can try a version during labor as long as your amniotic sac hasn't ruptured yet.

Because a version can be complicated, you need to have fetal monitoring during and after the procedure. If the baby becomes tangled in the cord or experiences fetal distress, your doctor needs to be ready to do a cesarean on the spot. You should consider trying a version if

- ✔ **Your baby isn't engaged or already settled into the pelvis.** After the baby is engaged, he's much harder to move.

- ✔ **This isn't your first pregnancy.** Your baby has more room to maneuver, so to speak, if you've been pregnant before.

- ✔ **The amniotic sac is intact, and you have enough amniotic fluid.** This fluid cushions the baby during the version and reduces the risk of complications.

- ✔ **You're carrying only one baby.** Twins are too complicated to try to turn in the uterus. Unless twin A is head down, you're unlikely to have a vaginal delivery, anyway, and some doctors insist that both babies be head down before they'll allow a vaginal trial of labor. Even when both babies are head down, the second twin can shift after delivery of the first, meaning you could end up delivering one twin vaginally and the other by C-section, a scenario that coauthor Sharon has seen more than once.

## Trying other turning methods

In some cases, lying head down and feet up (you, not the baby) for a certain amount of time each day can turn a stubborn baby. Don't try this technique unless your medical practitioner gives you the okay, and be sure to follow her instructions for how to position yourself carefully. Putting yourself in a position where your feet are too far over your head could make you dizzy.

Another option is simply to talk to your baby. Some people strongly believe in the power of suggestion, even if the person you're making the suggestions to can't speak yet. But if you want to try sitting quietly for a period of time each day and softly suggesting to your baby that now is the time to make a turn for the better, go for it! It can't hurt to try.

## Trying some alternative turning techniques

If a version doesn't appeal to you, you can look into some alternative methods of getting your baby to face the world the right way (which is actually upside-down in this case). Although only external version has a greater than 50 percent documented success rate, several other methods — including one chiropractic method, a homeopathic remedy, and one traditional Chinese medicine remedy — may help. Keep in mind, though, that before 34 weeks of pregnancy, your baby may well decide to turn on his own. If he doesn't, consider the following options.

The Webster chiropractic technique uses light force on the spine as a type of spinal adjustment. In a study on this technique, 82 percent of practitioners reported success with this method, which can be done only by a chiropractor. However, in 59 of the 112 cases reported, breech presentation was not documented by ultrasound before the procedure.

Talk to your medical practitioner before trying this technique.

Moxibustion is traditional Chinese medicine that utilizes the burning of herbs, in this case placed near the base of the little toenail. A 2009 Swiss study found no benefit to the procedure, but previous studies have reported a benefit. It certainly wouldn't hurt to try it.

If you're into homeopathic medicine, some practitioners use Homeopathic Pulsatilla to "even out" the muscle fibers in the uterus and help the baby to turn. Take this only under the guidance of an experienced homeopathic practitioner.

Positioning yourself in ways to help the baby turn may get your recalcitrant little one in the right position. See the website www.spinning babies.com for numerous suggestions on ways to encourage a breech baby to turn.

## *Handling herpes*

Genital herpes isn't a topic that women like to discuss, even with their health practitioners. Having genital herpes doesn't mean you have to have a cesarean delivery, but it does mean you need to be aware of your outbreaks. After all, if your water breaks or you go into labor when you have lesions, the infection could travel up into the uterus and affect your baby. For this reason, most practitioners suggest a C-section if you have an outbreak at the time of delivery.

Another option may be taking antivirals in the month prior to your due date. Research studies have found that it reduces the risk of lesions appearing, which will allow you to have a vaginal delivery instead of a C-section. Be sure to discuss this option with your doctor early in pregnancy so you can start the medication on time.

## *Having an elective C-section*

If you've had one cesarean birth, your healthcare provider will likely suggest that you have a scheduled C-section with your next baby. Technically speaking, this reason for a C-section falls under the category of elective C-section because, in many cases, there's no reason to have another C-section unless you have a similar issue to the one that lead to your first operative delivery.

Doctors often discourage women from having a *vaginal birth after cesarean,* more commonly known by the term *VBAC* (pronounced v-back). The reason has to do with liability and the small risk that your uterus could rupture at the site of the old scar during vaginal delivery. In practice, this occurrence is extremely rare, affecting less than 1 percent of laboring moms who've previously had a C-section. But because doctors prefer to minimize the chance of any complications in pregnancy, they often prefer to turn to the scheduling book instead of giving labor a second chance.

If you do want to have a VBAC, you have the best chance for success if

  ✔ Your first C-section was for abnormal position or fetal distress rather than failure to progress or for maternal-health conditions.

  ✔ Your second labor isn't being induced or augmented with drugs that can cause overly strong uterine contractions, which are more likely to cause uterine rupture.

  ✔ Your first incision is low transverse rather than vertical (refer to Figure 14-1). Vertical incisions on the uterus are more likely to rupture.

  ✔ You have had only one previous cesarean birth.

If you want to go the VBAC route, bring the topic up at your very first appointment with your medical provider. She may want to look through your medical records for information that can help her determine whether you're a good candidate for VBAC. Approaching this subject early on also gives you time to seek a second opinion if your first doctor turns down your VBAC request.

In many parts of the world, truly elective cesarean has caught on as an option to avoid labor. In this scenario, women who have no medical reasons for C-section choose this option simply to avoid going through labor. Not as many doctors in the U.S. support this decision, although some do perform elective C-sections on request. Review the list of risks in the section "Explaining the risks" earlier in this chapter for a laundry list of why this really isn't a good idea.

# Deciding on the date for surgery

Although picking the date for your baby's birth may seem like a bonus of a scheduled C-section, your medical provider has as much input — if not more — into your baby's birthdate as you do. Most doctors don't do scheduled surgery on the weekends, so although Saturdays or Sundays may work well for your partner's work schedule, they probably won't work well with the doctor's — and you can guess who holds the most cards in this situation.

You may have strong preferences about whether to schedule your birth or let nature take its course and dictate the day. Either way, talk to your doctor about your options and find out which ones she's willing to consider for your situation.

### Picking the day

In some cases, you may want to wait until your baby's official due date before you schedule his arrival time. But your doctor may not like this idea because it increases the chance that you'll go into labor first, probably in the middle of the night. For this reason, most doctors schedule your D-day for a week or so before your official due date. This approach walks the fine line between delivering a baby who's slightly early and taking a chance that labor will start before the big day.

The advantage of not scheduling your delivery until after your official due date is that you don't have to worry about the baby being born a bit too early because of a miscalculation of the due date.

### Picking the time

If you have any say in the matter, always choose to be the first scheduled C-section of the day at your hospital. If you're scheduled for later in the day, you have a good chance of being "knocked off" the schedule by laboring women who need cesareans for more pressing issues. Whether those other laboring women are your doctor's patients doesn't make much of a difference because most hospitals have just one or two operating rooms that they use for cesarean deliveries.

Your turn will come eventually, but if you happen to hit a busy day in labor and delivery, you may have to sit through several other cesareans first. To top things off, you won't be able to eat or drink anything and you'll be hooked up to an IV (and probably feeling extremely frustrated) during the wait. Take it from us: Grabbing an early C-section time is worth getting up early for. You probably have to get up at the crack of dawn to go to the bathroom anyway at this stage of pregnancy.

### Allowing labor to begin first

Allowing your body to choose the day of your C-section — by waiting for contractions to begin rather than scheduling the day ahead of time — is one way to ensure your baby isn't born too early. Plus, the body releases hormones during labor that help prepare the baby to be born. For instance, your body releases catecholamines during labor, which help prepare the baby's lungs.

If you have strong feelings about letting your baby choose his own birthday by waiting until labor starts, you may have to do some heavy persuading to get your doctor to agree. Obstetricians have their sleep interrupted often enough for unscheduled labors and deliveries; most prefer not to have scheduled cesareans wake them up in the middle of the night, too. Obviously, your baby's health should come before your doctor's convenience, but be prepared to argue your side.

Waiting for labor to begin isn't always safe. If your baby is in a position that could cause complications, your doctor may prefer that your water not break before your surgery. In the case of genital herpes, the infection has a small chance of traveling to the baby after the membranes rupture if herpes lesions are present. If your baby isn't positioned correctly down in the pelvis, the umbilical cord could *prolapse,* or fall below the baby's head, if your water breaks.

# Facing an Unscheduled C-Section

It's one thing to know, plan for, and write your birth plan based on a scheduled cesarean birth; it's quite another to get into labor — sometimes nearly all the way to the end — and then find out you need to have a C-section. Knowing that about 32 percent of all women end up having an operative delivery (a number much higher than the 5 to 10 percent that the World Health Organization suggests as the optimal number) likely won't make you feel any better, although you may be too tired or too worried about your baby to care when the moment arrives. The following sections go through the main reasons why you may end up having an unscheduled C-section after labor begins.

## Reacting to failure to progress

*Failure to progress* is one of the most commonly cited reasons for cesarean birth. This term can mean just about anything your doctor wants it to mean, but what it should mean is that, after an adequate trial of labor (which normally means strong contractions without any labor progress over a period of two to four hours), you didn't dilate or give birth to your baby within the prescribed norms. Here are just a few examples of when your doctor may diagnose you with failure to progress:

> ✔ You were induced when your body really wasn't ready. (This scenario isn't always avoidable if induction was necessary due to the baby's medical condition or yours.)
>
> ✔ Your pelvis isn't large enough to accommodate your particular baby. (This scenario is also rare, occurring in just 1 in 250 pregnancies, or just 0.5 percent.)
>
> ✔ An epidural slowed your labor and stalled your baby's progress through the birth canal, and it's taking too long to get things going again, especially if you've developed a fever and your baby's heart rate is a little too fast.

Of all the diagnoses for cesarean, failure to progress is the one most negotiable with your doctor. Of course, no mom is going to argue to try laboring for a few more hours if her baby is in distress. But you can argue — or your partner or doula can, if you're not up to the task — for a little more time to beat the failure to progress diagnosis if you and your baby aren't having any major issues.

If you had pain medication that slowed down your progress for a few hours but your baby's head is nicely down, you can argue for an extra hour or two of labor with a change of position to get things moving again. For instance, you can try walking the halls if you're able or sitting in the birthing pool to help you relax.

## Responding to fetal distress

Fetal distress is the most frightening of reasons for a cesarean birth; it's often accompanied by a frantic rush down the hall after a quick prep, a brief explanation, and a feeling of urgency. Obstetricians and labor and delivery staff generally don't panic easily, so if they think your baby needs to be born right now, don't argue.

*Fetal distress* usually means that your baby's heart rate has dropped below 110 beats per minute or is dropping dangerously with each contraction and not recovering by the end of the contraction. A loss of variability (the normal change in heartbeat over time), or a so-called "flat" heartbeat, can also indicate that your baby isn't tolerating labor well (see Chapter 12 for more on fetal heartbeats).

If you run a fever during labor, your baby can also develop a fever, which usually increases his heart rate just as it increases yours. If you run a fever, your baby could also become infected. A rapid heart rate can also be dangerous for your baby. If you're still a long way from giving birth, your doctor may decide to deliver your baby now via C-section so she can start giving him antibiotics.

# *Treating maternal complications*

Besides failure to progress and fetal distress, you can develop a few other serious complications during labor. In most of these cases, your doctor can't wait for you to continue to labor without putting you and your baby at risk, so you have to have an immediate C-section.

### *Placental abruption*

*Placental abruption* is the premature separation of the placenta from the uterine wall. This separation can happen during labor if your contractions are too strong because of augmented labor, if you have very high blood pressure, or if you use street drugs such as cocaine.

When part of the placenta detaches from the uterine wall, your baby gets less oxygen and you can bleed. Most of the time, placental abruptions are small, in which case you may be able to continue to labor, but a large abruption means you need an immediate cesarean.

### *Preeclampsia*

Severe pregnancy-induced hypertension can lead to *preeclampsia,* a life-threatening condition that leads to seizures that threaten the life of you and your baby. The only cure for preeclampsia is delivery of the baby. If you aren't in labor and very close to delivery, your doctor will likely want to do an immediate C-section.

### *Other possible complications*

Most moms don't become really ill during labor, but it is possible. For example, complications from chronic diseases such as diabetes or heart disease could lead your doctor to do an immediate delivery. In these cases, you have little room for argument, because your well-being and possibly your baby's are at stake.

# *Asking questions before your doctor makes the first cut*

Most of the time, an unscheduled cesarean isn't an emergency. So you have a chance to ask questions and make your wishes known about who will be in the operating room with you and whether you want to have your baby with you right after birth (as long as neither you nor the baby has life-threatening complications requiring immediate care). When your doctor says she wants to do an unplanned C-section, consider asking these questions before she wheels you down to the operating room:

✔ **Why are you recommending a cesarean now?** Although you probably already have some idea, you'll feel better if you get your doctor's input firsthand. Make sure she discusses both the pros and the cons.

✔ **Can we try any other options first?** These options can include getting in a different position, walking up and down the hall, simply giving labor a little more time, augmenting your labor to strengthen your contractions, turning the dose down (or off) if your baby appears to be stressed, or waiting for your epidural to wear down a little.

✔ **Is my baby in immediate distress?** In most cases, if your baby is in distress, you'll know it by the flurry of activity in your room. If your room is still fairly quiet, ask your practitioner what she feels the risk to your baby is at this time.

✔ **Am I in danger?** Again, if you are, you'll probably know it by the activity level around you. If the danger isn't immediate, ask your doctor for an explanation of why a C-section is the best option for you right now.

✔ **What kind of anesthesia will I have for the surgery?** The anesthesiologist may talk to you about the pros and cons of putting a higher dose of medication in your epidural for the surgery versus putting in a spinal. One benefit of using the epidural is that you can use it for pain medication after your surgery.

✔ **Can I hold my baby right after the surgery?** If your baby isn't in immediate distress, this should be an option.

✔ **Who can come into the operating room with me, and where will they be?** Hopefully you decided ahead of time (and put in your birth plan) your first choices. But if you've been in labor for a while, you may have a clearer idea of who's a good choice and who isn't.

✔ **How long will the surgery take and what type of incision will I have?** Keep in mind that the incision on the uterus and the incision on the skin may not be the same. (See the earlier section "Reviewing the process" for details on the different types of incisions.) The baby is usually out within five to ten minutes, but putting everything back together again can take up to an hour.

# Receiving Pain Medications for a C-Section

Obviously, you can't have a cesarean delivery without some type of pain medication, and a few waves of narcotics through your IV aren't going to cut it. Most hospitals use regional anesthesia that numbs you from the chest down, meaning a spinal or epidural; general anesthesia, which puts you completely to sleep, is used in rare cases.

# Having spinal anesthesia

Spinal anesthesia goes into the spinal space on your back. Unlike an epidural, spinal anesthesia results in immediate numbness from the chest down. You should still be able to breathe on your own with spinal anesthesia because the area the anesthesiologist injects starts with the nerves just below your lungs. If you have spinal anesthesia, you can expect the following to happen:

1. You sit up for the spinal, which the anesthesiologist does exactly like an epidural, with you curling up to widen the spinal space.

   The spinal isn't placed until you're in the operating room (OR).

2. As soon as the spinal is placed, you lie back down with the help of the staff.

   Your legs and abdomen go numb right away. If they don't, tell your anesthesiologist, but rest assured that she'll check to make sure you're numb before your doctor starts the surgery.

3. The staff places a strap around your legs so they don't fall off the OR table.

   Because your legs are completely numb, you can't feel them fall off. But you can suffer nerve damage from compression on the nerves if your leg falls and the staff doesn't notice it.

4. Your hands are strapped at your side so you don't contaminate the sterile field.

After a spinal, you may not feel yourself breathing as you normally do, which may make you panicky. Keep in mind that if the anesthesiologist is sitting quietly, you're breathing just fine. She'll reassure you about your breathing. If for some reason the spinal medication goes too high and you really aren't breathing, your anesthesiologist will place a tube that breathes for you, but this situation is extremely rare.

After your baby is born, the numbness in your legs will slowly wear off. Your anesthesiologist probably won't release you from the recovery area until you can move your feet. You won't be able to walk yet, so a nurse will move you to your room by stretcher, and she'll need to be with you the first few times you get out of bed so you don't fall on the floor.

# Beefing up the epidural

If you already have an epidural in place and your doctors aren't in a mad rush to do your cesarean, your anesthesiologist may just give you a stronger dose of medication through the epidural. You don't have to sit up for this procedure because the catheter is already in place.

The disadvantage of this method is that it takes about ten minutes for you to get completely numb. The other disadvantage is that you must have a good epidural for this to work. If you have *hot spots* — areas where the epidural isn't working well — you may be better off with a spinal.

## Undergoing general anesthesia

General anesthesia puts you to sleep, so if you have it, you won't see your baby be born. Doctors prefer not to use general anesthesia for deliveries because it also puts the baby to sleep, and sleeping babies often don't breathe on their own right after delivery. Having general anesthesia is also more dangerous for you; maternal mortality increases with general anesthesia.

In some cases, general anesthesia is the best choice because it can be initiated very quickly. If your situation is critical and you don't have time to lose in getting your baby out, general anesthesia may be the best choice. If you have general anesthesia, here's what you can expect to happen:

- ✔ **You won't have anyone in the operating room with you.** Doctors allow support people in the OR for cesareans as support for you; in most cases, if you're asleep, no one else is allowed in.

- ✔ **You'll get medication through your IV that will put you to sleep.** Then the anesthesiologist will place a tube down your throat to breathe for you. During the procedure, you'll receive anesthesia gas through a mask, but you won't be aware of it.

- ✔ **When you wake up, you'll be in more pain than if you'd had regional anesthesia, which lasts for several hours after surgery.** You may have a medication pump that delivers constant doses of narcotics, which can make you sleepy.

- ✔ **You may have nausea and/or vomiting from the anesthetic.** Your doctor can give you medications to help combat these side effects.

Your baby can come into the recovery room with you as long as he's not having any problems. You need a support person there with you because you may be too sleepy or too uncomfortable to hold the baby without help.

General anesthesia is never a doctor's first choice for doing a cesarean. If you do get general, realize that it's for your safety or your baby's.

# Considering Your Options in the Surgical Room

If you know you're having a cesarean, you can plan in advance for all the possible contingencies and write them into your birth plan. But even if you're planning to have a vaginal birth, we recommend that you consider your options for a C-section ahead of time and include them in your birth plan, too — just in case.

## Bringing along your partner or doula

Hospital operating rooms aren't all that big, and much of the space is filled with people who are essential for the surgery, such as the anesthesiologist or anesthetist, your doctor, her assistant, the scrub nurse, the circulating nurse, and often a physician or nurse to take care of your baby after delivery.

Because of the tight quarters, you may be allowed to have only one person with you in the operating room for the actual surgery, though some hospitals allow your doula plus one more person. Right before you get wheeled into the room is no time to try and decide who's going with you, so think about this ahead of time and write in your birth plan who is going into the OR with you if you have a C-section.

Your partner probably seems like the most logical choice, but he may not be the best, depending on how he handles stress, blood (although he really won't see much), and the whole OR scene. When deciding whether your partner is OR material, consider the following questions:

- ✔ **Does he want to be there?** Some people really do have a fear of surgery, maybe from a bad tonsillectomy experience as a child or maybe from watching too many TV medical shows.

- ✔ **Will he be a help or a hindrance?** If you think he's going to make you more nervous or drive the doctors crazy, he may not be the best choice. Also, if you want to try breast-feeding on the operating table, consider whether your partner will be able to help you or whether someone else would be better for this task.

- ✔ **What's his cultural perspective?** Some cultures, even today, don't buy into the idea that Dad has to be at the delivery. Although he may have been willing to be there for your sake at a vaginal birth, being in the OR may be way out of his comfort zone.

> ✔ **Do you have an alternative?** For example, you may have a doula, or your mom may really want to accompany you into the OR. Of course, your mom could be a worse choice than your partner if she's the type to drive your doctor — and you — crazy. See why you need to make this choice ahead of time? You won't have the strength to argue effectively with your mom in the labor room.

Whomever you choose to accompany you into the OR will have a chair to sit on (because no one wants him falling down and disturbing the sterile field), and he'll be positioned close to your head so he can support you throughout the surgery.

## Lowering the curtain for delivery

Normally, doctors place a drape that blocks your view of the surgical field — a nice way to describe your pregnant belly! — during the actual surgery. They do this for two reasons:

✔ So you don't have to watch what's going on

✔ To keep the field sterile, reducing your chance of developing an infection after surgery

If you want to watch the birth, you can ask to have a portion of the drape lowered so you can see the baby being born, or you can ask to have the drape eliminated altogether (as long as you promise to keep your hands where they belong). Write your preference in your birth plan and ask about moving the drape as soon as you get into the OR.

## Seeing your baby right after the birth

Your chances of the hospital staff giving you your baby right after birth and leaving him in your arms for the duration of the surgery are slim. After all, assessing the baby right after birth is another part of the hospital's attempts to avoid lawsuits down the road — and, of course, you also want your baby checked out to make sure he's okay. A cesarean delivery is more stressful for your baby than a vaginal birth, and if he had fetal distress before birth, it's especially important to make sure he's doing fine now.

Even so, depending on why you're having a cesarean birth, you should be able to see your baby right after he's born — even if only briefly. Your doctor hands your baby off to the circulating nurse, who stays outside the sterile field during the surgery, and she hands the baby off to you.

This process isn't quite as easy as it sounds, though, because one of your arms has an IV in it and may be strapped to a board attached to the table. Your other arm may also be strapped down, although your anesthesiologist can undo it so that you can hold your baby. You can ask in your birth plan for one arm to be free for the baby. Otherwise, your support person will hold the baby next to you.

If your baby needs immediate care (besides just the routine post-birth assessment), the nurse probably won't take the baby out of the room; she'll just take her a few feet away, where the warming table and resuscitation table are located. Most of the time, your baby can come back to you as soon as he's stable. At that point, you can hold him, with your support person's help, and start nursing if you want to (see the next section).

If the circulating nurse takes care of the baby after delivery, keep in mind that she also has to answer the phone, get the scrub team whatever they need, get things ready to move you to recovery right after delivery, keep equipment functioning, and do the sponge count and needle count with the scrub nurse. She's happy to help you with the baby when she can, but your support person is the most important person in the room for helping you hold the baby and start nursing, if you want — a good reason to choose ahead of time whom to take into the OR with you.

## Nursing the baby on the operating table

In many cases, you can hold the baby skin to skin and start nursing right after the nurses complete their initial post-birth assessment, as long as you have your support person there to help. You can't sit up, so positioning the baby close enough to reach the nipple takes an extra set of hands. Have your support person hold the baby, face down, near the nipple. He needs to watch closely to make sure the baby can still breathe in this position.

Don't worry if you can't nurse your baby as soon as he's born. Not establishing nursing in the first few minutes after birth doesn't mean you're doomed to have an unsuccessful nursing experience. The majority of women who deliver in hospitals don't get to nurse immediately after birth and many still go on to nurse successfully. Babies are resilient and not having this experience doesn't equate with failure.

# Settling into Your Recovery Room

As long as your baby isn't having any problems, he'll likely get to go with you to the recovery room, which often isn't a room at all, but rather a portioned-off area in a larger room. You still have an IV and a cardiac monitor during this initial recovery time, but you can hold the baby and start breast-feeding, with help, if you want to.

One benefit of starting to nurse in the recovery room is that you'll still have some abdominal numbness. After the anesthesia starts to wear off, holding the baby near your incision becomes more uncomfortable, and you may need to try alternative positions, such as a side-lying position. You may need help the first few times to pull it all together. To nurse in a side position, follow these steps:

1. **Carefully roll to one side and put pillows behind your back for support.**

2. **Place a small pillow or blanket over your incision area to protect it from the baby's kicking.**

3. **Place your baby on his side so you're chest to chest and use one hand to steady him so he doesn't roll back.**

4. **Line up the baby's mouth with your nipple.**

You can usually have support people visit you in the recovery room, although you may prefer to take that time to rest and just enjoy your baby with your partner. Your nurse should be in the room with you most of the time, so take advantage of her expertise and ask any questions you have about your baby or the cesarean recovery process.

If you're breast-feeding, remind your nurse to let the maternity floor staff know that you don't want them to give your baby any supplemental bottles or water without discussing it with you first.

# Part V
# It's All About the Baby

The 5th Wave                    By Rich Tennant

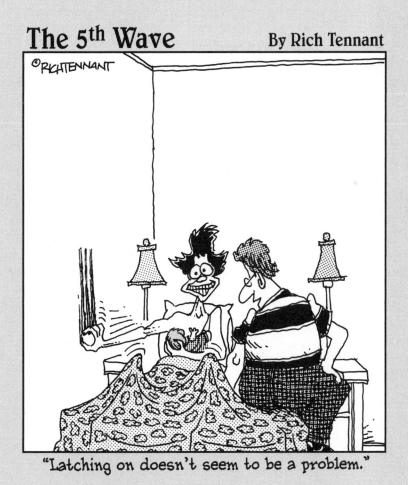

"Latching on doesn't seem to be a problem."

# In this part . . .

In this part, we talk about the most important part of the whole pregnancy process — your baby! From how to initiate bonding to what to feed your baby, these chapters guide you through the first few days of parenthood. Knowing what to expect when you meet your long-anticipated arrival will help you through the hormone-ridden days after delivery. We also help you create a birth plan that will ensure that your baby's first few days of life are all that you want them to be, from feeding preferences to where your baby sleeps.

# Chapter 15

# Welcoming Your Baby
# to the World

· · · · · · · · · · · · · · · · · · · · · · · · · · · · · · · · · · · · · · · · · · · · · · · · · · · · · · · · · · · · · · · · · · · ·

· · · · · · · · · · · · · · · · · · · · · · · · · · · · · · · · · · · · · · · · · · · · · · · · · · · · · · · · · · · · · · · · · · · ·

**N**othing in the world can match your first look at your new baby. Here she is — a little person that you're going to know for the rest of your life. She's part of you and, at the same time, completely her own person. It's enough to bring tears to your eyes — and often, to everyone else's eyes too, no matter how many deliveries they've seen.

In this chapter, we explain the wonders of the moments of birth and help you decide how best to hold and cherish them in your heart and memory forever. Because when your child is a teenager, you're going to need these wondrous moments to look back on — we guarantee it. We guide you through the decisions involving final delivery that you'll want to consider in advance, because you're not likely to be able to think about anything besides your baby when she's actually being born. We also let you know what to expect in the first minutes after delivery. Go ahead and put your thoughts and wishes for a perfect birth in your birth plan so that when the time comes, you can feel free to wax sentimental over every moment.

## Birthing Your Baby Your Way

This is your baby and your birth, so have it your way. Easier said than done, sometimes. By the time you get to the actual birth, you may be tired, hot, irritable, hungry, and sick of your entire birthing team, including the person responsible for putting you in this position. Yes, you'll probably say it at least once.

Even so, the actual moment of the birth of your baby is likely be one of the most exciting moments of your life. The decision to watch that moment in a mirror, capture it on film, or just experience it in a serene environment is up to you, so we help you think through your options in this section.

## Keeping things quiet

To a certain extent, the members of your birth team determine how noisy your birth is. You're not usually the one making all the cheering and yelling noises, although you may be doing your fair share of grunting and groaning. But the actual chatter, attagirls, and general hubbub in the birthing room usually comes from other people, not you. Talk to your medical practitioner, support people, and nursing staff if you'd like your baby to emerge into a quiet and calm world — even if she will immediately shatter the quiet with a piercing wail. If you want a quiet birth atmosphere, include the following points in your birth plan:

- ✔ **How much cheerleading you want going on:** Coauthor Sharon has been at deliveries that sounded more like the final moments of a close Super Bowl game than the birth of a new person. The yelling and encouragement may be just what you need to keep going in the final moments of childbirth, but if they're not, say so.

- ✔ **Who announces the sex of the baby, if you don't know it already:** If you don't want your nurse yelling, "It's a girl!" before your partner gets to say a word, make that request clear.

- ✔ **If you want a certain song playing during the delivery:** Sharon remembers one OB who played a well-known classical piece during every delivery, but you don't have to abide by your OB's music choices.

Some religious groups, such as Scientologists, practice silent birth, a technique that discourages all noise in the delivery room at the time of birth. No studies have proven the benefit of this method, but if it's your choice, make sure you include it in your birth plan and remind the nursing staff and your doctor about the request.

## Dimming the lights

A few decades ago, birthing in a dimly lit room was all the rage, and it still may appeal to you for the following reasons:

- ✔ **A dimly lit room seems to bring the noise level down a notch and facilitate a quiet, calm atmosphere.**

> ✔ **Your baby is more likely to open her eyes right away if she isn't blinded by the light.** Remember, she's been living in a fairly dark environment for nine months, and even a dimly lit room will seem quite bright to her.

If having the room dimmed for the delivery is important to you, note it in your birth plan. If you're delivering in a hospital, be sure to also talk over the possibility of dimming the lights with your doctor. He can shine a light down on the parts he needs to see most, and most delivery rooms have several sets of lights, so you should be able to work out with the doctor how you can dim most of the room but still allow him to see where needed. If any type of emergency arises, of course, you can expect the lights to be flipped on so everyone can clearly see what they're doing.

If you're birthing at home or in a birthing room, you can generally have the lighting any way you'd like it. When you're arranging a birthing area at home, consider whether the natural and artificial light is to your liking. You can find soft lighting that works for illumination but isn't too harsh. Dimmer switches allow you to put the lighting at exactly the level you'd like.

## Watching the birth

You may or may not want to watch the birth of your baby in the mirror (or simply by looking down, if you're sitting up enough). Managing to see your baby arrive with your own eyes is often rather difficult. If you're giving birth in the hospital, the staff will try to position a mirror so you can see well, but then your medical provider will plop himself down on a stool between your legs and ruin the view. Depending on how flat you're lying — hopefully not completely flat! — you may have a hard time seeing around your stomach to watch the birth.

The other difficult part about watching your baby emerge is that you're often pushing at the time, and when you push, you may involuntarily close your eyes or scrunch them up. Fortunately, many practitioners don't want you to push at the moment of delivery, because they want to control the baby's exit to minimize tearing and, of course, to avoid having the baby shoot out like a torpedo. Seeing is easier if you're panting rather than pushing.

If you want to watch the baby's actual birth, address the following points in your birth plan:

> ✔ **Your desire for the mirror to be placed where you can actually see into it:** Most hospitals have moveable mirrors; if yours doesn't, ask if you can bring one in. Some hospitals have an overhead mirror, which makes seeing easier. If there's no mirror, bring a mirror that your partner can hold so you can see.

✔ **Your desire to not lie flat on your back during the delivery:** This position ensures that you won't be able to see anything and also decreases the blood supply to your baby. Note in your birth plan that you want to sit in a semi-upright position or squat during the birth so that you can view a mirror. (Of course, you may change your mind about what feels comfortable when you're actually delivering your baby. Check out Chapter 9 to read up on all your position options.)

## Taking pictures

Most hospital staff today understand that many delivering mothers and their partners want to have photographs and video of the baby's birth. Some nurses and doctors may request that they not appear in any pictures, which is their right. Your doctor may also request that you not photograph certain parts of the delivery. Although the reasons for his request may not be clear — after all, he isn't the one revealing private parts of his anatomy in living color — you have to bow to his wishes.

Normally, you can film just about any part of the birth you feel comfortable showing. If you deliver outside the hospital, you can drag in an entire video crew if you want. To ensure that you get the best pictures of the first moments of your baby's life, plan ahead by taking care of the following preparations:

✔ **Appointing a photographer:** Although all your support people will likely have their cameras and phones ready to snap pictures, you want good pictures, not just any pictures. Choose the best photographer out of the group and loan her your best camera. Show her how to work the video camera ahead of time; you won't feel like explaining it to her when the baby's coming out.

✔ **Discussing what shots you want:** If you want to avoid crotch shots, make that very clear. If having your practitioner in the pictures is a must, make that clear too. You may want to ask your photographer to err on the side of more pictures. You can always delete certain pictures if they're more graphic than you expected, but you can't go back and get those shots later.

✔ **Considering someone other than the dad as the photographer:** Even if he's the best photographer, you may prefer to have him in the pictures rather than behind the lens. Although dads often relish this task because it gives them something to do, explain you'd rather spend your first few minutes as a family together, with someone else taking your pictures.

✔ **Scoping out the setting:** Before labor gets too intense, look around and assess the lighting and the angles you have to work with and give your photographer some suggestions. If you take the world's worst pictures and don't know a lens from a compact mirror, assign the task to someone else and let him wander around looking for ways to best capture the moment. You could also consider hiring a professional birth photographer.

# Catching the Baby

Babies generally exit the birth canal without much help, but in some cases, your medical practitioner will have to guide the baby out by either giving a little tug to facilitate delivery of the shoulders or by slowing down her exit if she's coming out too fast. In either case, if you're using a doctor for your birth, he may not want to share the birthing tasks with your support person, just in case anything goes wrong.

## Can Dad catch?

If Dad really wants to help deliver the baby, talk to your medical practitioner — and have your partner talk to him, too. Midwives are more likely to allow this assistance. Your medical doctor may say no, mainly for liability reasons, although he may veto your plan for any of the following reasons:

- ✔ **Sometimes babies come out too fast and need a controlled delivery.** Your doctor knows how to control the situation without hurting the baby; your partner doesn't.

- ✔ **Some babies, especially large babies, don't come out without some guidance.** Again, your doctor knows how to help without hurting the baby; your partner doesn't.

- ✔ **Some dads think they want to help deliver the baby right up until the moment they pass out into the placenta bucket at the doctor's feet.** No one has time to take care of Dad at the moment of birth.

- ✔ **Emergencies can arise very quickly at the time of delivery.** Although emergency situations are rare, you want someone in place who knows how to deal with a cord wrapped around the baby's neck, a sudden hemorrhage, or other last-minute crisis.

However, if you really want Dad to participate, he can help your medical practitioner guide the baby out by placing his hands on the baby. Not all practitioners will agree to this, so ask ahead of time.

## Helping deliver your own baby

If you'd like to, you can reach down and help bring out your own baby. Because you can't really reach your own vagina very well during birth, you would be assisting or putting hands on the baby as she emerges rather than actually delivering her. Because you won't interfere with his job, your medical practitioner may be open to this idea. Midwives are very likely to agree to it.

To help deliver your baby requires the following things:

- ✔ **Proper positioning:** You need to be in a semi-sitting position. If you're lying down, you can't reach your vagina over your stomach, because the baby is still be in there. If you're giving birth in a birthing pool or squatting, reaching down for the baby is much easier.

- ✔ **Concentration on your part:** When the actual moment of delivery comes, your attention may be focused on your medical practitioner's directions on whether or not to push, the burning sensation in your vagina, or the feeling that you're about to have a massive bowel movement rather than where to put your hands.

- ✔ **A willing practitioner:** Your doctor or midwife will need to help place your hands; you don't want to poke your baby in the face trying to get your hands around her.

- ✔ **A controlled delivery:** Some babies come out very quickly without time for much direction or guidance.

If you'd like to help guide your little one into the world, talk to your practitioner and your delivery-room nurse about the logistics beforehand and write your wishes in your birth plan.

# Cutting the Cord

Having dad or another support person cut the umbilical cord after the birth has become a time-honored tradition in the hospital. You can also do it yourself. Because you really can't hurt anything as long as you cut exactly where your practitioner tells you to, most doctors are quite willing to let you or a designated person do the honors.

## Cutting correctly

Who gets to cut the cord is one of the issues that your birth plan should definitely discuss. Most medical practitioners have no problem with this, as long as they know you want to do it or have someone else do it.

To prepare the umbilical cord for cutting, your medical practitioner will place two clamps on the cord. The nurse or practitioner will hand you or your designated person scissors, and you cut between the clamps, which prevent blood loss from you or your baby if the blood hasn't clotted off in the cord yet. The cord is tougher than you may think, and some are thicker than others, so cutting through it takes a little effort.

As long as you cut between the two clamps, you can't possibly do any harm, so don't worry. You may see a spurt of blood, but it isn't coming from you or the baby; it's just blood trapped in the cord.

# Delaying cord cutting

In the hospital, where time is often at a premium, your practitioner may clamp the cord immediately and cut it so the nurse can take the baby to the warming table and assess and weigh him immediately. But if you want to hold the baby skin-to-skin or start nursing right after giving birth, you can ask your practitioner to delay cord clamping and cutting until the cord stops pulsating so that your baby gets a little extra blood volume. The cord generally stops pulsating within one to five minutes after birth.

Many doctors just clamp and cut the umbilical cord immediately after birth, which is probably what they were taught to do in medical school. However, delayed cord cutting has the following benefits:

- **A little extra blood and higher iron levels for the baby:** Extra red blood cells increase iron stores, which can help prevent *anemia,* or low iron levels.

- **Possible boosting of the immune system and other health benefits:** Some researchers think that the delayed cutting of the cord and transfer of stem cells and T cells in cord blood may help protect the baby against respiratory illness, brain hemorrhages, and other problems in infancy.

On the other hand, not everyone thinks delayed cord cutting is beneficial. The World Health Organization lists the following possible risks of delayed cord cutting:

- **Polycythemia, a condition caused by an excess of red blood cells, can cause lethargy, seizures, tremors, stroke, apnea, and respiratory distress:** Delayed cord clamping can increase the risk of your newborn developing polycythemia or it worsening if she's born with the condition. However, it's unlikely to occur unless your baby has an underlying risk of polycythemia.

- **Jaundice from an increased red blood cell count:** In several studies, delayed cord clamping led to a significantly higher percentage of infants needing phototherapy to resolve neonatal jaundice.

Most babies who don't have their cord cut immediately do fine. But so do most babies who do. Talk to your practitioner about the possibility of delaying cord cutting and its pros and cons and then decide if you want to put it in your birth plan. If you do, remind your practitioner, who is very likely to clamp the cord immediately out of habit. After the cord is clamped, the blood clots, and unclamping doesn't restart the blood flow.

# Saving the cord for cord banking

Many parents these days save their baby's cord blood in case she needs the stems cells from it later in life. Although cord-blood stem cells have limited application — they don't cure all types of cancer or disease and can't do anything for a broken leg — they may have some benefit if your baby develops certain childhood cancers or diseases characterized by immune problems or bone-marrow disorders. Cord blood can also be used for a sibling or other family member, in some cases.

Cord blood can be saved indefinitely, at least in theory, in a cryogenically frozen state. However, to save your baby's, you need to plan ahead and act fast after the delivery. Cord blood must be removed from the cord within 15 minutes after delivery and processed within 48 hours after delivery. Take these steps if you want to arrange cord-blood banking:

1. **Talk to your practitioner about saving cord blood and write your wishes in your birth plan.**

2. **Choose a storage facility accredited by the American Association of Blood Banks to store the cord blood.** The company will send you a kit to be used to collect the cord blood at the time of delivery. Your doctor or nurse will collect the blood sample. A courier will come to the hospital to pick up the cord blood.

3. **Pay the storage fees.** Initial freezing fees can run from $1,000 to $2,000 and around $100 per year after that. The collection kit and courier service can also run a few hundred dollars.

There is no risk of contamination or transfer of any diseases to either of you because blood is drawn directly from the cord. Cost is the only drawback to cord-blood storage, unless you are planning to ask your practitioner to delay cord clamping. Because cord blood clots fairly quickly, you can't do both cord-blood banking and delayed cord cutting.

If you don't want to store your baby's blood, consider donating it to a cord-blood donation site. Donating is free, but the donation remains anonymous, so you won't be able to retrieve your baby's sample at a later date if she becomes ill. Contact the American Red Cross or check the National Marrow Donor Program's list of registered cord-blood facilities to find one near you.

You can have cord blood saved during a vaginal delivery or cesarean section. However, often less blood is saved during a cesarean delivery because the staff is busy doing other things after the baby is out and cord-blood collection is delayed.

# Give Me That Baby!

Making the baby's mom wait in line to hold her baby after she's born seems ridiculous. Unfortunately, in many hospitals, that's exactly what happens. Your baby emerges and is handed off to a nurse, hurried over to a warmer, and then given to Dad, Grandma, or another support person to hold before you get your hands on her. This scenario doesn't seem right to us, and it doesn't have to be that way for you.

If you give birth in the hospital, especially if you have a C-section, you may have to fight for first dibs, but unless your baby is having health problems, the doctor shouldn't have any valid reason why you can't hold her before anyone else does.

## Getting to hold the baby first

Talk to your practitioner about delaying the immediate baby care such as weighing, cleaning off, and giving eye drops until after you've had a chance to hold and nurse the baby. Studies have shown that an unmedicated, healthy newborn left to her own devices will crawl up her mom's chest and start nursing. Skin-to-skin, mother-baby interaction is obviously nature's intention, and hospitals break up mom and baby right after birth strictly for convenience of the hospital staff.

The initial assessment of the baby's skin color, breathing, muscle tone, reflex irritability, and heart rate can be done by a staff member at the bedside (see the next section). A baby who has breathing problems, has poor muscle tone, or is turning blue is usually quite evident. To get to know your baby from the moment of birth, we recommend the following tips:

- ✔ **Make skin-to-skin contact with her.** It allows her to hear your heartbeat, a sound she's familiar with. Your rhythmic breathing will also help her breathe more easily and rhythmically. Skin-to-skin contact also helps with temperature stabilization.

- ✔ **Have the staff cover you and the baby with a blanket from the warmer, because you will probably shiver after the delivery.** Most women shiver, and it can be uncomfortable and distracting. Your body heat helps warm the baby, though. Dry the baby gently, because fluid on her skin will evaporate, which can lower her body temperature.

- ✔ **Talk softly to the baby and gently stroke her skin.** Encourage everyone to keep their voices low so as not to startle the baby.

- ✔ **If you're allowing antibiotic eye drops to be used, ask the staff to wait until you've had a few minutes to let the baby look at you without ointment in her eyes.**

If you're having a cesarean, holding the baby is more difficult because your doctor will still be performing an operation on your abdomen, but it can be done. Check Chapter 14 for the details.

## Conducting initial exams while holding the baby

Most assessments don't require much more than looking at the baby. However, staff members may also need to take the baby's temperature and listen to her heart rate. Ask that they warm the stethoscope with their hands before placing it on the baby's chest. Taking the temperature is tricky if the staff wants to do a rectal temperature, which is the most accurate reading. Ask if they can wait a few minutes before getting the baby's temperature.

Bracelets with the baby's vital information need to go on your wrist and on the baby's ankle before the two of you travel to another room, but attaching the bracelets shouldn't be too disruptive. If your baby needs warming, your skin is an excellent warming agent, but expect the staff to prefer putting the baby under a warmer. Talk to your doctor or your chosen pediatrician about this possibility ahead of time and write your wishes to keep the baby skin-to-skin unless there's a pressing medical reason for removing her.

If your baby needs to be checked out by the pediatrician, he can usually carry out his examination while you hold the baby. An added advantage is that you can ask questions as he goes along.

## Breast-feeding for the first time

Unless your baby is sick, you can breast-feed right after delivery — if not immediately after giving birth, then within a few minutes. Although the first breast-feeding is important for you and the baby, don't feel bad if things don't go very well with the first nursing. Think of it as a practice session and a way for the two of you to establish yourself as mother and child.

Many things can make the first nursing difficult, including the following:

✔ **Getting stitches:** If you tore or had an episiotomy, your doctor will take time to place stitches. This procedure can pull or hurt, distracting you from nursing. And if your legs are in stirrups while your doctor sews, you may not be comfortable enough — or agile enough — to situate yourself or your baby the way you'd like to.

✔ **Shivering:** New moms, especially those who have had epidurals, often have violent shivering after delivery. The warm blanket will help but may not completely eliminate the physiological response to the physical and hormonal changes after giving birth.

> ✔ **A disinterested baby:** Babies aren't hungry right after being born, because they were still getting fed right up until the time of delivery. And medications, including epidurals, can make the baby somewhat lethargic and not very interested in nursing.

You have a better chance of things going well with breast-feeding if your hospital supports breast-feeding by following the guidelines of the 1991 Baby-Friendly Hospital Initiative introduced by UNICEF and WHO, two organizations heavily invested in the health of moms and infants. These guidelines recommend initiating breast-feeding within 30 minutes of birth, training staff to help new breast-feeding moms, and not offering formula or pacifiers to a newborn if you're establishing breast-feeding. Visit `www.babyfriendlyusa.org` to learn more about this initiative and consult a map marking Baby-Friendly hospitals around the United States.

Don't have a Baby-Friendly hospital in your area? There are still many things you can do to successfully breast-feed. Best for Babes (`www.bestforbabes.org`) is an excellent resource for beating breast-feeding roadblocks. See Chapter 17 for tips on establishing breast-feeding in the first hours and days after giving birth.

# Cleaning Up

Both you and the baby will need to be cleaned up after delivery. You will actually need cleaning up before she does, because you'll have amniotic fluid, blood, and often stool on your nether regions. Your nurse won't leave you in a mess, though; your cleanup will come shortly after you give birth.

## Washing you up

You won't be heading off to the showers right away after delivery, because you may be shaky and prone to falling. Blood loss has made many a new mom faint on the bathroom floor, so a staff member will accompany you to the bathroom if you deliver in the hospital.

Before you get up, your nurse will probably wash you off and put what feels like a gigantic diaper on you, often held in place by one-size-fits-all mesh underwear. Don't disdain these unattractive garments; when they get bloody (and they will), you can simply throw them in the trash or wash them out easily in the sink.

The fresh hospital gown you'll get is also a convenience, even if it's not the height of fashion. It's easy to remove, and better yet, because it's open in the back, doesn't get all bloody if you experience a gush now and then (which you probably will). If you really want to wear your own nightclothes, bring them with you to the hospital but save them for the day after delivery, when you won't be bleeding as heavily and your IV will be out. Nursing gowns that you bring from home aren't much more chic than hospital gowns, but the openings in the front are more practical.

The pièce de résistance of your new outfit will be the ice pack, sometimes made from a glove filled with ice chips wrapped in a soft towel. It helps keep the swelling from your stitches or tears down. You'll come to cherish your ice pack. Make sure to let your nurse know if you have a latex allergy so she can use non-latex gloves, which many hospitals now use exclusively due to the rise in latex allergies.

If you've had an epidural, urinating for the first time can be very difficult. Hearing the sound of running water or pouring warm water over your perineum can help get you flowing. Going with someone else in the room can be hard, but your nurse probably won't leave you in the bathroom alone no matter how much you beg; it's too much of a liability if you hit the floor.

If you've had a cesarean, you'll get the same cleanup treatment, although you may not be able to feel it or be able to help much by moving your legs. Your Foley catheter will probably remain in overnight or for a few hours after delivery so you don't have to get out of bed to use the bathroom.

## Cleaning up the baby

Your birth plan requests don't have to stop with the birth of the baby. You may have preferences about the baby's care after birth, particularly her first bath. The white coating called *vernix* that covers the baby absorbs into the skin and protects it, so you may not want the staff to wash it off in the first bath. Gently massage the baby's skin to rub it in.

The baby's hair may be coated with amniotic fluid, blood, or worse after birth. If you want to give the baby her first real bath, ask the staff if they can just wash off her hair rather than giving her a full bath without you. Or wash her head gently with a soft, warm cloth and dry it thoroughly. A baby's head makes up a large proportion of her total body surface area, so she loses more heat from the top of her head than an adult would.

# Chapter 16

# Making Decisions about Shots, Drops, Snips, and Newborn Tests

*A*s soon as your baby's born, you become his chief protector and decision maker for the next 18 years, and that job requires quite a few big decisions in the first few days of life. We recommend that you make many of these decisions during pregnancy when you can research them and give full weight to the pros and cons of each option. To help you get started, we dedicate this chapter to looking at the practical decisions you'll need to make — and spell out in your birth plan — before you leave the hospital. They're not as much fun as picking out a name, but their consequences can be just as long lasting and important.

## Preventing Infection with Antibiotic Eye Drops

One of the first decisions you have to make after your baby's birth is whether you want to put antibiotic eye drops in his eyes. Because you're going to have a lot on your mind at that point, think through this decision beforehand and make sure to clearly write your preference in your birth plan.

What are the eye drops for? Many hospitals routinely give antibiotic eye drops to babies to protect them against vaginal infections such as gonorrhea or chlamydia, a leading cause of blindness in some undeveloped countries.

(You can have gonorrhea without any noticeable symptoms 20 percent of the time, and 70 percent of women with chlamydia, the most common sexually transmitted disease in the U.S., have no symptoms.)

Years ago, hospitals used drops made of silver nitrate, which often caused severe eye irritation. Nearly all babies looked Asian because their eyes closed to mere slits for several days after they got the drops. Today, the drops contain erythromycin or tetracycline, antibiotics that cause much less eye irritation and swelling. But they can still cause a chemical conjunctivitis, with redness and swelling that lasts 24 to 36 hours, in some cases.

Some parents — and you may well be one of them — object to having their babies receive the drops. Their reasoning goes like this: If you know you don't have a vaginal infection, why subject your baby to an invasive procedure minutes after birth? If you want to opt out of eye drops for your baby, you may want to be tested for chlamydia and gonorrhea before delivery.

If you deliver in a hospital, you may have to sign a medical waiver, refusing to authorize eye drops for your newborn. Most hospital staff administer the drops so routinely that you'll probably have to remind your nurse several times, including before she takes your baby to the warmer to be weighed and checked out.

# Debating Vitamin K Injections

In 1961, medical providers in the U.S. began giving all newborns born in hospitals an injection of vitamin K shortly after birth to help with blood clotting. But because only 0.2 to 1.7 percent of newborns have trouble with blood clotting after they're born (a disorder known as *vitamin K deficiency syndrome* or *classic hemorrhagic disease of the newborn*), you may decide you don't want your child to receive this injection. The choice is up to you.

Symptoms of vitamin K deficiency syndrome include severe bleeding from lack of clotting factors in the first week of life, but a late-appearing form of the disease can occur between the ages of 2 weeks and 12 weeks. Baby formula contains added vitamin K, so this disorder mostly affects newborns who breast-feed exclusively.

The injectable form of vitamin K can also be given in oral form, which is an option you may want to consider if your main concern is the pain your baby will experience during the injection. The drawback of the oral form is that you have to give it to your baby for a total of 13 weeks and it's not always effective.

If you don't want your hospital-born baby to receive vitamin K, write it in your birth plan, but be aware that you'll probably need to sign a waiver and remind your nurse about your decision in the hospital.

If you choose a pediatrician before your baby is born, talk to her before your baby's birth about the pros and cons of the vitamin K injection.

# Considering Hepatitis B Immunization

Immunizations are another major hot-potato topic among new parents in the U.S. Although the American Academy of Pediatrics states that immunizations aren't linked to autism or any other disorder, some parents remain suspicious. Some parents don't think the benefits of vaccinations outweigh the risks. Other parents want their babies to receive immunizations but prefer to delay the shots until their kids are older.

The only immunization you're likely to have to make a decision about in the hospital is one that protects against *hepatitis B,* a viral infection that attacks the liver. The infection can be transmitted through blood or bodily fluids, so if you have hepatitis B, the baby could pick it up during pregnancy. For many parents, however, giving a hepatitis B injection to a baby when you know that you don't have hepatitis B is overkill.

The Centers for Disease Control and Prevention (better known as the CDC) recommends that all newborns receive the hepatitis B vaccination, which is just the first in a series required for full protection from the infection, for the following reasons:

✔ It protects infants whose mothers carry the virus but haven't yet shown a positive result, which can take several months.

✔ It protects infants against contracting the virus from other carriers through exposure to blood or other body fluids.

✔ Infants who receive the first vaccination in the hospital are more likely to get the rest of the vaccinations in the series for full protection.

✔ The rate of new hepatitis B infections in children has dropped since the introduction of the vaccine for newborns and infants.

✔ Children who contract hepatitis B before they're 12 months old have a higher risk of developing a chronic infection and resulting health problems, including liver failure, during their lifetime.

If you don't want your newborn to receive this vaccine, you'll need to sign a waiver if your baby is born in the hospital. Also don't forget to note it in your birth plan.

# Circumcision Decision

One of the biggest decisions you have to make if you have a baby boy is whether or not to have him *circumcised,* which refers to having the foreskin of the penis removed (see Figure 16-1). This procedure is irreversible, so don't rush to make the decision. Although many babies are circumcised before they leave the hospital, you can have this procedure done at a later date.

Circumcision has both religious and cultural significance. If you're Jewish or Muslim, your baby boy will likely be circumcised, although the procedure often occurs in a religious ceremony rather than in the hospital.

Circumcision has fallen out of favor as a cultural mandate in the U.S. Although nearly all baby boys born in the U.S. were circumcised in 1960, only about 54 percent are circumcised today.

We cover the pros and cons of circumcision in the following sections. Whatever you decide, make sure you include this decision in your birth plan.

**Figure 16-1:** The difference between a circumcised penis (a) and an uncircumcised penis (b).

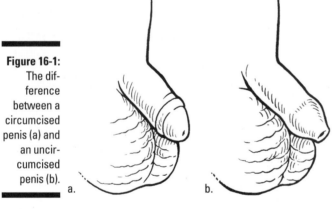

a.          b.

*Illustration by Kathryn Born*

## Choosing circumcision

Consider the following points when deciding whether or not to have your son circumcised:

- ✔ Circumcised men have a lower incidence of cancer of the penis, although penile cancer is very rare in any case.
- ✔ Women with circumcised partners have a lower risk of cervical cancer.
- ✔ Circumcision can reduce the incidence of urinary tract infection in boys, but the incidence of urinary tract infection in boys is low; 1 percent or less.

✔ Circumcision later in life is an extremely uncomfortable procedure.

✔ Circumcision makes cleaning the penis easier to do. If you don't have your baby boy circumcised, you may have to gently push the foreskin back so it doesn't adhere to the tip of the penis, although this often isn't necessary.

✔ Dads who are circumcised may want their sons to look like them.

## Deciding not to cut

Be sure to consider the following reasons for not having your baby boy circumcised, as well:

✔ Circumcision is a surgical procedure with few proven benefits.

✔ The difference between circumcised and uncircumcised men's risk of cancer and other health problems is slim.

✔ The procedure causes pain; local anesthesia is generally given today.

✔ The foreskin protects the head of the penis, and removing it can cause some degree of desensitization.

✔ Complications — usually minor bleeding or infection — occur in between 0.5 and 3 percent of circumcisions. More serious long-term complications can occur, but they're rare.

## Settling some details

Even if you've decided you want your son to be circumcised, you may not want to have the procedure done in the hospital right after birth. You can wait until your baby is a few weeks old to make sure he doesn't have any bleeding problems before you have his foreskin cut off. Or you may want to plan a religious ceremony for the procedure. Then again, you can just take a few more weeks to think about it if you still haven't made up your mind by the time you go home. Because circumcision is a permanent surgical alteration, you can't go back and change your mind later. Take your time if you need it.

# Understanding Newborn Testing

All parents-to-be have fleeting moments during pregnancy when they fear that something might be wrong with their baby. Because you can minimize some problems by effectively treating them right after birth, mandatory blood testing for certain genetic disorders is part of many hospital routines.

Different states have different regulations about what genetic disorders hospitals must test for, but some test for as many as 30 genetic disorders in one blood test called the *tandem mass spectrometry*.

## PK who? Deciding on PKU testing

*Phenylketonuria* (often called *PKU*) is a genetic disease that affects about 1 in 25,000 infants in the U.S. Babies with this disorder inherit the gene from each of their parents. You can carry a recessive gene for PKU without knowing it because carriers have no symptoms. Although it occurs most commonly in people of Northern European and Native American ancestry, people of any race can have PKU.

A baby with this disorder lacks *phenylalanine hydroxylase*(PAH), an enzyme that breaks down *phenylalanine,* a part of protein found in most foods. As a result, phenylalanine builds up in the baby's bloodstream over time, affecting mental development, including intelligence and behavior.

Babies with PKU appear perfectly normal at birth, but they begin to develop symptoms by the time they reach 3 to 6 months. Symptoms include lack of interest in their surroundings, irritability, and developmental delays, and most children with this disorder have lighter hair than their siblings. A special diet that includes no milk, including breast milk, in infancy can help prevent symptoms.

To test for PKU, a nurse takes blood from your baby's heel. If the test is done before your baby is 24 hours old, your doctor may suggest doing a second test at 1 to 2 weeks of age.

All states require PKU testing on newborns. If you want to opt out of testing for any reason, you have to sign a religious waiver. Discuss your reasons for refusing the test with your medical provider before doing so, though.

## Other commonly tested genetic disorders

Although PKU is the genetic disease most commonly tested for, hospitals often add other genetic testing to the tandem mass spectrometry. Tests that your state requires as part of genetic blood testing for newborns may include

 ✔ **Congenital adrenal hyperplasia:** Babies with this inherited disease don't make enough of the hormone cortisol. The disorder affects the baby's ability to maintain blood pressure, blood glucose levels, and energy levels and his ability to deal with physiological stress. About 1 in 15,000 babies inherits it, and most states do routine screening.

✔ **Congenital hypothyroidism:** This disorder is the most common one detected in newborn screening tests; about 1 in 4,000 babies has this disorder at birth. It can cause growth retardation and developmental delays. Giving the baby thyroid hormone prevents the complications of this disorder. All states require this testing for newborns.

✔ **Galactosemia:** This genetic disorder affects 1 in 60,000 to 80,000 newborns. These babies lack an enzyme that breaks down *galactose,* a milk sugar, into glucose. As a result, galactose accumulates in the body, causing organ damage, blindness, severe developmental delays, growth retardation, and even death in some cases. All states test newborns for this disease.

✔ **Medium chain acyl-CoA dehydrogenase deficiency:** This disorder can cause sudden death in infancy and severe developmental delays in survivors. About 1 in 20,000 babies inherits this disease. At least eight states tests for this disorder.

✔ **Sickle cell disease:** Sickle cell disease affects the red blood cells. Babies who have the disease have some abnormally shaped red blood cells that don't carry oxygen as well as normally shaped cells. The abnormal cells can accumulate in the kidneys and lungs, damaging the organs. Although African Americans have the highest incidence of the disease (1 in 500 babies are affected), Hispanics, Asians, and people of Mediterranean descent can also inherit this disease. Most but not all states mandate sickle cell testing.

Nearly all states also test newborns for hearing loss, which affects 3 to 4 out of 1,000 babies. Hearing tests are noninvasive, though, and they don't require drawing blood. You can request that the hearing test be done in your room in your birth plan.

## Sugar blues: Testing for glucose

You may wonder why your baby, who hasn't lived long enough to develop a sweet tooth, would need his blood sugar tested. Surprisingly enough, babies can have trouble regulating their blood sugar levels and can have levels that fall suddenly, causing *hypoglycemia,* or low blood *glucose* (another name for blood sugar). Symptoms of hypoglycemia include tremors, shrill cries, irritability, poor feeding, trouble breathing, or in severe cases, seizures.

If your baby has conditions related to blood-sugar regulation and starts to develop symptoms, the medical staff may want to test his blood glucose levels, which they can do in several ways. A blood sample can be obtained through a heel stick or be drawn from a vein, and then it's tested by using a glucometer or by sending it to the lab for verification. If your baby's blood sugar levels are low, your doctor may suggest giving him sugar water or formula to raise his levels quickly. If you're trying to establish breast-feeding, you may not want to give your baby either of these solutions without getting a thorough explanation of why it's necessary and what your alternatives are. There's no reason not to breast-feed to bring your baby's glucose levels up. Be sure to cover this issue in your birth plan.

Several conditions increase your baby's risk of having problems regulating his blood sugar, including the following:

- ✔ **Infection:** Babies who have an infection often have difficulty keeping their blood sugar within normal levels.

- ✔ **Cold stress:** Keeping your baby warm and dry, either wrapped or skin-to-skin, helps prevent cold stress from lowering glucose levels.

- ✔ **Maternal diabetes:** If you have diabetes or develop gestational diabetes in pregnancy, your baby may also have a higher-than-normal blood sugar. That's why diabetic moms sometimes have very large, or *macrosomic,* babies. After birth, your baby no longer has access to your high sugar stores, so his blood sugar plummets.

- ✔ **Prematurity:** Premature babies often have difficulty regulating their blood sugar levels.

- ✔ **Small size:** Like very large babies, very small babies can also have trouble maintaining their blood sugar.

- ✔ **Genetic disorders:** Babies who have genetic disorders may have difficulty regulating blood sugars (see the previous sections for details on genetic disorders).

- ✔ **Drugs to stop early labor:** If you were given drugs to try to stop premature labor, your baby may be at increased risk for hypoglycemia.

Nursing your baby often is the best way to prevent hypoglycemia, but if you're breast-feeding, your milk supply may not be well established yet. In this case, you should nurse more frequently. The more you nurse, the more milk you produce. For bottle-fed babies, giving them sterile water containing glucose or formula is the fastest way to raise their blood sugar.

In some hospitals, large babies automatically have their blood sugar levels tested after birth. Ask your doctor about the hospital's policy and write in your birth plan that you want hospital personnel to discuss routine testing and supplementation with you before doing any testing or giving your baby any supplements.

# Chapter 17

# Nourishing Your Baby

. . . . . . . . . . . . . . . . . . . . . . . . . . . . . . . . . . . . . . . . . . . . . . . .

## In This Chapter

▶ Understanding the benefits of breast-feeding for you and your baby

▶ Increasing your chances for breast-feeding success

▶ Pumping breast milk

▶ Bottle-feeding your baby

▶ Deciding to bottle-feed and breast-feed

. . . . . . . . . . . . . . . . . . . . . . . . . . . . . . . . . . . . . . . . . . . . . . . .

*D*eciding how to nourish your baby is one of the most socially charged issues related to childbirth and newborn care in the U.S. and other developed countries. Everyone from your sister to complete strangers on the street will offer you their opinion on how you should feed your baby.

In the end, however, the decision of how you nourish your baby is yours to make. Although breast-feeding has numerous benefits for you and your baby, it isn't right or possible for everyone. Even if you're completely dedicated to the idea of breast-feeding, it may not come easily because of medical issues, hospital policies, or misinformation from family and friends. Fortunately, your birth plan can help you address some of the possible roadblocks you may face when establishing breast-feeding if you choose to go that route.

In this chapter, we look at what benefits breast-feeding offers, how you can increase your chances for success, and how to get help if you need it. We also discuss why some women may need to pump breast milk and why some may not be able to breast-feed at all. Finally, we cover the decision to bottle-feed exclusively as well as the decision to use a combination of breast-feeding and bottle-feeding.

## Deciding to Breast-Feed

When your baby is nestled inside the womb, your body provides all the nourishment she needs. After she's born, you can continue to be the exclusive source of her nourishment through breast-feeding for at least the first four to six months. Even after your baby starts eating solid foods, you can continue breast-feeding. In fact, the American Academy of Pediatrics encourages mothers to breast-feed for at least one year and longer if they'd like, while the World Health Organization encourages moms to breast-feed for at least the first two years. Breast-feeding is good for your baby and you; we tell you why in this section.

Many of the benefits of breast-feeding increase when the baby is exclusively nourished on breast milk and breast-fed for several months. However, breast-feeding is beneficial even if you do it for only a short while. If you know you don't want to or can't breast-feed long-term, don't let that stop you from nursing for just the first few days or weeks. You and your baby still get plenty of benefits from the experience!

## Benefits of breast-feeding for the baby

Although formula companies love to claim that their particular brands are the "closest" to breast milk, nothing beats the real thing. Research has proven that babies reap many benefits from receiving their mother's milk, including the following:

- **Increased immunity:** Breast milk provides your baby with loads of antibodies, which help her fight infections. The first milk you create, called *colostrum,* is especially rich with germ-fighting cells, though mature milk continues to give your baby an immune boost. Whenever you get sick, your breast milk passes antibodies on to your baby to fight the infection. It's like giving your baby an immunization shot each time you catch the flu.

- **Fewer ear infections:** Breast-fed babies get significantly fewer ear infections. This may be because they get fewer colds and respiratory illnesses due to their better immunity (see the previous bullet), or it may be because breast-fed babies are fed in a more upright position.

- **Lower risk of many diseases:** Research has found that breast-fed children are less likely to develop some childhood cancers, Crohn's disease, ulcerative colitis, juvenile diabetes, and multiple sclerosis.

- **Lower risk of obesity:** A study published in the *Journal of the American Medical Association* in 2001 found that children who were predominately fed breast milk for the first six months of life were 22 percent less likely to be overweight as children. Because overweight children often become overweight adults, breast-feeding also lowers the risk of obesity in adulthood.

- **Lower rates of asthma and allergies:** Breast-fed babies are less likely to develop asthma and allergies as they grow older.

- **Higher intelligence:** Research has found that children who were breast-fed have on average 7 to 10 higher IQ points when compared to the average formula-fed baby. Breast-fed babies are also more likely to have higher grades in school. This may be because of the brain-building fats, like DHA and cholesterol (which are good for growing brains), contained in breast milk. It may also be due to the increased amount of touch and interaction that breast-fed babies receive, because they require feeding more frequently than bottle-fed babies.

✔ **Lower risk of dying from SIDS:** Breast-fed babies are less likely to die from sudden infant death syndrome (SIDS). Researchers theorize that this may be because formula-fed babies sleep more deeply than breast-fed babies, who are more likely to awaken if they stop breathing for too long. Another theory is that the immunity-boosting power of breast milk somehow protects babies from SIDS.

✔ **Fewer tummy troubles:** Breast-fed babies are less likely to have gastro-intestinal problems like reflux and diarrhea. Breast milk changes as your baby grows, adjusting to your baby's changing needs, giving her small amounts of colostrum during the first couple of days and then greater amounts of milk as she needs it.

# Benefits of breast-feeding for the mama

Breast-feeding isn't good only for babies; it's also good for you! The benefits of breast-feeding for mothers include the following:

✔ **Reduced rates of breast cancer:** Breast-feeding can reduce your risk of developing breast cancer by up to 25 percent. The percentage increases the more months or years a woman breast-feeds over her lifetime.

✔ **Reduced risk of uterine and ovarian cancer:** Women who breast-feed are less likely to develop uterine or ovarian cancer. This may be due to the lower levels of estrogen in your body while breast-feeding.

✔ **A vacation from menstruation:** Women who exclusively breast-feed — no bottles at all — are likely to get an extended break from their periods. You can even use breast-feeding as a natural birth-control method, as long as you nurse your baby on demand (including through the night), you don't use any bottles or pacifiers, you haven't yet gotten your first period after birth, and your baby is younger than 6 months old. Some women may not menstruate for more than a year postpartum while breast-feeding.

✔ **Increased feelings of happiness and calmness:** Breast-feeding lowers your risk of suffering from postpartum depression and anxiety. Breast-feeding mothers get a dose of the love hormone oxytocin every time they nurse, which helps them feel calmer and increases their ability to bond with their baby. This love hormone also gets into your breast milk, which is why babies frequently fall asleep at the breast and why nursing is such a great way to calm a crying baby.

✔ **Healthier bones:** Women who don't breast-feed are four times more likely to develop osteoporosis when they're older.

✔ **Less hassle and mess:** After you get the hang of breast-feeding, you may find that it's significantly easier to deal with than bottle-feeding. No cleaning out bottles or preparing formula, and when you go out, all you need to bring to feed the baby is yourself! No coolers with prepared formula required.

✔ **Lower costs:** Breast-feeding is less expensive than bottle-feeding. When taking into account the extra cost of food for a breast-feeding mother (just 500 extra calories a day), the American Academy of Pediatrics estimates that a breast-feeding family saves up to $400 in the first year of the baby's life. This doesn't account for saved money on doctor's visits, since breast-fed babies are also less likely to get frequent illnesses.

✔ **Easier postpartum weight loss:** Although you have to consume more calories to help produce breast milk, you're more likely to lose your pregnancy pounds if you breast-feed. Researchers have found that one month after birth, mothers who breast-feed have more reduction in their hip circumference and more body fat reduction when compared to formula-feeding moms. This is likely because your body stores extra fat during pregnancy to help produce breast milk after the baby is born. Breast-feeding taps into these fat stores. Newer research has found that for every six months of breast-feeding, a woman's weight is more likely to be in the healthier range even decades later!

# Getting Off to a Great Start with Breast-Feeding

The early days of breast-feeding are the most crucial for you and your baby. You need as much support as possible, and your baby needs access to you and your breasts as often as she desires. Although breast-feeding is the most natural way to feed your baby, it doesn't always come naturally to mama and baby right away. The first few days or weeks are a time of learning for both of you.

Lucky for you (and your baby), your birth plan can help you avoid some early breast-feeding problems. Despite the push for more baby-friendly hospitals — those that follow specific protocols meant to help breast-feeding mothers and babies — most hospitals in the U.S. aren't considered breast-feeding friendly. But just because your chosen birth place isn't certified as baby friendly doesn't mean you can't take steps to increase your chances for success. In this section, we give you the lowdown on how to make breast-feeding work for you in the early days.

Not every birth goes according to plan, and not every mother and baby get what they need most in terms of breast-feeding in the first hours or days. If you and your baby are separated for long periods of time or your baby gets an extra bottle or two of formula at the hospital, don't panic. You can recover from a bad start, though you'll likely have more difficulty than if the mishaps hadn't occurred. Coauthor Rachel had a very difficult start with her twins, including hours of separation and far too many bottle-feedings, but after she and her babies got out of the non-breast-feeding friendly hospital, she was able to fix the damage. About two months after birth, with the help of two amazing lactation consultants, the twins were off bottles and exclusively breast-feeding. So don't give up if you really want to go the breast-feeding route!

## *Putting baby on the breast within the first hour of birth*

Research has found that putting the baby to the breast within the first hour after birth increases the chances of successful breast-feeding. At this point, your baby is likely in a calm and alert state, ideal for learning how to suckle. Keeping your baby skin-to-skin on your chest, whether you're nursing or not, helps your baby stay warm and regulates her heartbeat and respiration rates. Even if your baby doesn't latch on in the first hour or so, the skin-to-skin contact is beneficial for both of you.

Just after birth you may feel euphoric thanks to your post-birth hormones, so it's a great time to stare into your newborn baby's eyes and start a relationship with her. Nursing within the first hour of birth also helps signal to your breasts to begin to boost milk production, and your baby's sucking causes your uterus to contract, reducing postpartum bleeding. (Not to mention, the thick yellow-white milk, called colostrum, that comes in first is full of nutrition and immunity protection that will help your baby's body confront the new world.)

Unfortunately, mothers and babies in hospitals don't always get this early skin-to-skin time. Nurses may take your baby away to be weighed, cleaned up, and swaddled in thick blankets, which discourages the skin-to-skin contact that's so vital. Sometimes nurses take babies away so the moms can rest, though most mothers have difficulty resting when their babies aren't by their side. This separation happens less frequently than it did in decades past, but if your hospital still follows antiquated policies, speak up and insist that your baby stay with you unless a sound medical reason prevents it.

You can request in your birth plan that your baby be handed to you immediately after birth unless a medical emergency occurs. You can also request that the nurses wait until you've had at least an hour of bonding time with your baby before they weigh and clean your baby. There's really no reason why the baby has to be weighed and cleaned right after birth, and your chest is an ideal baby warmer. Even if you have a C-section your partner or nurse can hold your baby right after delivery and start encouraging her to suckle. (See Chapter 14 for details on breast-feeding on the operating room table.) Your baby should also be able to stay with you as you move from the operation room to the recovery room and eventually to the postpartum floor.

Ask your nurse or midwife to help you get your baby to latch onto the breast. Although you may have seen photos of nursing moms cradling their newborns in the crook of their arms to breast-feed, in practice, this isn't the best position to use in the early days. Instead, using the football hold or cross-cradle hold is best for getting a great latch, and most nurses can help you learn these easier positions. Getting a good latch takes practice, so don't feel embarrassed to ask for assistance. Many hospitals employ lactation consultants who should be available to help you; take advantage of their help while you can. If your hospital doesn't have them, ask a breast-feeding-friendly nurse to help you at each feeding. Just be aware — not all maternity nurses are proponents of breast-feeding.

## Rooming-in and remaining in contact with your baby

One of the most essential keys to breast-feeding success is staying in almost constant contact with your baby. Now we don't mean you can't go to the bathroom or take a shower! But separation from your baby for more than a couple of hours during the early days and weeks can be detrimental to your breast-feeding success, and breast-feeding through the night is important in establishing your milk supply. In the first week after your baby is born, expect to nurse your baby 10 to 12 times per 24 hours.

Most hospitals in the U.S. encourage *rooming-in,* that is, remaining with your baby around the clock. If you plan to breast-feed, be sure to state in your birth plan that you want full rooming-in.

When you're with your baby 24 hours a day, you may also be able to pick up on subtle signals. For example, you may wake up in the night just before your baby begins to stir and show signs of wanting to suckle. If your baby is in the nursery, the nurses won't notice these early signs, and often, your baby will be crying before she's brought to you. Getting a crying baby to latch properly can be stressful for you and your baby.

## Avoiding nipple confusion and unnecessary formula

"Just one or two bottles won't hurt" is a refrain that many mothers hear in the first few days after their babies are born. A nurse may say this as a way of encouraging the mother to sleep while the baby stays in the nursery over-night, or the mother's partner or one of the grandmothers may say this in hopes of giving the new mother a break. Usually, the person making the offer means well, but the truth is that one bottle can cause issues for some babies and mothers, especially in the very early days. Here are some of the possible negative effects of early bottle-feeding:

- **Unnecessary formula fills up the baby's tummy, leading to less suckling.** Babies aren't designed to eat a lot in the first few days after birth. Plus, formula is more difficult for the baby's digestive system to process, so the baby goes longer between feedings. Nursing also stimulates production of breast milk, so if the baby doesn't nurse, the breasts produce less milk. As a result, you may find yourself switching to bottle-feeding sooner than you'd planned due to decreased milk production.

- **The nipple on a bottle requires completely different sucking techniques than the breast.** While an older baby can switch between breast and bottle, a newborn may not be able to make the transition easily. Some babies who use bottles in the first few weeks after birth develop *nipple confusion,* which makes latching onto the breast difficult. A bad latch leads the baby to get less milk, which leads the mom to produce less milk in the breast. A downward spiral can quickly take over. (See the later section "Splitting the Difference: Breast-Feeding and Bottle-Feeding" for details on the ideal time to introduce bottles to newborns if you want to use both methods.)

Although formula supplementation is medically necessary in some cases, these situations are rare, and you should always check with your doctor (not only the nurse!) for guidance before you add formula to your baby's diet. If you have to supplement with formula, use a breast-feeding-friendly feeding method, such as one of the following:

- **With a cup:** Even your newborn baby can use a cup, though not the same way you would! Hold a small sized cup — like the ones used to measure out medication — up to your baby's lips. Don't pour the milk into her mouth, but instead encourage the baby to lap up the milk like a puppy drinking milk from a bowl.

- **With a spoon:** As with a cup, hold a spoonful in front of the baby's lips and let her lap up the milk. This method can be messy and may not be appropriate for long-term supplementation.

- **With a syringe:** You can use a plastic syringe, like the kind used to measure medication for children, to feed small amounts of formula or breast milk to your baby. The baby sucks on the end of the syringe while you very slowly squirt tiny amounts of formula into her mouth. Sometimes this method is done while also placing a finger alongside the syringe (see Figure 17-1), but it's only beneficial if suck training is required.

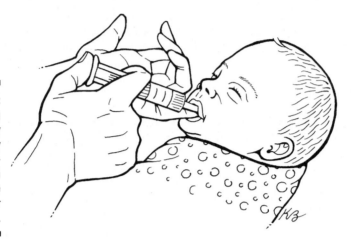

*Illustration by Kathryn Born*

**Figure 17-1:**
Giving
medically
necessary
supplemen-
tation via
a syringe
with a finger
alongside.

✔ **Through tubing that's taped to a finger:** A thin, small tube runs from a bottle or cup of formula or breast milk alongside your finger. You place your finger, nail side down, on the baby's tongue, and the baby sucks on your finger with the tubing, which brings the milk to the baby's mouth (see Figure 17-2). Make absolutely sure you wash your hands to avoid introducing dangerous bacteria.

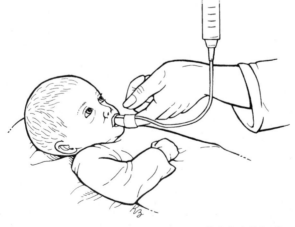

*Illustration by Kathryn Born*

**Figure 17-2:**
Giving
medically
necessary
supplemen-
tation via
tubing taped
to a finger.

✔ **With a supplemental nursing system (SNS):** An SNS includes a bottle that hangs around your neck with tubing that goes from the bottle alongside your breast and nipple. With an SNS, the baby gets the milk or formula from the bottle, but the breast is still being stimulated to produce more milk and the baby is still latching on normally. See Figure 17-3.

You can include in your birth plan a request that your baby not receive any bottles, pacifiers, or formula unless medically necessary. You can also state that you prefer a breast-feeding-friendly method if supplementation is required.

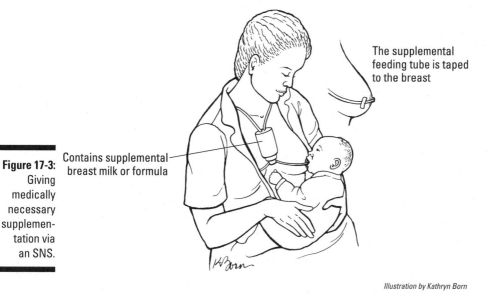

The supplemental feeding tube is taped to the breast

**Figure 17-3:** Giving medically necessary supplementation via an SNS.

Contains supplemental breast milk or formula

*Illustration by Kathryn Born*

**REMEMBER**

If your baby does get one or two bottles of formula, don't panic! Just nurse more frequently for a day or two, and if you have any trouble with getting the baby to latch, ask a nurse or lactation consultant to help you. If your baby gets multiple bottles even though you wanted to exclusively breast-feed, consult with a lactation consultant on how to proceed.

## Tackling common early breast-feeding challenges

Images of breast-feeding usually include smiling, calm moms and satisfied, suckling babies. They make it look so easy! Although one day you may fit the happy-breast-feeding-mama image, don't feel discouraged if your early days look and feel far from it. This section addresses some common early breast-feeding challenges and offers some advice for how to tackle them.

### Getting your baby to latch on

A common misconception is that babies suck on the nipple when breast-feeding. This isn't quite true; they should actually be sucking on the areola, the darkened area around the nipple, because that's where the milk reservoirs are located. Imagine a circle drawn around your areola with your nipple at the center. Your baby's gums should be about one inch away from the nipple, with your nipple toward the back of the baby's mouth. See Figure 17-4 for an illustration of what a good latch looks like. Dr. Jack Newman's website hosts breast-feeding videos of how to get a good latch at www.nbci.ca.

Look for the following signs to check if your baby is latching on properly:

✔ Your baby's chin should be against your breast. If it isn't, she hasn't taken in enough of your breast.

✔ Both of your baby's lips should be turned out like a fish. If your baby's lips are flipped in or if she seems to be sucking on her upper or bottom lip, the latch isn't quite right.

Getting your baby to take in enough breast to latch on properly takes practice. You may need to firmly but gently press the baby to your breast to get her to take in enough of the areola. If she doesn't latch on deeply enough, you can carefully break the suction by sneaking one finger into the corner of your baby's mouth between your breast and her lips and then gently take the baby off and try again.

Inverted nipples or engorgement can make getting a good latch even trickier. Expressing a little milk by hand, if you're engorged, or gently teasing out the nipple, if you have inverted nipples, can help.

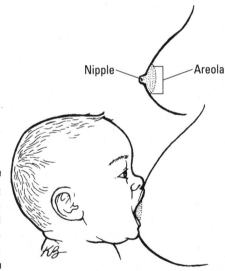

Nipple — Areola

**Figure 17-4:**
Proper latch
is essential
to breast-
feeding.

*Illustration by Kathryn Born*

### Treating tender nipples

Tender nipples are a common early breast-feeding challenge. Although many breast-feeding advocates claim that tender nipples are due to poor latch technique, during the first days of breast-feeding, even the best latch can be uncomfortable. Your raging hormones and unaccustomed nipples contribute to the tenderness. The good news is that the tenderness will go away after a week or so, as long as your baby's latch is good.

If your nipples are tender, try these tips to help soothe them:

- Put lanolin or another edible oil on the nipples between feedings.

- Expose your nipples to air and sunlight (like from a window) between feedings.

- If one side is more tender than the other, start nursing from the less tender side first, because your baby sucks harder at the first breast.

- Dab a little breast milk on each nipple and let it dry; breast milk helps heal sore and cracked nipples.

Keep in mind that tender nipples are not the same as sore nipples, especially if they are cracked, bruised, bleeding, or blistered. Very sore nipples can be caused by a bad latch, and a bad latch prevents your baby from getting enough milk. Speak to your nurse or a lactation consultant if you need more help with sore nipples or if you develop any visible sores.

## Staying confident in your breast-feeding abilities

Staying confident is a major key to having breast-feeding success. Getting started isn't easy, so don't feel as though you're not meant to breast-feed just because your first days are difficult. Rest assured; most mothers and babies face the same early challenges.

One of the most common (and often unnecessary) worries new breast-feeding moms have is that they're not producing enough milk. In actuality, however, not producing enough milk is relatively rare, so even if you share this worry, you're likely providing for your baby perfectly.

To help boost your confidence and make sure your baby is getting enough milk, try tracking your baby's diapers during the early days. Speak to your nurse about how to track diapers and keep in mind that, in general, a newborn breast-fed baby should produce the following dirty diapers:

- ✔ **Day 1:** One barely wet diaper and one black stool

- ✔ **Day 2:** Two wet diapers and two blackish stools

- ✔ **Day 3:** Three wet diapers and three brownish to green stools

- ✔ **Day 4:** Four wet diapers and four greenish-yellowish stools

- ✔ **Day 5 and on:** An average of five soaking wet diapers and three yellowish stools daily

If your baby isn't producing these exact diapers, don't panic, as some variation is normal. Just be sure to speak to your doctor or a lactation consultant for guidance on tracking diapers to make sure your baby is getting enough to eat.

Hospitals unintentionally sabotage breast-feeding mothers by sending them home with several packages of free formula. These freebies have been shown to decrease breast-feeding rates. If you're breast-feeding, don't even take the formula home. Leave it behind at the hospital before a moment of doubt (which all mothers have!) leads to an unnecessary bottle of formula.

# Pumping Breast Milk

If you plan to return to work after your baby arrives, pumping breast milk is a great way to continue providing your milk to your baby even when you're not with her. After a few weeks postpartum, you may also want to pump so you can enjoy a night out with the girls or your partner. However, in the early days and weeks, try to exclusively nurse your baby from the breast to properly stimulate your milk production and help your baby learn to latch.

Ideally, you should wait until breast-feeding and your milk supply are well established before you start to pump. However, some medical situations require mothers to pump breast milk from the beginning. In this section, we discuss when pumping may be required and how you can boost your chances for success.

If you know you may need to pump in your early days after birth, be sure to note your intentions in your birth plan. Request to use a breast pump right after the birth, ideally within the first hour. Even though you won't get much, if any, milk at this first pumping, it's important for stimulating your milk supply. You may also want to note in your birth plan that you hope to provide your baby with as much expressed breast milk as possible.

# Checking out why you may need to pump

Although pumping may not be the ideal vision you had of breast-feeding your baby, sometimes it's the only way to feed her your breast milk. Other times, moms use pumping in addition to direct breast-feeding. Here are a few reasons why you may need to pump breast milk in the early days:

- **Your baby is born prematurely.** If your baby is born before 37 weeks, she may not be able to breast-feed directly for some time, depending on how small or unhealthy she is at birth. Pumping from day one can help you build a milk supply and eventually provide your preemie with breast milk, something premature babies greatly benefit from.

- **You and your baby are separated for medical reasons.** If you or your baby are in different hospitals, perhaps because one of you needed special care that wasn't available where you delivered, you may need to pump at first.

- **Your baby can't latch properly, possibly because of a medical issue like cleft palate.** If no medical reason explains why your baby can't latch well, be sure to consult your nurse or lactation consultant for guidance. You may just need help with latching technique.

- **You need to take a medication that's dangerous to your baby.** Your doctor may tell you to *pump and dump,* which means throw away the pumped milk. This is rare, however, so don't pump and dump unless your doctor specifically tells you that you need to. If your doctor suggests you *pump and dump* "just to be safe," speak to a lactation consultant who may be able to offer more information to you or your doctor on safe medications.

- **You need to increase your milk supply.** True low milk supply is relatively rare, but if a doctor or lactation consultant finds that your milk supply needs help, you may need to pump for a period of time after every breast-feeding. Don't go this route unless you're under the care of a lactation consultant, however, as it can boost your supply beyond what your baby needs, leading to painful engorgement.

Not being able to breast-feed your baby directly can be a disappointment, and understandably so. You may feel cheated out of the full breast-feeding experience. Remember, however, that you can still exclusively provide breast milk via pumping, and you and your baby still benefit. Some mothers who start out exclusively pumping may even be able to switch to regular breast-feeding when medically possible. Speak to a lactation consultant or your baby's nurse for guidance and support.

## Increasing your potential for success

Babies are born to get the milk from your breasts, but pumping isn't always as effective. Here are some ways to boost your pumping success:

- ✔ **Use the right pumping equipment.** The pumps sold in most stores are meant for occasional use and can be great for working mothers or those who are occasionally expressing milk. But to build supply and provide breast milk for your baby in the early days, you need a hospital-grade pump with a double collection kit. A *double collection kit* allows you to pump from both breasts at the same time, which is more effective and saves you tons of time. Most hospitals offer pump rentals.

- ✔ **Use the right size flanges.** The *flanges* — the plastic cup-like things that go over your breasts — need to be the right size for you, or they can cause pain and be less effective. A lactation consultant can help you find the right fit.

- ✔ **Pump at regular intervals.** If you're pumping solely to produce breast milk, you need to do it as often as a nursing baby would breast-feed. That's every two to three hours for at least 20 minutes. If you're pumping to build supply, ask your lactation consultant how long and how often you should pump.

- ✔ **Pump next to your baby.** Seeing your baby helps you produce more milk. Most NICUs allow mothers to pump right next to their baby's incubator. If you have help and good coordination, and your baby is well enough, you may even be able to have the baby skin-to-skin on your chest while you pump. If you can't always pump next to your baby, even looking at a picture of your baby can help.

- ✔ **Take care of yourself.** Pumping can be stressful, and many of the situations that require pumping, like going back to work, can be stressful. Be sure to take care of yourself; eat well, stay hydrated, and rest when you can.

- ✔ **Don't concentrate on how much milk you're producing.** If the amount stresses you out, you can cover the collection bottles with paper or a plastic bag. Especially if you're pumping to build supply, don't assume what you collect is a representation of your milk supply. Your baby is more effective than a pump at getting the milk out.

# Asking for a Lactation Consultant's Help

A *lactation consultant* is trained and certified to help mothers with breast-feeding, especially when they encounter problems. Many hospitals have one or more certified lactation consultants on staff, but they may or may not be available every day. As long as you're a patient in the hospital, you should be able to see the staff lactation consultant free of charge.

You can include in your birth plan a request to see a consultant, even if you don't have problems with nursing. She can help you with positioning and make sure your baby is latching on well. Just let the staff know as soon as possible after the birth that you'd like to see the consultant to increase the chances of her getting around to see you.

After you're out of the hospital, hiring a lactation consultant privately can be pricey — anywhere from $50 to $150 per hour of consultation. You may be able to privately hire the hospital's lactation consultant, or you can find one on the International Lactation Consultant Association's website, www.ilca.org.

You may want to consider contacting your local La Leche League (LLL). LLL volunteers can speak with you at no cost, and LLL leaders can help with many breast-feeding basics, like getting a good latch. If you need the professional help of a certified lactation consultant, the LLL volunteers can refer you to someone. Find a local LLL leader online at www.llli.org.

# Deciding to Bottle-Feed

Although breast-feeding from the start is ideal, not everyone can or wants to do so. In this section, we explain why you may not be able to breast-feed, even if you'd hoped to do so, why some women choose to bottle-feed, and how to deal with bottle guilt or disappointment.

## Understanding why you may not be able to breast-feed

Although breast-feeding is usually best for you and your baby, exceptions exist. Here are some reasons why you may not be able to breast-feed:

- ✔ **You need to take medications that are unsafe for breast-feeding.** Your doctor should be able to provide breast-feeding-safe medication options in most situations, but doing so isn't always possible. (However, some women wean their babies only to discover they really didn't have to. Be sure to speak to a lactation consultant as well as your doctor.)

- ✔ **You're HIV positive.** If you're HIV positive, you could pass the virus to your baby through breast-feeding.

- ✔ **You've had breast reduction surgery.** This type of surgery may have compromised your milk supply, though you should speak to a lactation consultant to see if any level of breast-feeding is possible before you decide to bottle-feed exclusively.

✔ **You take street drugs or have a serious drinking problem.** Drugs like cocaine, heroin, and methamphetamine, as well as alcohol, pass through breast milk and can be extremely dangerous for your baby.

✔ **Your baby has galactosemia.** *Galactosemia* is a rare metabolic enzyme deficiency, occurring in about 1 out of 85,000 births. Babies with galactosemia can't be breast-fed and must receive specialized formula.

✔ **You've had a double mastectomy.** Breast cancer survivors who have had a double mastectomy are unable to breast-feed. Reconstructed breasts don't produce milk.

✔ **You don't produce enough milk.** Insufficient milk production occurs in about 1 in 1,000 women. It may be due to hormonal or physical conditions, like insufficient glandular tissue (IGT). In some cases, pumping along with lactation-inducing medications like domperidone can help a mother with low milk supply breast-feed her baby partially or fully.

If you can't breast-feed, you don't necessarily have to feed your baby formula. You could purchase breast milk from a donor bank; however, this option isn't workable for everyone, especially because of the expense. Don't accept milk from just anyone, though, as certain diseases can pass through breast milk. If you decide to use donor milk, get it from a milk bank, not your friends.

## Choosing to bottle-feed

Women choose not to breast-feed for a variety of reasons, including the following:

✔ Some women are nervous about needing to breast-feed in public, so they choose not to nurse at all.

✔ Others know they want to return to work soon and aren't interested in starting something they can't continue.

✔ Mothers who have had previous difficulty with nursing in the past may choose not to breast-feed with subsequent children. (Remember that every baby is different, though, so you may still want to try nursing to see whether it goes better this time.)

✔ Some women decide not to breast-feed because they don't like the way it feels, or they can't handle the physical discomfort of the early days.

✔ Others are just uncomfortable with the idea of breast-feeding, possibly because no one in their family or friendship circle breast-feeds.

If you have chosen to bottle-feed, be sure to note this in your birth plan. Some nurses are likely to encourage you to breast-feed anyway, and if you're comfortable with doing so, you may want to go ahead and nurse once or twice so your baby can get the colostrum, the early milk that gives your baby an immunity boost. But you can certainly decide not to breast-feed at all. It's your choice.

## Dealing with bottle guilt and disappointment

Formula isn't the ideal baby food, but it's more than good enough. You're not harming your baby by giving her formula, and plenty of babies thrive and grow strong on only formula. In fact, you or your mother may even have been fed formula exclusively — and you turned out okay, right?

Bonding is a big topic related to breast-feeding and bottle-feeding, with some saying that bottle-feeding mothers have more difficulty bonding with their babies. Breast-feeding does cause a physiological reaction in both the mother and the baby that increases feelings of connection and love, but your body also secretes the love hormone oxytocin when you hug another person. So holding your baby close as often as possible or even giving her bottle-feedings while skin to skin can help you bond just as well with your baby as any breast-feeding mother.

People may criticize you for choosing to bottle-feed, and that criticism can be especially painful if you wanted to breast-feed but couldn't. Although it's unpleasant, try to think of it as just one of many parenting decisions you'll be judged for over your lifetime as a mother. Keep reminding yourself that bottle-feeding doesn't make you a bad mother — because it doesn't.

# Splitting the Difference: Breast-Feeding and Bottle-Feeding

Maybe you intended to breast-feed but had problems you couldn't completely overcome, or perhaps you always intended to bottle-feed but then felt a pull to try a little breast-feeding. After your baby is taking mostly bottles, you can't switch back to exclusively breast-feeding because you won't produce enough milk. However, assuming you and your baby don't have any medical concerns, you can still nurse your little one occasionally.

Breast-feeding is more than providing your baby with nutrition; it can also be a source of comfort and connection. Plus, your primarily bottle-fed baby can still receive a small immunity boost from the breast milk she does take in. You may decide to breast-feed a few times a day or when your baby is extra cranky, or you may nurse your baby after a bottle-feeding to help put her to sleep for a nap. Just make sure you don't rely on your breast milk to nourish your baby after you've mainly given her formula.

After you've started bottle-feeding, you may have difficulty getting your baby to latch properly during nursing, which can be painful for you, but not every baby has this issue. You can try out some of the newer bottles that are made specifically to cut down on nipple confusion, but the verdict is still out on how well they work.

If you hope to mainly breast-feed but would still like to give your baby an occasional bottle, try to wait to introduce bottles of breast milk for at least 3 to 4 weeks and not introduce formula until at least 6 to 12 weeks. This way, your body has a chance to establish a strong supply of breast milk, and a bottle every now and then won't seriously impact your supply.

# Part VI
# Putting Your Plan in Writing and into Action

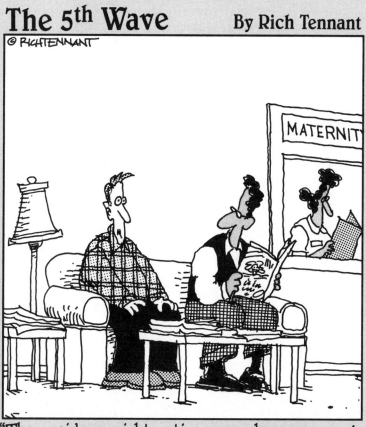

The 5th Wave    By Rich Tennant

"They said we might notice some changes a week before she went into labor. Sure enough, 5 days ago, gas prices went up .06 cents at the pump, my lawn mower stopped working, and the guy across the street had his house painted."

# In this part . . .

Writing a birth plan is an exciting but sometimes overwhelming task. If you're not sure where to start and what sorts of information to include, this part helps you figure it out. Composing a birth plan that makes your desires known requires careful thought; it's not a job to be dashed off in a day. Instead, your birth plan should be a work in progress that can change right up until the time you give birth. The chapters in this part help you not only write your birth plan but also present it to your birth team and get their support.

# Chapter 18

# Writing Your Birth Plan

*T*hroughout this book, we explain the pros and cons of your birth options in detail. In this chapter, we get down to the nitty-gritty writing of your actual birth plan. Some prefer to call it a *birth wish list* or an *ideal birth plan,* leaving room for the uncertainty of childbirth. Whatever you call it, its purpose is the same — to lay out your requests for the birth and immediate postpartum period. Your birth plan lets the medical-care team know what you want, and it also helps your support people — your partner, doula, or other labor attendant — advocate for you and provide you with what you need during labor and birth.

In this chapter, we explain how your big birth decisions shape your birth plan, what issues are generally included in a birth plan, and how to write a plan that will be understood and accepted. We also provide a couple sample birth plans to guide you as you write your own.

# Deciding on the Big Birth Issues First: Location and Attendants

Understanding the impact of your big birth decisions — like where you give birth and who your birth attendants are — is vital to creating a successful birth plan.

Although we cover many different birth options throughout this book, we don't intend to imply that all options are on the table for every woman. Your options are limited not only by your pregnancy and birth situation but also by your birth location and medical practitioner. If you hope for an intervention-free childbirth but choose a medical practitioner who is in love with routine interventions, you're going to be in trouble. If you've dreamed of a very hands-off home birth but hire a midwife who is heavy handed, your birth wishes may not be followed.

Birth location can also affect your birth plans. If you'd love a water birth but choose a birth center or hospital that doesn't have birthing pools — unless you rent one (*and* get permission to bring it with you, *and* get approval from your medical practitioner for a water delivery) — you're not going to have a water birth. If you want to try for a VBAC (vaginal birth after cesarean) but your chosen hospital or doctor does not allow VBACs, that's going to be an issue.

Your choice of birth location also affects your postpartum and baby-related requests. For example, although most hospitals in the United States allow full rooming-in (meaning the baby stays with you throughout the night instead of going to the nursery), some smaller hospitals may not, which can be an issue if you want to keep your baby with you night and day. On the other hand, if you hope to send your baby to the nursery at night but your hospital insists on full rooming-in for healthy babies, that policy can also interfere with your birth plans.

At the start of pregnancy, when you're first choosing your medical practitioner, you may not know what you want at the birth. As your knowledge grows along with your belly, your desires may change. Changing your mind is common and totally normal, but remember that your medical practitioner won't be changing as you change. Toward the end of pregnancy, you may need to reconsider who you've chosen as your birth attendant and what kind of birth location you want. See Chapters 3, 4, and 5 on choosing birth attendants and birth location.

Be sure to discuss your birth plans with your medical practitioner before labor begins — ideally a few months before your due date. Approach the meeting as a way to discuss your requests in a nonconfrontational manner. If you go in expecting a fight, your medical practitioner is probably not the right one for you, and you're bound to create more harm than good. A doctor who has been approached in an aggressive way may feel defensive, leading to tension in the relationship. This can then lead to tension in the labor room, which you do not want. Discussing your birth hopes early also gives you a chance to switch practitioners, if necessary.

After you discuss the birth plan with your medical practitioner, you may want to ask her to sign it, under a phrase stating "I have read and understand this birth plan." This signature is not a promise or guarantee that you'll get what you want, but it may help later at the hospital, especially if your plans don't match the hospital's routine policies.

# Breaking Down the Sections of a Birth Plan

Although your birth plan will be unique to you because it will contain your personal requests, most birth plans follow a general format and target specific issues. In this section, we list the main components of most birth plans and touch on your various options.

This section is just an overview of possible requests people make in their birth plans. It is by no means a "must have" list, nor does it include every person's birth wishes. If some issues here don't apply to you or you just don't have a strong preference, leave them out. On the other hand, if you have an issue that's not included — like a special medical or religious situation regarding your baby, you, or your partner that you want the staff to know about — be sure to write it into your plan.

## Listing guests and the birth team

At the very top of your birth plan, you should include the names of guests who will play an important role at the birth. This list of course includes you, your partner, and your medical practitioner but also includes other support people, like your doula.

If you plan for your kids to be present during the actual delivery, this detail should be included in your birth plan. You may also want to include one line explaining why you've made this decision and one line on how you've prepared them. Whoever is your child's support person (the person looking after him or her while you and your partner are busy with labor and delivery) should also be listed. (See Chapter 6 for more details.)

Further down in your birth plan, you can also state your hopes for guests attending the birth who are not part of your support team. Do you want your mother and sister in the room for the actual delivery? Say so. Do you want it to be only you and your partner? Write that.

You may also include your preferences for medical and nursing students. You can ask they have no part in your birth and delivery, permit them to be present but not do cervical checks or hands-on care, or leave the issue out completely if you're not particular about their participation.

See Chapter 6 for guidance on who to invite to the birth and Chapter 19 on dealing with your guests and hospital staff.

## Wanting a natural birth

Beneath the basic facts at the very top of your plan, state your overall approach to your birth. If you're planning a natural childbirth, this is the spot to say so. Because a natural childbirth tends to set the tone for your overall birth plan, placing it front and center makes sense. If you're planning to get an epidural or use other pain medications, you can skip to the next section, "Choosing medication or questioning a nonmedicated birth."

Although you can simply state that you intend to have a natural childbirth, *natural* means different things to different people, and your birth guests and nurses will be able to better advocate for you if they really understand what you want. Your natural-birth statement may also include:

- ✔ **What you mean, exactly, by *natural:*** If you mean to use natural soothing techniques instead of pain medications, say so. If you mean you'd like to avoid any routine interventions, say so.

- ✔ **Why you've chosen natural childbirth:** Don't write an essay — this isn't the place to reference all the research you've done! — but one or two sentences of explanation show you're serious and committed to your choice. Whether you've chosen natural childbirth because of a previous bad birth experience, a previous bad epidural reaction, or because your research on the issue has convinced you this is what you want, say so in your plan.

- ✔ **How you've prepared:** Have you studied a particular childbirth method? Taken classes? Gone under hypnosis? Including how you've prepared reassures your nurse that you have the tools to make it through a natural birth. State this briefly in your plan; just a sentence is enough.

After your natural birth statement, you should list the ways you intend to cope with labor, including movements and labor positions you hope to use. This information not only reassures your birth attendants that you actually have a plan of action but also can serve as a cheat sheet for you and your labor support team. See Chapter 8 for natural methods of coping during labor and Chapter 9 for your movement and position options.

Some hospitals offer natural birthing rooms or natural birthing centers, which are pre-equipped with birthing tools and even staff committed to supporting you. If your birth location has this kind of room or center and you'd like to use it, be sure to include that in your birth plan.

You may also want to request that staff not offer you pain medication, and ask that they wait until you request it. Staff may or may not strictly abide by this request — not because they don't support natural childbirth, but because they hate to see you struggle! But having it in the plan can be helpful because your labor-support partner can reference your birth plan if staff offers too frequently.

Until you're in labor, you may not know how you'll cope — even if you've given birth before. Writing in your birth plan that you want a natural childbirth doesn't mean you can't change your mind. Even if you deliver at home or at a birth center, you can still change your mind. (You'll just need to transfer to a hospital.) Your birth team should respect your decisions, and you're not a failure if you change your mind. See Chapter 20 for more on birth-plan changes and dealing with disappointment.

## Choosing medication or questioning a nonmedicated birth

If you're unsure if you want to go through labor without pain medications — or you're *certain* you want pain medication — be sure to include these details in your birth plan at the top. You don't need to be absolutely sure about wanting a natural childbirth or an epidural, and plenty of women wait until labor begins to make a decision. As long as you're prepared for either scenario, that's no problem, and you can include this uncertainty in your birth plan.

Even if you plan to use pain medication, you may still want to list natural soothing techniques, along with labor positions and movements, which you plan to use before you get an epidural.

You can also include specific medication requests, preferably based on discussions you've had with your medical practitioner before labor. See Chapter 11 for details on your options. Here are some drug-related requests you may include in your birth plan:

- **Wanting an epidural as soon as possible:** Depending on your doctor and hospital's policy, you may need to wait until you've dilated a certain amount before getting an epidural, but maybe not.

- **Wanting an epidural only after you've dilated to 5 centimeters:** Waiting until 5 centimeters may avoid unintentionally stalling labor.

- **Wanting — or not wanting — certain narcotic pain relief:** If you had a bad experience in the past with a particular drug, state that in your birth plan.

- **Wanting a walking epidural:** Some hospitals offer walking epidurals, which theoretically allow you more movement and numb you less.

- **Asking for the epidural to be turned down when it's time to push:** Having more sensation may help you push more effectively, but it may also mean more discomfort.

- **Asking for position changes or gravity-friendly positions after the epidural is in:** Whether you have a walking epidural or a regular one, you should change position every so often to help labor along. You can make this request in your plan.

If you have any known allergies to medications, be sure to write them in your birth plan. The hospital staff will likely ask you about allergies anyway, but it doesn't hurt to repeat the information.

## Listing comfort tools and props

Whether you're doing natural birth or planning on an epidural, your birth plan should also list any comfort tools and props you hope to use, like music, a birth ball, aromatherapy, or hot and cold compresses. (See Chapter 8 for more ideas.) When you're admitted to the hospital or birth center, be sure to mention any requests that require birthing equipment, like a squat bar, birthing stool, birthing pool, or shower. Some rooms may have easier access to these birthing tools, so speak up before you're settled into a room.

## Setting the scene: Birthing-environment requests

Your surroundings during birth can deeply affect your experience. Some birthing methods require or encourage a specific mood, like diming the lights just before the baby is born. Following are some topics you may want to address:

- **Lighting:** Do you prefer the lights to remain dim as you labor? Or during the actual delivery? State that in your birth plan.

- **Noise level:** You can ask that staff use quiet voices when possible. You can ask that the door to your room remain closed so hallway activity doesn't distract you.

- **Crowd control:** You can ask to have as few people as possible in the room.

- **Music:** Your hopes for playing relaxing music or, alternatively, upbeat tunes during labor can be included in your birth plan.

You may also have specific requests about the lighting and noise level in the room as the baby is born. If you plan on having a water birth, be sure to include this intention in your birth plan. See Chapter 15 for more on delivery environment requests and Chapter 8 on water birth.

## Laying out desires for interventions and monitoring

Requests regarding interventions may be considered the heart of the birth plan and the main reason why many women choose to write one. In this section, we go over the typical interventions addressed in a birth plan. As with all birth plan topics, don't feel obligated to include every possible intervention option. Only include issues most important to you and your partner.

You can't possibly cover every intervention situation in your birth plan. However, you can include a request that your medical practitioner explain the reason for any intervention to you before carrying it out, assuming there's no emergency. For example: "Before carrying out any nonemergent intervention, please answer these questions so we can make an informed decision: Is this intervention necessary for my or my baby's health? What are the risks? The potential benefits? What happens if I decline?" You can also request that the staff allow you time alone, when possible, to make a decision. See Chapter 22 for more on handling unexpected situations.

### Eating and staying hydrated

In Chapter 10, we explain your various options for staying hydrated and nourished during labor, including the pros and cons of routine IV fluids. Food, drink, and IV policies vary widely, and your choice of practitioner and birth location play a big role in your available options. With that said, your birth plan may include any of the following points:

- ✔ **Acceptance of routine IV fluids:** In some situations, IV fluids are required, like if you get an epidural or require IV medication during labor. You may also prefer to receive IV fluids if you feel dehydrated or have been vomiting.

- ✔ **Refusal of routine IV fluids:** You may write that you prefer to remain hydrated by taking in clear fluids instead, though some hospitals only allow ice chips.

- ✔ **Acceptance of heparin or saline lock:** Some hospitals allow you to forgo IV fluids but ask you to have a saline lock — an IV placed in the arm without the tubing — to allow for quick medication delivery in the case of an emergency.

- ✔ **Intake of light foods and fluids:** Some, but not all, hospitals allow you to eat lightly during labor (foods like toast or applesauce). You will likely need your medical practitioner's permission to eat during labor. See Chapter 10 for more on your nourishment options.

### Performing cervical checks

In Chapter 12, we give a rundown of the pros and cons to cervical checks. You may want cervical checks as often as permitted, because you're curious about how you're progressing. In that case, you can leave out the topic of cervical checks from your birth plan. If you hope to limit them, state that you only want cervical checks when deemed medically necessary (and not just for curiosity's sake). You may also ask that cervical checks aren't done unless there are other signs of labor progression, like a sudden change in mood or the urge to push. You can also request that no medical or nursing students perform cervical checks.

## Monitoring the fetus

Fetal monitoring, covered in detail in Chapter 12, may be required depending on your medical situation. The policies of your birth location and practitioner also have a strong impact on your options. That said, here are some ways you may address the issue in your birth plan:

- ✔ **Consent to continuous monitoring:** Continuous monitoring of fetal heart tones and contractions is the routine in most hospitals and is required in some situations, like during an induction or if you have an epidural.

- ✔ **Initial monitoring followed by intermittent monitoring:** If you hope to remain active during labor, you may want to consent to initial monitoring (usually 20 to 30 minutes) and then only to intermittent monitoring. Speak to your medical practitioner about your options.

- ✔ **Doppler for intermittent checks:** Doppler may be most useful when laboring in water, so you don't need to completely come out of the water every time they want to check the baby.

- ✔ **Telemetry monitoring:** Not available in all hospitals, this monitoring uses radio waves so you can remain active. It's useful for inductions, when continuous monitoring is required.

- ✔ **Fetoscope:** This device works like a stethoscope, except it's made for listening to fetal heart tones. Although many midwives are familiar with fetoscopes, most doctors aren't comfortable using them and prefer a printout on the fetal monitor that can be used as documentation of the fetal heart tones.

## Inducing and speeding up labor

Induction is discussed before labor begins, so your "big birth plans" — like when to do the induction and how to start things — are usually decided with your medical practitioner before you get to the hospital. In Chapter 13, we discuss induction options in detail. For a scheduled induction, your birth plan should cover all the regular issues while also taking into account the higher risk of induction. For example, you'd need continuous monitoring, so requesting intermittent monitoring would be inappropriate.

If you're not having a scheduled induction, your birth plan should cover the topic of speeding up labor if labor stalls, slows down, or isn't going as quickly as your medical practitioner prefers. Following are topics you may address in your plan:

- ✔ **Allowing labor to progress on its own schedule:** Assuming you and the baby are well, you may ask that labor be allowed to slow, stall, or speed up without interference.

- ✔ **Asking that your water not be broken prematurely:** Some doctors routinely break the bag of waters to get things moving along, without specific medical reason. You can turn down this option.

✔ **Trying movement and position changes before drugs:** You may request a chance to try moving around to speed up a slow labor.

✔ **Using nondrug methods to speed up labor:** Besides movement and position, you can try nipple stimulation or breaking your water.

✔ **Request oxytocin (Pitocin) be used at a slow pace, at the lowest dose:** You can ask that induction medications be started slowly and only increased after allowing time for a low dose to work.

### Receiving an episiotomy

Your birth plan can indicate whether you prefer an episiotomy or prefer to tear naturally. If you request not to be cut (the most common request), include in your birth plan any preparations you've done — like Kegel exercises or perineal massage — along with anything you want to do to prevent tearing. Tear prevention options may include:

✔ **Pushing from particular positions:** A side-lying position is the least likely to cause tearing, but squatting is more effective and may work better during a slow-pushing stage. You may also consider pushing in a hands-and-knees position, which allows a modified squat with a lower perineal trauma rate. See Chapter 9 for more options.

✔ **Warm compresses:** A warm compress against the perineum during the pushing stage may help prevent tears and discomfort.

✔ **Perineal support:** Either with or without a warm compress, gentle counterpressure may prevent tears.

✔ **Application of lubricating oils:** Often along with gentle massage of the perineum, you may request lubricating oils be applied by your medical practitioner during the pushing stage.

✔ **Allowing time for the perineum to stretch:** You may ask your medical practitioner to advise you when to pause during pushing to allow the skin to stretch.

You may also request a shot of local anesthetic for stitching any repairs. The pros and cons to episiotomy and natural tearing can be found in Chapter 13.

## Accounting for cesarean section

If you're planning a vaginal birth, cesarean section might be the last thing on your mind when writing a birth plan. But in case your situation changes and a C-section becomes necessary, you should consider your options before labor begins. And if you know ahead of time that you're having a cesarean, you can write your birth plan specifically from that perspective.

Many aspects of your birth plan will affect your overall risk of C-section. For example, a scheduled induction or use of epidural increases your risk. You can try to avoid a cesarean by including the following points in your plan:

- **No time limits on labor and birth:** Some practitioners push for a cesarean section if labor is moving too slowly or doesn't finish within a set number of hours. Assuming mother and baby are well, with no indications of infection or fetal distress, you can note in your birth plan that you prefer to ignore arbitrary time limits.

- **Request alternative actions before cesarean:** Depending on the reason for C-section, you may ask that you first be given a chance to change pushing positions, turn down the epidural, or attempt an assisted vaginal delivery, such as with forceps or vacuum. See Chapter 13 for more on the risks of assisted vaginal delivery.

If you do need a cesarean section, as long as it's not a major emergency, you have options you can address in your birth plan. Chapter 14 goes over your options in detail. Your doctor and hospital policy have a strong impact on which options are open to you, but requests you may make include:

- **Who will be with you:** You can usually bring one person with you into surgery, and sometimes one person plus a doula.

- **Which anesthesia will be used:** In most cases, your doctor will choose for you, but you may be given a choice between a spinal or epidural. Chapter 14 discusses these options.

- **Lowering the drape:** You may ask that the drape be lowered or removed altogether so you can see your baby being born. A few doctors have allowed mothers with gloved hands to help deliver the baby, but this opportunity is rare due to risk of contamination of the sterile field.

- **"Gentle cesarean":** A gentle cesarean can include anything from soft music playing in the background to a slower delivery of the baby from the incision. This concept is relatively new, and few doctors offer it, but you can ask if it's an option for you.

- **Keeping one or both arms untied:** Usually, both arms are tied down during surgery. You may be able to request that one or both arms remain free, if not throughout surgery then at least after the baby is born so you can touch him easily.

- **Taking photos or video:** Few doctors allow videos or pictures of the actual surgery, but they may allow a camera that remains behind the drape.

- **Requesting double-layer sutures:** Cesarean sections are closed up by a variety of sutures. Double-layer sutures are required by some practitioners in order to qualify for a VBAC in the future.

✔ **Requests regarding the baby:** Many common birth-plan issues — like who cuts the cord, who announces the sex of the baby, and delaying weighing and washing — can be applied during cesarean birth, assuming the baby is healthy and breathing normally at birth.

✔ **Nursing the baby on the table:** Assuming the baby is well, you may request to breast-feed the baby while your incision is closed. You'll need help from your partner or a nurse to do so, however.

✔ **Asking to keep the baby with you:** You may request that the baby stay with you through the end of surgery, as you're moved into a recovery room and eventually into your hospital room.

# Pushing time!

In Chapter 9, we discuss your choices for pushing positions, and in Chapter 15, we address some of your options as the baby is delivered. Following are some requests you may make in your birth plan regarding pushing stage of labor:

✔ **Choosing instinctive instead of coached pushing:** Coached pushing means the birth team tells you when to push, possibly counting as you push, and (often) asking you to hold your breath. Coached pushing can have negative consequences, like an increased risk of tearing and early exhaustion. Instinctive pushing is pushing according to your natural urges.

✔ **Laboring down:** If you have an epidural, you may ask to labor down until you feel pushing sensations. *Laboring down* means allowing the contractions to do the work of pushing the baby.

✔ **Use of a variety of pushing positions:** You may ask to switch between a variety of pushing positions. Even if you have an epidural, you can try different positions, like lying on your side.

✔ **Ask to use pushing props:** You may request a squat bar, a birthing stool, or a long sheet or rope to tie to the squat bar. You may ask to use stirrups while pushing or ask not to use stirrups.

✔ **Request no artificial time limits on pushing:** Many doctors limit how much time they'll allow a mother to push before strongly suggesting a C-section. You may ask that no artificial time limits be used as long as there is progression, even if it's slow, and as long as you and your baby are tolerating the pushing stage.

✔ **Other ways to participate during pushing:** You may ask to watch the birth in a mirror, or to reach down and touch your baby's head just before he's born. You may request that your husband "catch" the baby, or for yourself to help deliver the baby (often easier to do during a water birth).

# Attending to your new baby

All your efforts through pregnancy and childbirth come down to one special person (or more, if you're having multiples!): your baby. In this section, we list the issues in your birth plan that relate to your baby.

### Announcing the gender

Most people assume the doctor will announce the sex of the baby at birth, but you can write in your birth plan that you or your partner would like to announce the gender instead.

### Cutting the cord

The umbilical cord — that direct link between you and your baby — is a hot topic in some circles, especially the debate on when to clamp or cut the cord. Chapter 15 covers cord issues in detail. Your birth plan may address any of the following cord-related issues:

- ✔ **Who cuts the cord:** Traditionally, the dad cuts the cord, but he's not the only option. You can cut the cord, an older child at the birth can cut the cord, or you can opt for the birth team to cut the cord.

- ✔ **When to cut the cord:** You may request in your birth plan that the cord not be cut or clamped until it stops pulsating.

- ✔ **Saving the cord:** If you've made arrangements prior to the birth for cord-blood banking, be sure to indicate them in your birth plan.

### When can I have my baby?

Finally, the baby is here! But whether he goes directly into your arms or is whisked away depends partially on his condition at birth and partially on your request. More details are in Chapter 15 and 16. Your birth plan may request any of the following:

- ✔ **Placing the baby directly on your chest after birth:** You can ask that the baby be placed right onto your chest and into your arms straight out of the oven, with no clean up.

- ✔ **Performing initial screening and Apgar's while the baby is in your arms:** Early tests performed at the first and fifth minutes of life evaluate the baby's adaptation to life outside the uterus, the baby's breathing, heart rate, muscle tone, reflexes and skin color. As long as your baby is not in distress, the team can evaluate the baby's health while he's in your arms.

- ✔ **Requesting that no suctioning be done:** Routine suctioning of the baby's mouth and nose may be done as the baby emerges from the birth canal or be delayed until he's fully born. You may request in your birth plan that no suctioning be done unless medically necessary, that suctioning wait until he's delivered, or that your partner do the suctioning.

✔ **Delaying or rejecting eye drops:** Hospital born babies are routinely given eye drops, meant to prevent blindness if the mother has gonorrhea. You can ask that the drops be delayed until after initial birth bonding or forgo the drops altogether.

✔ **Delaying weighing, cleanup, and other routine procedures:** You can request that the baby not be taken away for weighing and cleanup until you've had an hour or two to bond together.

✔ **Asking for weighing and cleanup before baby is handed over:** You may ask that the team finish with their routine weighing and cleaning before the baby is handed to you. You can also request that your baby not be bathed at all, choosing to keep the vernix coating as long as possible.

✔ **Breast-feeding and skin-to-skin contact right after birth:** Your birth plan may indicate that you'd like help with breast-feeding right after birth, that you'd like the baby placed skin-to-skin on your chest, or that you'd like to allow the baby to naturally find his way to your nipples after being placed on your chest. See Chapter 17 for more on breast-feeding in the first hour after birth.

### Feeding preferences and rooming-in

Your birth plan should address how you plan to feed your baby and where you want your baby to sleep. Whether you intend to breast-feed, bottle-feed, or a little of both, make sure your choice is in your birth plan. Your birth plan may also include:

✔ **No medically unnecessary supplements:** If you're breast-feeding, you may ask that hospital staff not give your baby formula or sugar water without discussing the situation with you first or without medical reason.

✔ **No artificial nipples for supplementation:** If medical supplementation is necessary, you can write in your plan your preference to use breast-feeding-friendly methods, like cup feeding, syringe feeding, a tube on the finger, or an SNS system. See Chapter 17 for more information.

✔ **No pacifiers:** Whether pacifiers cause nipple confusion is up for debate, but some mothers prefer to avoid them altogether for a variety of reasons.

✔ **Request to see the hospital lactation consultant:** Often available without charge, you can request a quick check-up with a lactation consultant as soon as possible after birth.

✔ **Request hospital pump rental:** If you know you'll need to pump, you can request a rental as soon as possible after birth. You can also indicate in your birth plan that you prefer your baby receive pumped breast milk, when available.

✔ **Requesting full rooming-in or partial rooming-in:** Full rooming-in means your baby stays with you all day and all night, whereas partial rooming-in means your baby sleeps in the nursery. Your options depend on your hospital's nursery policies.

### Shots and circumcision requests

Your baby's first shots are often given at the hospital, and circumcision is also usually done before discharge. Chapter 16 covers these issues in detail. Clarify your wishes on the following options in the birth plan:

- ✔ **Allowing all routine shots:** You can accept all routine shots. If you plan to allow them, you can probably leave this statement out of your birth plan.

- ✔ **Delaying shots:** You can choose to delay some or all vaccines. See Chapter 16 for more details.

- ✔ **Stating vitamin K shot preferences:** You may turn down vitamin K or ask that it be given orally or by injection. (Not all options are always available.)

- ✔ **Requesting that your partner be present for all tests and shots:** You can ask that you or your partner be present when your baby is given shots or examined.

- ✔ **Accepting or refusing circumcision:** Your birth plan should address whether you want the hospital to perform circumcision or not.

## Making requests about the placenta

Yes, you even have options regarding the placenta! Chapter 13 covers many of these issues in detail. Your birth plan may cover any of the following:

- ✔ **Allowing placenta to be delivered naturally:** You may ask that controlled cord traction not be used.

- ✔ **Requesting or turning down routine oxytocin (Pitocin):** You may ask to delay routine oxytocin as long as placental bleeding remains under control, or to try other methods first, like uterine massage or breastfeeding, to help the uterus to contract. Or, alternatively, you may request oxytocin.

- ✔ **Asking to see or save the placenta:** You may ask if you can see the placenta or even take a photo. You can ask if you can bring the placenta home, for burying, creating a placenta print (see Chapter 22), or for creating placenta pills (said to help with postpartum depression). However, some state laws prohibit hospitals from allowing families to take home the placenta due to public health concerns.

## Planning for home birth and birth centers

If you're having a home birth or delivering at a birth center, your plan may look very different than a hospital birth plan. You may be able to focus less on interventions and more on birth preferences, like wanting your partner to catch the baby or desiring a water birth. Don't assume, however, that a home birth or birth center practitioner will be as hands-off as you'd like — always discuss routine interventions with your practitioner before the birth, no matter who she is.

Be sure to address emergency transfer in your birth plan. Your plan may indicate which hospital you want transferred to, whether you want your midwife to stay with you at the hospital (as your doula, instead of as your medical practitioner), and if you want a particular doctor called.

You may also want to include roles for the various birth guests. For example, who will be watching your other children? Do you want your birth guests present the entire labor or to be "invisible" until the big moment? Your midwife may also want information on where the birth team can park their cars, where they can rest (when they aren't actively needed), and what food and drink is available for them.

You may also want to write a separate birth plan for hospital transfer. Although you may not want to think about the possibility of transfer, it's better to be prepared. Get more details about home birth in Chapter 5.

## Taking photos or video

If you plan to take photos or video of the birth, include this point in your birth plan. Because of lawsuits and liability, your medical practitioner or place of birth may have rules about when and whether photography is allowed. Be sure to check before labor, and if any paper work is required, complete it and bring it with you along with your birth plan.

In Chapter 22, you can find more ideas for preserving birth memories, including tips for taking great childbirth photos and videos.

# Writing the Birth Plan

Many women create their birth plans using online templates that allow you to check off choices from a list and then print your finished plan. We can certainly understand the allure of these templates — they're much easier to use than writing one from scratch. However, handing to your birth team a checklist you printed off the Internet isn't as powerful as using one you've written yourself. Writing your own plan shows you've given careful thought to your wishes, and if you appear more serious about your plans, your birth team will take you more seriously. In this section, we provide tips to keep in mind as you write your plan.

Just writing your plan down doesn't mean your requests will be heard and followed. Especially in a hospital, your birth team is likely attending to many women; keeping everyone's requests straight can be difficult. Don't be afraid to speak up. See Chapter 19 for more on advocating for yourself.

Be sure to print out multiple copies of your birth plan. This way, if the nursing shift changes and your plan gets lost in the shuffle, you'll have additional copies to hand out. Your birth plan can also serve as a cheat sheet for you, your partner, and any other birth guests, so have enough copies for yourselves as well.

## Using honey, not vinegar, to get what you want

You may want to open your birth plan with statement making clear that you know birth doesn't always go according to plan but that these requests are for your ideal birth. This explanation may help with hospital staff who find birth plans pretentious. (Not all health practitioners have embraced the idea of birth plans.)

Avoid writing a birth plan that is aggressive or deeply critical of other birthing choices. For example, if you're planning a natural childbirth, don't bash medication or women who choose medication in your birth plan. Some members of your birth team have likely given birth themselves, and possibly insulting their choices isn't going to get them on your side!

Instead, be assertive but polite. Use phrases like "I plan," "I intend," or "I request," instead of "I refuse" or "I insist." On the other hand, don't be too wishy-washy either. For example, don't write, "If it's okay with you, I'd like to avoid an episiotomy." Instead write, "Do not give me an episiotomy unless medically necessary. I prefer to tear naturally instead."

Try to be as positive as you can. Instead of saying, "I want to avoid all pain drugs," you can say, "I plan to labor and deliver using natural coping techniques." On the other hand, if there's no way to phrase a request in the positive, just state your wish clearly. For example, "Please don't offer me pain medication; I will ask if I feel the need for it."

## Focusing on your most important wishes

Although you may be tempted to include every possible birth-plan option you find in this book (or on the Internet), if you don't feel strongly about an issue, leave it out. Without unnecessary details in the plan, your birth team can focus on what's most important. Plus, an extremely long list of requests is less likely to be read and taken seriously.

Another downside to including requests you don't really care much about is that if your birth team asks you about an issue in your birth plan and you respond, "Oh, I don't really care about that," then they may consider the rest of your plan optional.

To emphasize your requests, add some personal information when possible. For example, if you want an epidural right away because a previous birth went traumatically too fast, write that in your plan. Staff is more likely to remember your request, too, because people remember stories better than lists.

## Knowing your birth location's policies and capabilities

When deciding on your preferences, you need to keep in mind what options are and aren't available at your birthing location. If your doctor absolutely won't allow something or the hospital has a policy against it, don't bother asking for it in your birth plan. (Keep in mind the points we raise in the earlier section "Deciding on the Big Birth Issues First: Location and Attendants.") If you write in your birth plan that you want a water birth but your chosen birth location doesn't have birthing pools or doesn't allow water birth, you will be disappointed and the staff will get the impression you haven't done your homework. This conflict will reflect poorly on the rest of your plan as well.

## Considering fonts, photos, and other practical details

Creating a birth plan out of collage pictures you cut out of magazines may seem like a creative and fun activity, but that isn't the best way to clearly make your requests to the birthing team! Here are some nitty-gritty details to consider as you write your plan:

- ✔ **Keep your plan to one or two pages:** A one-page plan is best, and a two-page plan is the upper limit. The less there is to read, the more likely staff is to take the time to look through it.

- ✔ **Put your basic information at the very top:** Your name, your partner's name, your medical practitioner's name, and any essential birth guests, like your doula's name, should appear at the very top of the plan.

- ✔ **Use standard, clear fonts:** Stick to fonts that are easy to read, like Times New Roman or Arial. An elaborate font may look super cool, but your goal is readability — not artistic expression.

- ✔ **Use as few words as possible:** Although you should say what you need to be clear, avoid writing long paragraphs. A birth plan is not a research paper! Each paragraph should be concise, with just two to four sentences, for easy reading.

✔ **Consider using bullet points:** Bullet points can make reading your birth plan easier. You may also use bold font to emphasize your most important requests.

Although it's not required, attaching a small photo of yourself and your partner can be nice touch.

# Reviewing Sample Birth Plans

Checking out sample birth plans can help you write your own. You can find hundreds (and probably thousands!) of birth plan examples on the Internet; just search for "birth plan examples" or "sample birth plans." Here, we provide two sample birth plans to help you write your own. Remember that your plan will be unique to your situation and your preferences, and these sample birth plans aren't the "ideal" — they're just one way of doing them.

## Sample natural-birth hospital plan

**Mother and father's names:** Jane and John Smith; **Doula:** Rebecca Birthhappy; **Doctor's name:** Dr. Joe Shmoe

**Our ideal birth wish:** We plan to use natural soothing methods to cope with labor and delivery. Our wish is to allow birth to progress with as little intervention as possible. I had a beautiful natural birth in the past, and I hope to have another. Thank you in advance for your help and cooperation.

**How we plan to cope:** I have studied Lamaze and the Bradley Method. Comforting methods I hope to use include: music, imagery, massage, aromatherapy, movement and position changes, water therapy, natural breathing, hot and cold packs, and deep-relaxation exercises.

**Monitoring and cervical checks:** I want to remain as active as possible throughout labor. I consent to an initial monitoring strip for 20 minutes and then once every hour for 10 minutes, as I've discussed previously with my doctor. I consent to a cervical check upon admission and then further checks every four hours, or upon my request, by nonstudent hospital staff only.

**Labor augmentation:** I wish to labor without arbitrary time restrictions. I do not want my bag of waters broken prematurely. If birth must be sped up, I prefer to try movement and nipple stimulation before Pitocin. If Pitocin is necessary, please start at the lowest dose possible.

**IV fluids and hydration:** I consent to a saline lock; I do not want IV fluids unless medically necessary. I intend to drink clear fluids throughout labor, including sports drinks, herbal tea, and water. My doctor has approved this plan.

**Pushing stage:** I intend to push in a position that feels right at the time, possibly supported squatting with the help of my doula and partner. I wish to push instinctively, and I prefer quiet voices and dim lights as I push. I wish to tear naturally, and I do not consent to an episiotomy, unless medically necessary.

**Baby's birth:** I want my baby placed on my chest or in my arms immediately after birth and all initial evaluations performed while in my arms. My husband wishes to announce the gender of the baby. Please don't give my baby a bath. I want to cut the cord; please do not clamp the cord until it stops pulsating.

**Baby shots:** I do not want my baby to receive the hep-B vaccine or antibiotic eye drops. Please discuss with me any other tests and shots.

**Baby feeding and rooming-in:** I intend to breast-feed my baby and want full rooming-in. Do not give my baby artificial nipples or formula supplementation without discussing the issue with me first.

**Cesarean section:** In a nonemergency situation, we want any suggestion of cesarean section explained to us in detail, giving us the risks, potential benefits, any alternatives, and an understanding of what happens if we decline. If cesarean section is necessary, I want my doula to be with me. I prefer the drape to be lowered so I can watch the birth, and as long as the baby is not in distress, I want to breast-feed my baby with my doula's help on the surgical table as soon as possible.

## Sample scheduled cesarean birth plan

**Mother and father's names:** Jane and John Smith; **Grandmother-to-be:** Sarah Parker; **Doctor's name:** Dr. Joe Shmoe

**Our birth wishes:** We wish for our scheduled cesarean section to go as smoothly possible for our baby and ourselves. We are nervous about the procedure and appreciate any staff support. Thank you.

**Birth guest:** I would like my mother, Sarah Parker, to be by my side during the cesarean section. Please inform my husband in the waiting area of the baby's birth and my well-being as soon as possible after the birth. I would like my husband and mother with me during recovery.

**Baby's birth:** Please don't announce the baby's gender; I would like to announce the gender myself. Please hand the baby to my mother after evaluating and cleaning him up. I request one arm free to touch my baby.

**Placenta:** Please save the placenta. We hope to plant the placenta in our backyard under a tree.

**Sutures:** Please use double sutures, to increase the possibility of having a successful VBAC in the future.

**Baby's feedings and rooming:** I plan to bottle-feed my baby along with some breast-feeding. I would like partial rooming-in, with my baby sleeping in the nursery the first night. Afterward, I would like full rooming-in.

**Baby's shots and circumcision:** We don't want the hospital to perform a circumcision. We are undecided on which vaccinations to give our baby. Please discuss with us any shots before you perform them.

# Chapter 19

# Advocating for Your Plan and Working with Your Team

*M*ost people don't want to deal with a lot of drama during labor. This time is filled with enough drama even without any complications. But any time you stand up for what you want, especially in the face of authority and rules and regulation, you may become anxious and upset. In this chapter, we show you how to have the birth you want without arguing with the other people going on this journey with you, whether they're hospital staff, friends, or family.

## Working with the Hospital Staff

When you're planning who should be at your baby's birth, the hospital staff, outside of your medical practitioner, may not even cross your mind. But hospital staff members, especially the nursing staff, can have a big impact on how your birth goes. A decade ago, few couples wrote birth plans and those who did might have been met with resistance. But birth plans are more common now, and hospitals today realize that patients are also consumers who should be allowed to have some say in their care.

Even so, getting what you want from the staff isn't always easy, but you'll certainly get more by working with the hospital staff, especially your nurse, than by coming in as an adversary.

## *Meeting your nurse*

Your nurse will be a big part of your labor team, and she — most labor and delivery nurses are women — is the one person you won't meet before the delivery or be able to personally choose. You can only hope that your personalities and philosophies mesh.

Many nurses work 12-hour shifts, which can be a good thing if you really like your nurse and not so good if you don't. If there's anything worse than having a nurse you've really bonded with go off-shift and meeting someone new just before you deliver, it's having a nurse who you don't like — and you're sure it's mutual — for 12 full hours.

Your best move is to get off on the right foot with your nurse, but that's not always easy when you're under stress. To make the most of your first meeting and help ensure that the rest of your time together goes well, remember the following basic facts:

- ✔ **Unless you have an unusual obstetrician, you'll be spending way more time with your labor nurse than with your OB.** If you have a midwife, she may spend more time with you than your nurse. (Most midwives in the hospital are also nurses.)

- ✔ **Your nurse understands that you're in labor.** She'll wait while you breathe through a contraction before asking another question. And she'll understand if you're not all that polite when answering them. There's nothing you can say that will scare her off.

- ✔ **Some questions only you can answer.** Hospitals may insist on you and only you answering certain things. In some hospitals, certain questions, like questions about spousal abuse, must be asked without your partner in the room.

- ✔ **Nurses are people.** They need to eat and hit the bathroom once in a while. Most have at least one other labor patient, and if things are really busy, maybe more than one other. If she's not in your room immediately when you need her, it's probably not her fault.

- ✔ **Most nurses really like their jobs and like laboring families.** They're prepared to meet you more than halfway to make your experience a positive one.

- ✔ **Many nurses don't like birth plans, for various reasons.** Don't let that stop you from presenting yours, with a positive and nonadversarial attitude. Birthing plans really make nurse's jobs a little easier, because they know what you want from the start, but they often don't realize that.

- ✔ **You don't have to be new best friends with your nurse.** If you have support people who will take care of many of your needs, you'll probably have less involvement with your nurse.

> ✔ **If you start off on the right foot, things will be easier for everyone.** Introduce yourself, say something nice if you have it in you during labor, and act confident but not belligerent about your birth plan. If you've ordered a birthing pool to be delivered ahead of your arrival, you can rest assured that the staff already knows who you are. Doing things outside of the normal procedures upsets some nurses, but that's their problem, not yours.

## Presenting your birth plan

You'll want to give your doctor or midwife a copy of the birth plan before you go into labor, but it's up to you to bring it in and present it to the hospital staff. Be sure to bring a few extra copies as well, for shift changes.

Mention that you have a birth plan when you first get to the hospital and hand a copy to the first person you meet in labor and delivery so your nurse knows your wishes from the beginning. When she begins asking you the usual hospital-stay questions about your childhood diseases and surgeries, check that she's received a copy. Don't act like you're giving her marching orders, but also don't act like your birth plan isn't important. If you're not up to the task, let your support person go over your birth plan with the necessary staff.

## Waiting for your doctor

When you get to the hospital, you may wonder where your doctor is. Although some OBs may appear at their patients' side as soon as they're admitted and stay there the whole time, we've never met one. Most doctors multitask, checking the patients who delivered yesterday and attending other patients in labor at the same time.

As soon as he arrives or has a minute, your doctor will be in to see you. If you go into the hospital in the middle of the night and you aren't in active labor, he may not arrive until the next morning. Getting to know your nurse is important, because she's your liaison and the advocate for you with your doctor. She'll tell him how your labor is progressing, how the baby's heart rate looks on the fetal monitor, and if you're asking for pain medication.

Nearly all doctors arrive in your room in time for delivery, but sometimes not much more. And occasionally they manage to miss a delivery because they're tied up elsewhere. Often, another doctor will fill in for your doctor until he gets there.

# Breaking the Rules (Nicely!)

Most hospital regulations aren't really laws; they're more like strong suggestions of what the hospital would really like you to do. For instance, no law says you have to have an IV in labor, but many staff members will say you need one like it's a legal obligation. You can refuse procedures you really don't want, but it pays to do so nicely and in a way that doesn't get you kicked out of the hospital.

## Turning down procedures

Most of the time, your doctor is the one who will want to do certain procedures, so you need to sit down with him beforehand to go over your list of procedures that you don't want unless absolutely necessary. The handling of routine procedures will probably form the bulk of your birth plan. The following procedures and regulations generate the most concern:

- **Placing an IV:** This procedure probably tops most laboring women's list of things they don't really want. Although your doctor may not be willing to forgo an IV altogether in case you need an emergency cesarean, he may be willing to compromise on a heparin lock, a device that goes into your vein and provides immediate access without the fluid bag and tubing.

- **Staying NPO:** *Nil per os* is Latin for nothing by mouth. Most hospitals cut off your food and drink supply and offer nothing more than ice chips until you've delivered your baby. The reasoning behind this policy is that you could aspirate if you need an emergency C-section under general anesthesia. (Do you get the feeling that everything hospitals do centers around C-section liabilities?) You may also vomit in labor, but many women vomit in labor anyway. Many women come into the hospital after just eating something; there's nothing magical about walking through the hospitals doors that precludes eating or drinking. See Chapter 10 for more on eating and drinking during labor.

- **Regulating visitors:** Visitor regulations are more likely to bother your friends and family than they do you. In most hospitals today, visiting regulations have been greatly relaxed in the last decade, but they still often limit the number of people in the delivery room and the age of visitors. Talk to both your doctor and hospital management if you want more visitors or younger visitors than hospital rules allow.

- **Monitoring the baby:** Most doctors want to monitor you for a period of time when you first arrive and at intervals thereafter, depending on whether you're high or low risk. Although some hospitals have new wireless technology that can monitor the baby without hooking you up to a cumbersome machine, this technology is expensive and not many hospitals have it. Negotiate fetal monitoring time with your doctor ahead of time and state it clearly in your birth plan. See Chapter 12 for more on monitoring labor.

✔ **Augmenting labor:** When your doctor shakes his head and says your labor isn't progressing and you need oxytocin (Pitocin) to get your labor moving, you may have difficulty refusing. After all, he's the expert in these matters, and you probably want this whole thing over quickly, too! In some cases, you may ask to forgo the oxytocin altogether for a couple more hours. See Chapter 13 for more on labor augmentation.

✔ **Breaking your water:** The only time that intentionally breaking your water is necessary is to put an internal monitoring clip on the baby's head. The procedure doesn't necessarily speed up labor, and it may make contractions more painful. Discuss this topic beforehand with your practitioner and put in your birth plan.

## Refusing student doctors and nurses

If you're delivering at a teaching hospital, you may have trouble getting away from student nurses, interns, or medical residents. They don't act without supervision, although teaching hospital residents often attend to patients overnight when private physicians go home. And if you go to a clinic, you're very likely to see more of the OB resident than the attending. In any case, contrary to what you see on TV, hospital residents do not push a baby's head back in and do an emergency cesarean in the ER when the baby's shoulder won't come out without an attending doctor present.

You don't have to allow the resident or a student nurse to practice her skills on you. Your doctor may ask the resident on call to check you and manage your labor until he gets there; ask your doctor ahead of time what his policy is on residents following his patients. If you'd rather not have the resident deliver your baby, even with the OB present, make that clear also. Or don't choose a teaching hospital.

Refusing to have a student nurse with you is a little easier. A student nurse won't be taking care of you without supervision from an experienced OB nurse, but you still may rather not have two sets of hands doing vaginal exams or suffer through the student nurse's newly learned IV skills. If you're a magnanimous and generous person who sympathizes with how hard learning a skill is without practice, you can agree to let a student nurse be there, but maintain the right to say when enough is enough.

Two IV tries and you're out. Many nurses follow this rule themselves anyway; both the nurse and the patient have lost confidence after two tries. You may also be agreeable to having one student nurse with you — but not the whole class.

## Getting along while getting your way

Most people want to be liked, even when they're in the middle of a trying situation such as labor. Some women in particular tend to be people-pleasers; they don't want to appear rude, and they don't want to make waves. If you're that type of person, let your birth plan do the talking for you rather than trying to explain what you want and why.

"That's in my birth plan" is all you have to say when someone tries to coerce you into something you don't want. If the birth plan doesn't talk loud enough, let your partner or other support person voice your wishes if you're not up to fighting about it.

On the other hand, if you're naturally aggressive and feisty, you might come across as an unlikeable troublemaker. You won't be neglected if the staff doesn't like you — you'll still get good care. But you may not get the little extras that can make labor more pleasant, such as an extra pillow or a blanket right out of the warmer.

Nurses are people, too, and the extra niceties take more time and effort on their part, maybe even taking away from their break or lunch time. Most nurses will go more than the extra mile for you if they like you. It's okay to be the squeaky wheel as long as you grease the wheel with honey.

# Dad-to-Be, It's Your Time to Shine!

As the dad-to-be, you may think you get off easy, and in many ways, you do. Giving birth to a baby is certainly harder than witnessing the birth! However, you're not completely off the hook, and some may argue you have a trickier role: to support and advocate for your laboring partner. Advocacy requires being vocal even when going with the flow may be easier, whether or not it's what you want. Supporting a laboring woman — especially if you're her partner — requires dedication and thick skin (to tolerate the curses that may come your way when she's deep in labor). In this section, we give you some guidance as you navigate these treacherous waters of labor and delivery.

## Advocating for the mom-to-be

Many dads-to-be wonder whether they have a real role during labor and may worry they'll feel out of place in the labor room. One vital role to take on is speaking up to make sure your partner gets the things she needs and isn't subject to procedures she doesn't want. Laboring women frequently struggle with advocating for themselves, given that 99 percent of their energy is going to labor. As the one who knows your partner best and loves her deeply, you can fill this important role with some determination and basic preparation. Here are many ways to be a great advocate for your partner:

- **Know the birth plan:** Hopefully you're not reading the birth plan for the first time on delivery day. Although you may be tempted to leave the birth planning to your partner, to best advocate for her you must know what she wants and why.

- **Support her when a change in plan is necessary:** Just as knowing the plan is important, so is remaining flexible to your partner's changing needs and desires. Maybe she hoped for a natural birth but now she's begging for an epidural. Your job is to support her change of heart. You're advocating for *her,* not for *the-original-plan-that-was-never-a-contract.*

- **Keep guests in check:** If guests are getting rowdy, you should take the reins and firmly but kindly ask them to leave for a few moments. When you have space and privacy, you can discuss with your partner whether she wants the guests back later or not at all. See later section "Politely Removing Troublemakers," for more.

- **Maintain the environment of the room:** Ensuring a good environment for your partner includes controlling the crowd and taking note of lighting and hallway noise. If your partner wanted hushed voices during the delivery, specific music played, or dimmed lights, make it your job to remember and request it from the birth team.

- **Be a squeaky wheel:** Not to your partner, but to the birth team. Especially if you're having a hospital birth, staff gets busy, and your request for the squat bar or an extra blanket may be forgotten. Kindly speak up and make sure your partner gets what she needs.

- **Ask questions with the plural** *we:* When a woman is deep in labor land, asking questions about possible interventions can be difficult. You'll need to ask questions, like, "We were wondering why you're suggesting this particular next step." You can also ask for time alone to discuss the situation (if it's not an emergency), allowing your partner unpressured time and space to think.

- **Remind staff of the plan at appropriate times:** If your partner wanted to delay weighing and cleanup of the baby and you see a nurse whisking away your healthy baby, kindly but firmly remind her of the birth plan. With so many laboring women, the birth team may unintentionally forget. Ask politely and most attendants will be glad you reminded them.

## Supporting your partner in labor

The other big role many dads-to-be play is supporting mom-to-be as she labors. You may be excited or wary about this aspect of labor and delivery. If you don't think you can handle supporting her, then hopefully you've discussed this together and assigned a doula or another person to the main role, or at least found someone to work together with you. Whether you're going at this alone or with some backup support, here are some labor-support tips to keep in mind:

- **Put away the whistle:** The term "labor coaching" is rather unfortunate, as it brings to mind personal trainers or football coaches. Unless your partner says this style of support is what she wants, please banish this image from your mind. You need to support her — not "train" her!

- **Tap into many resources to supply your comfort tool box:** Don't go into labor thinking you can figure it out as you go along. You need resources, like childbirth education classes (see Chapter 5). Be sure to check out the comfort and movement techniques in Chapters 8 and 9.

- **Practice labor-support techniques before the birth:** Childbirth education classes give you lots of techniques to try and a little practice time, but if you really want to feel comfortable during labor, practice at home, too. Practice can be intimate — massage, anyone?

- **Remain flexible to changes:** A cool cloth on her forehead may have felt great an hour ago, but if now she's screaming at you not to touch her, go with the flow. Some techniques that you tried out before labor may also not feel right during labor. Be open to change.

- **Encourage her to move and change positions:** When in pain, the instinct is to freeze and not move around, but this is the opposite of what's best during labor. Gently encourage her to move or at least change positions occasionally. See Chapter 9 for more on this. If she has an epidural, contact the nurse to help her change positions. (Don't do it yourself.)

- **Be her rock (even if you feel more like gelatin):** Everyone understands that childbirth isn't just a big time for Mom — it's also a huge moment for you! That said, when supporting your partner, try to put on a strong, confident appearance. Seeing you strong and steady will help her feel safe and more confident.

- **Offer verbal support:** Things like, "You're doing great," or "You look beautiful," or "Just keep breathing with me," can really help. If you're not sure what to say, just say, "I love you."

- **Don't take insults personally:** Many laboring mothers say things to their partners during labor that they later regret. That's not her talking; it's the pain and the hormones. Try not to take what she says personally.

- **Use a doula to your advantage:** Some couples hire a doula to act as the main support, but others hire a doula to help coach the dad-to-be to be a better support. Be sure to express to the doula before labor how you would like her to support you and your partner.

- **Take care of yourself:** You don't want to pass out from exhaustion or low blood sugar. Drink frequently, eat, and rest when possible. Having someone to stay with your partner while you lie down can be helpful.

- **Don't underestimate your simple presence:** You don't always have to be doing something to be supportive. Just sitting nearby can often be enough.

An epidural is not a replacement for your support and presence. Sometimes, after the epidural is placed (or planned for), the labor support team thinks Mom is fine and doesn't need encouragement, but she still does! Be there for her, whether for conversation or for moral support.

# Getting Assistance from a Doula

Doulas are experts at advocating and supporting laboring women, and if you have a doula by your side, research says you're less likely to have an intervention-filled birth and more likely to have a positive birth experience. Doulas can help advocate for you by reminding you of your rights, helping you ask questions you may not have thought to ask, and supporting your choices during labor. They can't give medical advice, but they can offer information on normal childbirth and common childbirth interventions so you can ask your medical practitioner better questions.

One great thing about doulas — they don't lose their cool. Both the laboring mom and dad-to-be are going through a major life change. They're also — obviously — directly confronting the challenges of childbirth! The doula, on the other hand, can be a calming presence.

Before the birth, many doulas will help you understand your options and write your birth plan. A few meetings before the birth are commonly part of a doula's service. These pre-birth meetings offer her time to get a better idea of the kind of birth and support you're hoping for. She may also share inside information on practitioners and birth locations.

Spending time with your doula also helps build rapport, and at least one of your meetings should be together with your partner. Whether your doula is your main labor support or working along with your partner, your doula and partner are a team. See Chapter 3 for information on hiring a doula.

The doula is there to support your birth choices — not her personal birth philosophies. Don't be afraid to change your mind during birth or hesitate to do something you assume your doula wouldn't "approve of." A good doula should remain impartial. If your doula turns out to be a bad apple, you can ask her to leave your birth at any time, just like any guest at your birth.

# Letting Family and Friends Help

Dads and doulas aren't the only ones who can support you — you can also get a little bit of help from your friends, as the Beatles so aptly said. In Chapter 6, we explain some ways to evaluate who to invite to the birth. Be sure to take into consideration the information in that chapter before assigning helping roles to particular friends and family members.

With that said, here are the many ways friends and family can support and advocate for you during birth:

- **Laboring support:** Labor coaching (sans whistle, of course) isn't only for dads! A friend, sister, or mother can also be a labor support person. Remember that having given birth isn't enough to make someone a good labor partner; taking a childbirth education class with you is important.

- **Supporting the dad-to-be:** Especially if he's taking an active role to support laboring mom, the dad-to-be needs support, too! He needs someone to grab him a sandwich, bring him a cup of coffee, or stand in while he runs to the bathroom or takes a much-needed power nap.

- **Taking photos or video:** Ideally, if you want to record your birth, a friend or family member should do the picture taking. It allows you and the dad-to-be to concentrate on what's most important — the birth itself! See Chapter 22 for more on recording the birth.

- **Watching after the older children:** In Chapter 6, we discuss the option of having your older kids attend the birth. Be sure someone is at the birth to support and watch over them. If your kids aren't attending, friends and family can hopefully watch them.

- **Playing gopher:** Friends and family can go get things that Dad or Mom need, like extra pillows, food and drink, support supplies, and so on.

# Politely Removing Troublemakers

Despite carefully deciding where to give birth, whom to hire, and whom to invite, sometimes guests and birth attendants don't behave. Thankfully, most of your choices remain open to you until the very end. If a friend or family member acts up, you have the right to ask her to leave. In this section, we give you tips on removing troublemakers from the labor room.

## Firing Nurse Ratchet or Dr. Do-Little

You're not likely to be in this situation, but you may get a nurse who really rubs you the wrong way — or vice versa. Maybe you started off on the wrong foot and, despite efforts on both your parts, you're still not on the same page. Or your nurse may be actively hostile to the type of labor you want. Whatever the reason, you may have to fire your nurse.

Getting rid of a nurse is never easy, and you may not know where to start. If you're at the end of your rope with Nurse Ratchet, try the following steps:

1. **Talk to the nurse:** Suggest a change in caregivers; it's easier for her to get a coworker to switch patients than it is to locate the labor-and-delivery

manager or nursing supervisor and demand a new nurse. This conversation can be painful and embarrassing, and it may take more energy than you have at the moment.

2. **Talk to your doctor:** If your doctor is in the hospital, you can ask him to do the dirty work. Doctors generally have no trouble marching up to the nurse's station and demanding that another nurse take care of his patient. He's also more likely to get his demands met than you are.

3. **Speak to the charge nurse, floor manager, or nursing supervisor:** If your doctor isn't there and you can't get your nurse to switch patients, one of these higher-ups can help you. The charge nurse makes the assignments and is the person most likely to be able to make a change. The floor manager and nursing supervisor can put pressure on the charge nurse, if need be, but things don't usually go so far.

If you feel a need to fire your doctor or midwife in the middle of labor, you're in a very difficult situation. Most doctors will not take on a patient in the middle of labor — they don't know you or anything about you, and they don't want to step on their colleague's toes. If your doctor has a partner who is willing to come and finish your delivery, you're very fortunate. If your hospital has a midwifery program, you can ask to have the midwife take over your care. If your hospital has an OB clinic, the clinic doctors will care for you just as if you had come into the hospital with no prenatal care. Keep in mind that some private practitioners also cover the clinic; you could end up back with your "old" doctor. Midwives are more likely to understand personality clashes and let another midwife take over.

Choose your practitioner carefully during pregnancy to decrease the possibly of ending up in this awkward situation.

## Asking difficult family and friends to leave

In Chapter 6, we lay out some guidelines to consider when deciding who to invite to the birth. Even if you've carefully considered your guests, the fact is that you can't know how they'll act in the labor room until they're there. Sometimes Ms. Cool-and-Collected becomes Ms. Ball-of-Anxiety when a moaning, laboring woman is on a bed nearby — especially if that woman is her daughter or very best friend.

You only need one reason to ask someone to leave the room: Their presence makes you feel uncomfortable in that moment. As discussed in Chapter 8, emotions play a key role in coping with childbirth, and even in how labor progresses. Many women's labors slow down when arriving at the hospital for this very reason, because those very moments can raise anxiety. Your comfort comes before the feelings of your guests.

If you need birth guests out of your room, you or your partner can kindly ask them to leave, perhaps saying you'd like to be alone now. Or you can ask your doula or nurse to deliver the news. A nice nurse may even be willing to tell them a white lie, claiming hospital policy requires them to leave now.

If you feel guilty about asking family or friends to leave, or worry that the decision will haunt you later, remember that tomorrow you'll hopefully have a brand new baby in your arms. Adorable babies tend to melt away previously hurt feelings, and your exiled guests probably won't mention the labor room incident at all.

## Kicking out the dad-to-be

The labor room is full of stress and hormones, and not just Mom's! While dads-to-be usually handle the labor room appropriately, a time may come when having Dad step outside, even if only for a moment or two, may be best for everyone. Following are a few reasons you or someone on the birth team may decide to kick out the dad-to-be:

- ✔ **He desperately needs a break but refuses to take one:** Some dads insist on being Super Dad, able to leap small hospital beds in a single bound. Even Super Dads need to eat and drink and use the bathroom sometimes. Having someone else there to support Mom while he takes a break can help, but sometimes Dad needs a firm but kind push out of the room. Reassuring him you'll survive while he's gone may help.

- ✔ **His anxiety is making you anxious:** Most dads have anxiety, and most moms can handle it. However, if the anxiety is out of control to the point where you want to rip his hair out, you may ask him to go for a short walk until he calms down a bit. Again, ask lovingly.

- ✔ **He's arguing — a lot:** Some men become argumentative when they get nervous. Not eating enough can also make dads agitated. If there's a lot of arguing back and forth, maybe Dad needs to take a break, grab something to eat, and come back when he's ready to behave himself.

- ✔ **He tries to force you (or prevent you) from making birth choices:** This unfortunate situation is uncommon, but some dads get really tied up in the birth options and forget (or want to forget) that Mom is having the baby — not him. If he's pushing you to do or not do something, remember that it's your body and your choice.

# Chapter 20

# Allowing for Flexibility in Your Birth Plan and Recovery

*Y*ou know what they say: Plans are meant to be broken. Although no one writes a birth plan with the intention of breaking it, thinking of your birth plan as your ideal wishes may help in the event that you change your mind or things go wrong. Some changes in plan are inconsequential — a decision to keep the lights bright instead of dimming them — whereas other birth-plan changes can have lasting impacts. A negative birth experience (which can occur even if your birth plan is followed) raises your risk of postpartum depression (PPD), and some traumatic births lead to posttraumatic stress disorder (PTSD). In this chapter, we discuss changing your birth plans in the moment, making difficult decisions during labor, coping with birth disappointment, and recognizing and treating PTSD and PPD.

## Changing Your Mind: The Plan Isn't Written in Stone

After spending so much time researching your options and writing your birth plan, you may be surprised that we tell you to view your plan as flexible. In fact, writing that very thing in your plan — that this plan is your ideal vision, open to change depending on circumstance — is a good idea. Critics of birth plans say there's no point putting so much energy into a document that's bound to be broken, but we say birth plans are not contracts but road maps. Would you fail to plan for a road trip if you knew you might take a few detours? Of course not.

Remember that your birth plan is not only your ideal birth hopes but also a way to research your options so that if and when you change your mind, you're making an informed decision. In this section, we give you some guidance on common changes of plan.

## Doing what feels right in the moment

You've spent months dreaming of a water birth, but when the time comes to push, you really don't feel like climbing into a birthing pool. You feel quite happy pushing in a squat on the floor. That's okay! How you imagine birth doesn't always turn out to be the experience you want in the moment. Even if you've given birth before, what worked great with baby number one may feel totally wrong with baby number two.

Here are some common issues that moms change their mind about mid-labor:

- **Pushing a certain way:** Squat bars sound cool in theory, but in action, they may not feel right. How to push is a decision best made in the moment, but by putting together your birth plan, at least you know all your options.

- **Having your kids at the birth:** You may have loved the idea of having your kids at the birth before labor, but when it starts, maybe the mere sound of their voices is making you crazy. That's okay. You — and your kid — can change plans at any moment.

- **Laboring or delivering in water:** Coauthor Rachel dreamed of laboring in water, but by the time the tub was ready, it was time to push and she didn't want to move. You may have planned to only labor in water but when you're in there decide (with your medical practitioner's approval) that you now want to deliver in water, too.

- **Having guests in the room:** Your fantasy of having your mother and grandmother by your side during labor may not play out as beautifully as you hoped. You can always ask guests to leave if things don't work out. See Chapter 19 on politely kicking out guests.

- **Having a natural birth or an epidural:** Many moms who hope for a natural birth decide in the end to get an epidural, though some women plan on an epidural but then decided to go all natural. We discuss more on this subject in the next section, "Wavering on natural birth plans — when to hold on, when to give in."

Not having the birth you dreamed of isn't a failure on your part. Sometimes you need to let go of your vision of how birth should have gone and hold onto the beauty of how the birth actually played out. A change in plans isn't a "bad birth" — just a different one.

## *Wavering on natural birth plans: When to hold on, when to give in*

If you change your mind about going au natural in the middle of labor, you're far from alone. Women change their minds about getting an epidural all the time, for a variety of reasons. Sometimes they just weren't prepared or supported well enough, but often they find that they can't cope with labor as well as they'd hoped. Because every birth is different, even a woman who had a great natural childbirth for one baby may decide the second time around it's too much to handle.

On the other hand, some women waver on their plans but decide to keep on going a bit longer, only to get a second wind and have the natural birth they planned on after all. Here are some things to consider before deciding to get the epidural:

- ✔ **Try to make it through just five more contractions:** Sometimes having a goal in mind makes it easier to keep going. You may find by the fifth contraction you're feeling more confident again.

- ✔ **Change your coping method:** You may find relief by trying a new massage, getting in the birth pool or shower, or just switching positions and taking a short walk around the room. A change can help.

- ✔ **Find out if you're almost done:** If you feel you just can't get through labor anymore, you may want a nurse or medical practitioner to check your dilatation. You may be in transition or just about ready to push. Knowing you're close to the end may renew your strength.

If you do decide to get an epidural, it doesn't make you a bad mother or mean you failed in any way. Deciding to get an epidural when you can't cope anymore isn't bad — it's smart. Don't let anyone tell you otherwise — including yourself.

# Making Important Decisions at an Impossible Time

Although everyone hopes to have a delivery that goes off without a hitch, problems can arise during labor and delivery. If it happens to you, you may be asked to make decisions at a time when you feel most vulnerable. Often your partner and other support people aren't much help. Your partner may not have taken the time to really learn about labor and delivery, and your other support people may have outdated or erroneous information about childbirth. At a time like this, a doula, a good nurse, and — most important of all — a medical practitioner you trust implicitly can help you make crucial decisions.

## Keeping calm

When the atmosphere around you is electric with tension, maintaining your cool is hard — especially when you're the one in labor. Some situations are true medical emergencies with very little time to discuss options, but most issues that arise in labor don't require immediate action.

If the situation you're in does require an immediate response, rest assured that your medical practitioner will make the urgency abundantly clear. If your baby's heart rate suddenly drops or you start bleeding heavily, the staff will roll you on your side, put an oxygen mask on your face, turn up your IV fluids and, in some cases, insert a Foley catheter in case you need a cesarean delivery. Your doctor may ask you to sign a consent for a procedure, such as a cesarean section, but if you or your baby suddenly develop issues that require immediate action, the staff will act quickly, telling you that they're putting in a breathing tube so the baby can breathe (or taking some other action) rather than asking.

 Keeping your cool in an emergency situation benefits you and your baby. Arguing about the procedures or demanding time to think about them can take valuable minutes — time you or your baby may not have. Although you deserve to know what's going on, long explanations or discussions can't always precede action. Having a medical practitioner you trust goes a long way in an emergency.

# Asking questions before agreeing to interventions

Because most situations that arise during labor don't require breakneck action, you have time to ask questions and clarify the pros and cons. The situation that occurs most commonly in labor is a decision to do a cesarean section. Most C-sections aren't done for emergencies like fetal distress but rather for "failure to progress," meaning your labor hasn't gone the way the textbooks say it should, or the way your doctor feels it should.

If your medical practitioner suggests doing a C-section or other intervention — and it's not an emergency — ask the following questions:

- **Is a C-section absolutely necessary at this moment for my safety or my baby's?** Obviously, if she says yes, you're not going to argue. A real emergency situation is usually quite obvious by the increase in the level of activity and tension in your room.

- **Can we first try some other intervention?** For failure to progress, you can try changing position, starting oxytocin (Pitocin), or walking to get labor moving. In some cases, getting an epidural could allow enough relaxation to bring your baby down.

- **What are the potential outcomes if we don't do it now?** Can you revisit the situation in an hour? What about longer than an hour? For example, if you develop a fever in labor, a not-uncommon side effect of a long labor and/or epidural anesthesia but also a potential sign of infection, you may ask how long is it safe to wait before doing a cesarean.

# Handling your worst fears: Stillbirth and birth defects

It's hard to imagine a worse feeling than entering the hospital in labor and watching the staff search in vain for your baby's heartbeat or facing a sudden silence in the delivery room after your baby's birth. Facing a stillbirth or news that your baby has a birth defect at the time you expected a joyous experience can tear at your heart like few other pains.

### Reacting to stillbirth

If your baby has no heartbeat when you reach the hospital, everything in your birth plan radically changes. You may opt for an epidural instead of delivering naturally. You also may consider labor augmentation to hasten delivery.

However your decisions change, take time to grieve in private and to make any decisions that need to be made in your own time. You may want close friends or family at the hospital so they can see the baby after birth, or you may instead decide to dismiss your support people so you and your partner can be alone with him. You may want to dress your baby in one of the outfits you bought and take time to hold him. Perhaps you want to take pictures, save baby footprints or handprints, or cut a lock of your baby's hair as a keepsake. No decisions are wrong in this situation; whatever feels right to you is right. And any decisions you make can be amended as you go through labor.

### Facing birth defects

Not all birth defects are evident before birth. If your baby is diagnosed with a birth defect right after delivery, you may go through a tumultuous cascade of emotions, including disbelief, shock, anger, and grief. You may even find yourselves temporarily rejecting your baby. These reactions are neither unusual nor abnormal. As with a stillbirth, you need to grieve the loss of your healthy baby and accept the reality of your baby's situation within a very short time period under very stressful circumstances.

Take your time, if you can; limit visitors, let a nurse take the baby to the nursery while you talk to your partner, and discuss with your medical practitioner and pediatrician any decisions that need to be made immediately. For example, a baby with a severe heart defect may need to be transferred to a different hospital and undergo immediate surgery. If at all possible, see if you can accompany him to whichever hospital he goes to. It's very difficult to get news long-distance and secondhand. If going with her right away isn't possible, ask your doctor how soon you can leave the hospital.

Your nurse can be a big help in sorting through things because most labor and delivery nurses have dealt with similar situations many times.

# When Birth Doesn't Go the Way You Hoped

Most of the time, when birth plans don't go exactly as planned, the good still outweighs the not-so-good. However, if your birth experience was especially difficult or traumatic — or the birth you imagined was far from the birth you got — broken birth plans may lead to a broken heart. In this section, we discuss the feelings you may experience after a difficult birth and how to cope with them.

## Accepting the feelings you may experience

The feelings you hope to have after childbirth are elation, happiness, and relief that it's all over. However, when birth is difficult, the positive feelings may be smothered by a mess of complicated and negative feelings. Emotions you may experience after a difficult birth include:

- ✔ **Guilt:** You may feel that the bad birth experience was your fault; that your choices or your inability to cope or give birth "properly" harmed you or your baby. You may also feel guilty for feeling disappointed about the birth experience.

- ✔ **Shame:** Feelings of shame are possible, as if the birth experience makes you a bad mother or less of a woman.

- ✔ **Anger:** You may be angry at yourself, your medical practitioner, your birth location, or just in general at the entire situation.

- ✔ **Sadness:** You may cry and be easily brought to tears, feeling like you've experienced a loss.

- ✔ **Failure:** You may see the difficult birth as a failure on your part and think you failed at Motherhood 101.

- ✔ **Regret:** You may experience regret, wondering whether you could have done something differently or questioning the choices you made.

- ✔ **Fear or anxiety:** Residual anxiety and fear are possible even after the difficult birth is over. You may experience feelings of panic when thinking about the birth and have anxiety over whether you're fit to be a mother if you "couldn't even give birth properly."

If these feelings are especially intense or last for more than a few days or weeks after the birth, be sure to discuss your feelings with your doctor and seek help from a counselor or therapist. You may be experiencing posttraumatic stress disorder, which you can read more about in the section "Why Can't I Forget? Posttraumatic Stress Disorder (PTSD)," or postpartum depression, covered later in this chapter in the section "Why Am I So Depressed? Postpartum Depression (PPD)."

## Coping with difficult feelings

Some well-meaning but uninformed people may suggest that the best way to cope with a difficult birth is to, "Look at the bright side, at least you and your baby are okay." This advice doesn't work, and it often makes you feel worse. Don't ignore your own feelings. Instead, consider these coping tips:

✔ **Allow yourself time to grieve:** It's okay to cry and feel upset, even when you and your baby are healthy in the end. Feeling like you should be happy when you're not doesn't make the feelings go away. Feeling relieved you and the baby are fine now *and* feeling sadness over the birth experience is perfectly okay.

✔ **Talk about the birth:** Research has found that being able to talk to someone about the birth experience, preferably within a few days of the delivery, lowers the risk of feeling anxious and depressed weeks later. Choose someone empathetic and patient, preferably not your partner because he may feel blamed for what went wrong (even if it's obviously not his fault), which makes listening without judgment harder for him.

✔ **Write your birth story:** Taking the birth and putting it into a sequenced story can help you sort the experience out in your head. A number of websites exist just for sharing birth stories, and knowing your story is being read by others can help you feel heard and understood. For example, you can share your story at www.thelaboroflove.com/birthstories or http://pregnancy.about.com/u/sty/birthstories/reader birthstories.

✔ **Surround yourself with supportive people:** Avoid the people who tell you to just get over it; instead, try to surround yourself with supportive friends and family. Now isn't the time to be a good sport and put up with negative friends or relatives. Take care of yourself and try to spend time with people whose company you enjoy.

✔ **Take care of yourself:** All new mothers should follow this good advice, but if you've been through a difficult birth experience, getting as much sleep as you can, along with eating right, is important. When the doctor approves, getting in some exercise — even if it's only a short walk around the block with your baby in the stroller — can help improve your mood.

✔ **Air your grievances:** If your medical practitioner's actions are responsible for your negative birth experience, consider discussing the birth with her, either during a postpartum checkup or through a letter. However, be prepared that she may not react sympathetically. You may want to consider writing a letter to the hospital or birth center telling your story and even suggesting how things could have gone differently with their help.

✔ **Seek counseling:** Speaking with a trained therapist, even if only for a few sessions, can be very helpful. You don't need to have postpartum depression or posttraumatic stress to speak to a counselor, and he may be able to help you feel better faster than if you try to cope on your own.

# Why Can't I Forget? Posttraumatic Stress Disorder (PTSD)

If you find yourself unable to stop thinking about a negative childbirth experience for weeks after the birth, so much that it interferes with your daily life, you may be suffering from posttraumatic stress. Research studies have found that up to 9 percent of mothers meet the criteria for posttraumatic stress disorder (PTSD) as a result of childbirth, with up to 18 percent of women experiencing some PTSD symptoms after a traumatic birth. PTSD can develop when a baby dies or is born with a birth defect, but it can also occur after a seemingly straightforward birth with a very healthy baby.

Because PTSD is often overlooked or misdiagnosed as postpartum depression, many women go untreated. PTSD is usually associated with war veterans, terrorist attack survivors, and victims of rape. Medical practitioners and even women themselves may not realize PTSD can develop from a birth experience even if nothing blatantly traumatic happened. Although most people understand how an emergency surgery or the death of a baby can be traumatic, few understand how powerful other birth traumas — like a long, difficult birth or pushed, unwanted interventions — can be to a mother. Trauma is in the eye of the beholder.

## Identifying symptoms of PTSD

PTSD can develop when a person goes through a frightening experience during which they fear they may die or become seriously injured, during which experience they have feelings of fear, helplessness, or horror. PTSD can also develop if a person witnesses someone else (like her baby) go through such an event. Dads can also develop PTSD after witnessing their partner or baby experience a traumatic birth.

Following are some symptoms of PTSD:

- **Remembering the birth as traumatic:** A new mom with PTSD may have an intense, fearful reaction to the birth, including feelings of helplessness or horror. Mothers who develop PTSD after childbirth may report feeling an extreme loss of control.

- **Trouble sleeping and hyperawareness:** PTSD may cause trouble relaxing or sleeping and feelings of tremendous anxiety and tension.

- **Numbness of emotions:** You may not feel anything about the birth, neither good nor bad; and have difficulty feeling good feelings like love.

PTSD may cause you to feel distant from others and have difficulty bonding with your baby.

✔ **Remembering and re-experiencing birth memories vividly:** You may experience flashbacks, nightmares, or frequent remembering of the events that may be easily triggered by reminders of birth, like a television show with a pregnant character. Even your baby can remind you of the traumatic birth.

✔ **Avoiding reminders of the traumatic event:** You may not want to look at photos from the birth or not want to discuss the birth at all. The idea of having another baby may be awful. Intense feelings of fear, panic, and anxiety arise when the topic of birth comes up.

✔ **Unable to stop focusing on the birth:** Although some women with PTSD avoid discussing the birth, others are unable to stop talking about the experience. They may become obsessed with trying to understand what went wrong and why.

## *Treating PTSD*

PTSD is usually treated with talk therapy. Cognitive-behavioral therapy, EMDR (eye-movement desensitization and reprocessing), and hypnotherapy are common psychotherapies used for PTSD. Medication may also be given, either antidepressants or antianxiety drugs, though drugs alone are not enough to treat PTSD.

Even if you don't have full-blown PTSD, if thoughts of the birth are affecting your everyday life or you are fearful of future pregnancy or childbirth, speak to a mental-health professional. You don't need to suffer with your memories alone, and therapy can help. Be sure to also check out the tips for coping listed in the earlier section "When Birth Doesn't Go the Way You Hoped."

PTSD is a normal response to an abnormal situation. PTSD is not your fault, nor is it a sign of weakness. Telling a mother who has experienced a traumatic birth to "get over it" or "just stop thinking about it" isn't helpful. Another common refrain — "The most important thing is you and your baby are okay" — doesn't help either. Whether your doctor or anyone else experienced the birth as traumatic is irrelevant. If you've been traumatized by the experience, then you need professional help to heal.

# Why Am I So Depressed? Postpartum Depression (PPD)

The baby blues are practically universal; as many as 80 percent of women experience emotional ups and downs in the first few weeks after birth. And no wonder — your hormone levels shift like sand and drop like rocks after the birth of a baby. The difficult part is separating the normal emotional highs and lows from true depression, when the world seems to turn gray and you find yourself less and less interested in anything, including your baby.

Like most depressive disorders, postpartum depression is hard to recognize when you're the one going through it. Other people may spot changes in your behavior long before you do. New moms have an especially difficult time recognizing postpartum psychosis, a rare but very serious potential complication of postpartum depression.

## Recognizing the baby blues

You may notice symptoms of the baby blues within a few hours after delivery. You're so happy, you just want to hug everyone, sing at the top of your lungs and shout to the world how wonderful your life is. Then a few hours later, you start crying because your partner brought in the wrong little outfit to put on for the baby's homecoming. Or because your pants still don't fit, or because they forgot your tea at breakfast, or because your mom said the baby's ears look like your second cousin's. Just about anything can set off happiness or sadness in the first few weeks. But baby blues rarely last longer than a week or two.

Symptoms of the baby blues, which can worsen if you're not getting enough sleep, include:

- ✔ **Weepiness over things that normally wouldn't bother you:** A glass of spilled milk or a casual comment from a friend may send you into a crying jag.

- ✔ **Irritability, restlessness, or anxiety:** You may obsessively worry about money, about whether the baby is developing normally, or even about the state of the world.

- ✔ **Trouble sleeping:** As tired as you are after giving birth, you wouldn't think this could be a problem, but hormone shift can interfere with sleeping.

- ✓ **Difficulty concentrating or getting things done that you would normally accomplish easily:** In the first few weeks with your baby, just getting dressed before dinner is an accomplishment.

- ✓ **Feeling inadequate about your mothering ability:** If you're having trouble breast-feeding or dealing with any physical problems after delivery, these feelings can intensify.

## Spotting symptoms of PPD and treating it

*Postpartum depression* is different than the baby blues, but you may not notice the general worsening of the baby blues until you slide into full-blown postpartum depression. Only around one in eight new moms develop postpartum depression, often called PPD for short. In addition to being more severe, postpartum depression starts later, even several months after birth and lasts longer than baby blues.

Symptoms of PPD include:

- ✓ **Sadness or anger that affect your ability to care for your baby or yourself:** You may lose your temper easily or, more likely, not care much about anything that happens in your life.

- ✓ **Feelings of inadequacy as a new mom:** You may feel that your baby doesn't like you or that other people can care for her better than you can.

- ✓ **Disinterest in activities you used to enjoy:** You may not feel like watching a favorite TV show or talking on the phone with a good friend. Hobbies you enjoyed in the past may not seem interesting anymore.

- ✓ **Difficulty making decisions:** Even the simplest decisions, like which shoes to wear, can throw you into an emotional tailspin. Deciding what to make for dinner — if you even have the energy to cook — is impossible.

- ✓ **Fears that you might hurt the baby, accidentally or on purpose:** Of all the symptoms you have, this one may scare you the most. You may also ignore the baby or fail to care for his needs or your own.

- ✓ **Changes in appetite:** You may not feel hungry and neglect to eat, or you may feel you can't stop eating.

- ✓ **Feeling like your baby and family would be better off without you:** You may make plans to leave your family because you believe you're a bad mother, or you may tell your partner he should "find someone else."

Don't ignore PPD or assume it will go away on its own within a few weeks. You may need to take antidepressants (some of which you can take while breast-feeding) and talk to a therapist. Ignoring PPD could cost you or your baby dearly and could color your relationship with your baby for months to come.

Having PPD doesn't mean that you don't love your baby or that you won't be a good mom. PPD is a temporary situation that can be helped with proper treatment.

Some circumstances can increase your risk of developing PPD. Following are some risk factors:

- ✔ A history of depression and antidepressant use, or previous PPD

- ✔ A history of stress in the last year, including job loss, previous infertility, pregnancy complications, financial issues, or relationship difficulties

- ✔ Problems with your partner or lack of support from friends and family

- ✔ Not having planned this pregnancy

Before you deliver, talk to your partner and friends about PPD. Ask that they let you know if they have any concerns about your behavior after you have the baby. Too many times, family and friends hesitate to say anything because they're afraid they'll hurt your feelings. Although this preparation isn't something to write in a birth plan, do prepare for the possibility of PPD (especially if you have any risk factors) by giving people who care for you advance permission to bring up their concerns.

## Dealing with postpartum psychosis (PP)

Postpartum psychosis (PP) goes far beyond postpartum depression, although many of the symptoms can be the same and this disorder can develop out of PPD. PP affects just one to two out of every thousand moms. The symptoms can be very similar to bipolar disorder or schizophrenia. You have a higher risk of developing PP if you have a history of bipolar disorder or schizophrenia, if your mom or siblings experienced PP, or if you have had PP in a previous pregnancy.

If you have any of these risk factors, your risk of developing PP is as high as 25 to 50 percent. Make sure your family and friends know the symptoms to watch for if you fall into a high-risk group. You're highly unlikely to recognize the symptoms on your own. You may experience

- ✔ **Manic behavior:** It can manifest itself as inability to sleep, talkativeness, racing thoughts, confusion, inability to concentrate on one thing, feeling like you can do anything, or feelings of power and grandiosity. You may lose your inhibitions, act impulsively, or spend large amounts of money.

- ✔ **Depression:** As with PPD, you may feel sadness, anger, inability to cope, or lack of appetite. Your interest in your baby may be little to none (alternatively, you may develop a fierce protection toward him).

> ✔ **Psychotic symptoms:** These symptoms include voices in your head, hallucinations or delusions, and paranoia. You may feel like someone is trying to take your baby or that people are following you.

Postpartum psychosis requires immediate medical attention to keep both you and your baby safe. You will very likely require inpatient treatment to prevent harm to yourself or to others. Although a unit where you could keep your baby with you would be ideal, such facilities are rare. Family and friends will probably have to care for your baby while you're hospitalized.

Hospital treatments include antipsychotic medications, antidepressants, and group and one-on-one therapy.

Complete recovery can take six months to a year, but the acute symptoms generally last between 2 and 12 weeks. Most women make a full recovery. Dealing with the aftermath of PP can take years; you may feel like you've failed your baby or that you can't build a close relationship after being separated for a time. This worry isn't at all true. Your baby won't remember this time, and with help you can form the same close bonds with him that any other new mom would.

# Part VII
# The Part of Tens

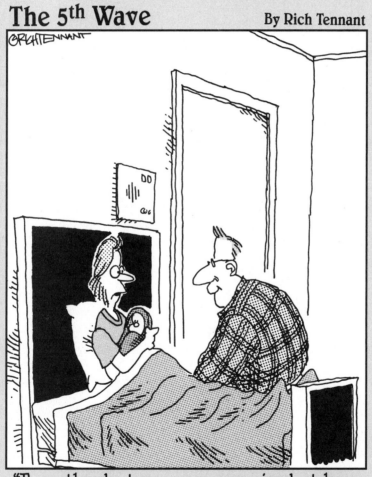

The 5th Wave          By Rich Tennant

"Even the doctors were surprised at how involved you were in there. Especially right near the end when you turned on that CD of the 'William Tell Overture.'"

## In this part . . .

For quick and easy reference, we throw out practical, fun, and interesting information about birth in small bites. In this part, we look at some techniques to try to increase the likelihood that your birth goes the way you want it to. You also get ideas for creating a record of your baby's birth that really captures the moment.

# Chapter 21

# Ten Tips for Creating a Workable Birth Plan

*W*hen faced with a blank sheet of paper and the task of creating a birth plan, your mind may go as blank as the paper before you. Why should you even have to do this? Women have been giving birth without birth plans for centuries — is this even necessary? It isn't, but it is incredibly helpful, if for no other reason than to help you clarify what you want in your own mind. In this chapter, we help you simplify the process by looking at the basic do's and don'ts of creating a birth plan and making important decisions about your baby's birth along the way.

## Do Research Your Options

What most women know about giving birth before they go through it is . . . very little. Women don't often give birth at home anymore, surrounded by female relatives. What you know about birth may be nothing more than what you've heard from your mom or your friends, all filtered through their positive or negative memories of the experience.

There's a whole big world of options for giving birth today; you're reading this book, so you're already ahead of the game! For additional information, you can search the Internet or check out a range of books available at your local library to learn about the variety of options so you know what kind of choices you should be making.

# Don't Write a Birth Plan That Reads Like a Research Paper

A birth plan should be user-friendly. The people who need to read it and follow it will not have the time to read a dissertation (or any interest in doing so) on why you want the type of birth you want and studies on different interventions. This sort of thorough document may interest you and help you make decisions, but keep your birth plan simple, easy to read, and not preachy or argumentative in any way.

# Do Discuss Your Options with Your Partner

When you're pregnant, you can easily forget that this whole experience isn't just about you. Your partner should also have some input into the birth plan. He may not be comfortable with certain choices, such as both of you slipping au natural into the birthing tub or him catching his newly born baby. He may want to be included in the whole birthing process, or he may prefer that you hire a doula to step in to coach labor and run interference.

# Don't Write Your Plan without Input from Your Other Team Members

Although having a birthing wish list is nice, you absolutely must make sure that your wish list dovetails with your medical provider's practices. There is no point in including choices that are never going to fly at your local hospital or with your doctor or midwife. Although your practitioner may be willing to deviate from his normal practices, he may have lines he won't cross. Find out where the boundaries are before you write your birth plan.

Discussing your wishes with your team also helps you evaluate whether or not you've chosen the right people so that you can change the lineup in advance. Labor is no time to realize that you've got the wrong doctor or have chosen the wrong hospital.

# Do Bring Copies of Your Birth Plan to the Hospital

Don't assume that your medical practitioner has sent copies of your birth plan ahead to the hospital so that the staff can memorize it and plan ahead for your birth. In some cases, he may have sent a copy over with your birth records, but then again, he may not have. Always bring several copies with you so you can hand them out to the people who will be following the plan — including your doctor or midwife.

# Do Give Your Nurse a Copy of Your Birth Plan

You spend more time with your nurse than any other hospital staff member, so make sure she has her own copy of your birth plan. Bring more than one for the nursing staff, because you may go through several shift of nurses if you have a long labor or your nurse gets tied up with another delivery. Present your birth plan in a positive way, without any tension or suggestion that your choices are written in stone and they'd better be followed — or else. Starting off in an adversarial position with the nursing staff will make following your birth plan more difficult. A simple, "Here's our birth plan; I've okayed everything with our doctor. Please ask if you have any questions" will suffice.

# Do Include the Obvious

Don't assume that anything goes without saying. You may think it's obvious that walking is good for you in labor and that you'll need to be out of bed and up to the bathroom whenever you want. But hospital policies may dictate otherwise. If you want to be able to eat during early labor, put that in your plan also, or expect that someone will remove your contraband food from your room, acting as if you had just tried to smuggle a dangerous criminal out of jail. Include information that you would assume everyone knows, because they may not.

# Don't Assume the Hospital Staff Will Follow Your Plan without Reminders

Hospital nurses often have more than one patient, and your doctor may also have more than one patient in labor. Although it's pleasant to think that you and your birth plan are so unique that people will remember the details without reminders, they probably won't. When Nurse Nancy appears with IV supplies piled in her arms, remind her that you're only getting a heparin lock, or no IV at all, or she'll have it in before you have a chance to protest. You don't need to yell — a gentle reminder will do.

# Do Adjust Your Plan as Needed

Giving birth requires flexibility. Circumstances change, emergencies arise, your birth tub isn't delivered or doesn't hold water, your doctor has to have an emergency appendectomy and you get the doctor's partner who doesn't believe that patients should have a voice in what happens to them — the list of things that can go wrong is endless. If things get a little mixed up or even royally messed up, do your best to keep your birth as close as you can to your ideal and don't fret if things don't go perfectly. The objective is to have your baby, not to check off all the items on your birth plan.

# Don't Assume Your Home Birth Team Will Do Whatever You Want

If you're having a home birth, don't assume that your midwife or provider has the same philosophies and views on birth that you do. Spell out the details the same way you would for a hospital birth, including who will cover if she can't be there, the option to go to the hospital at any time and the choices you have for getting there.

# Chapter 22

# Ten Ways to Preserve Birth Memories

## In This Chapter

▶ Documenting the birth through pictures and video

▶ Recording events in a journal, writing your story, or tweeting the details

*T*he birth of your child is a momentous occasion, and like other life events, you may want to record or create something to help you remember the details of this special day. In this chapter, we give you ten ways to preserve birth memories. Some are simple; some are more involved. Feel free to choose as many ideas as you like, or even combine a few together!

# Taking Photographs

Taking pictures may be the most common way to preserve birth memories. When you take pictures and how many you take is up to you. Some families decide to take the camera out only after the baby's born, whereas others want shots from the first contractions through to and including the delivery. To take great birth photos, consider the following tips:

- ✔ **Assign a photographer.** Preferably not Dad-to-be, as you'll want him in the photos and hopefully by your side. You may split the job between Dad and your doula, or give the job to a friend or family member attending the birth. Some couples hire a professional photographer for the birth, but it's essential that she know how to "fade into the background" and respect the mother's privacy.

- ✔ **Turn off the flash and take candid pictures.** The last thing you want are pictures that interfere with your birth flow. Flash can be distracting, so turn it off and tell your photographer not to ask you to pose.

- ✔ **Have two cameras with two sets of batteries and plenty of memory.** If you were hoping to get a few shots of the delivery, having a camera run out of batteries or memory at that very moment would be a big bummer! Having a second camera ready to go reduces the risk of that happening.

> ✔ **Remember that you can always throw pictures away.** Let your picture takers know whether you want G-rated, PG-rated, or X-rated shots of the birth, but remember that if the pictures come out too graphic for your tastes, you can always throw them away or delete them — but you can't go back in time and take a shot after the moment's gone.

# Recording Video

Making a video recording of the birth is a step up from taking only still pictures, and you can capture not just moments but the entire mood of the room. Video recordings can be simpler than still photographs because you can set up a tripod in a corner (in an area where the shot won't be blocked by someone's back or head!) and let it record. If you plan to record the actual delivery, you may need to get permission from your medical practitioner or birth location; because of lawsuits, some are hesitant to allow recordings of deliveries.

# Setting Out a Guest Book

For some women, birth is truly a family affair, and having friends and relatives present is part of the fun. If you're having a lot of guests at the birth, whether they're by your side or waiting down the hall, you may want to put out a guest book. You can purchase the kind of guest book used at weddings, or make your own by setting out a blank journal or notebook and pen.

You may want to write on the inside of the guest book what you'd like guests to share. Maybe you'd like them to share their blessings for you and your new baby, or maybe you'd like to hear what they will remember most from the day. Anything goes — it's your guest book!

# Making a Placenta Print

Here's something you've probably not heard of before — you can create a placenta print! The placenta is covered in veins, especially the baby/umbilical cord side, and they make a beautiful pattern on paper. You can even arrange it to look like a tree, with the umbilical cord representing the trunk.

To create a placenta print, you'll need to ask the birth team to preserve and give you your placenta. (Usually it's cremated.) Be sure to wrap the placenta in plastic wrap (bring some with you in your birth bag) and place it in the refrigerator or freezer until you're ready to make the print. You may also want to bring a gallon size plastic bag to transport the placenta home. The hospital is unlikely to allow you to keep the placenta in their refrigerator, so someone will need to bring it home shortly after the birth. (If law prohibits bringing home the placenta in your state, you can make the print in the hospital or birth center.) You'll also need: a large piece of high-quality art paper (watercolor paper works well), ink (you can use acid-free stamp ink pads, food dye, or create edible ink with beet juice), and gloves, if you don't want to get all inky.

When you're ready to make the print, unwrap the placenta and lay it out flat, veiny side up. Press ink pads along the surface until it's well covered, or gently apply food die or paints with a brush. You don't need to wash the placental blood off, as it adds color to your print! In fact, some people use only the natural blood on the placenta to create the print. Carefully press the paper down over the dyed placenta. Lift the paper gently and you have your placenta print. You can frame the print or hide it away in your closet, whatever feels right to you.

# Planting a Placenta Tree

Here's something else fun to do with your placenta: Plant it in the ground! Then plant a seedling tree in the spot where you bury the placenta. As your baby grows, the tree will also grow, a great reminder of the miracle of life and your child's birth day.

# Keeping a Journal

Especially in the early hours of birth, when you're still in the mood and head-space for writing, you may want to keep a journal. You can write down the bare birth facts, like the timing of contractions, along with your thoughts and activities. If you've planned a labor project (see Chapter 8), you can take pictures to later add to your journal entries.

You're not the only one who can keep a journal during the birth. Your partner, doula, or another birth guest to take their own notes, which you can later weave together to create one narrative. If you have a blog, you may want to post live as the birth progresses, filling in the blanks (and end, when you'll like be in no mood for blogging!) in the days after the birth.

# Collecting Mementos

Whether in a shoe box or a fancy stationary box, you can collect a number of birth-day mementoes: baby's first hat, booties, and pajamas; your ID tags from the hospital; the name card from the nursery bassinet; your labor project (or photos from your labor project); a photocopy of the birth certificate; a copy of the birth plan; your written out birth story. You can add pregnancy ultrasound pictures and even the positive pregnancy test stick, if you still have it. Some people even save the umbilical cord stump! (Because it's biodegradable, you may need to spray it with lacquer to preserve it.)

## Creating a belly cast

Creating a belly cast — a plaster model of your pregnant belly! — can be a messy but fun way to preserve pregnancy memories. Belly casts are made using supplies you can find in any craft store or pharmacy. Key supplies include rolls of plaster-casting material, petroleum jelly (to keep the cast from sticking to the fine hair on your belly), and gloves to protect your hands. After you create the belly cast, you can paint it or leave it as is. You can get complete instructions on how to make a belly cast online, or you can purchase a belly-casting kit, plus see a gallery of belly casts, at www.proudbody.com.

# Writing Your Birth Story

Writing your birth story while it's fresh in your mind can not only help you process the experience but also allow you to share it with others. You may not have time to write down the story in full in the first days after birth, so you may want to consider jotting down notes as events occur to help you remember the details. You can also write a letter to your baby about his birth day, sharing it when he's older.

If you'd like to share your story with the world, you can post and share birth stories on a number of websites. One site where you can share your story is http://pregnancy.about.com/u/sty/birthstories/readerbirth stories.

# Creating an Audio Recording

If keeping a written journal doesn't speak to you, you may consider keeping an audio diary. Consider recording your baby's first cry and first sounds as well. If you make a short audio clip of the baby's voice every so many weeks, after a year or more you can string the clips together and have a cool compilation of your child's changing voice.

# Tweeting Your Birth

Tweeting the details of your birth may be TMI (too much information) for some, but Twitter births are considered cool among birth junkies and birth activists. Pro-birth-Tweeters say it's a great way to be open and honest about real birth, and one way to share the juicy details with your online buddies. Use the hash tag #twitterbirth to include your non-followers in on the fun.

One thing to remember: Be sure to save all those tweets somewhere else as soon as possible, because Twitter isn't the most reliable storage space of information.

# Index

## • C •

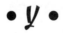

## ...ple & Mac

...ad 2 For Dummies,
...d Edition
...8-1-118-17679-5

...hone 4S For Dummies,
...1 Edition
...8-1-118-03671-6

...od touch For Dummies,
...d Edition
...8-1-118-12960-9

...c OS X Lion
...r Dummies
...8-1-118-02205-4

## ...ogging & Social Media

...yVille For Dummies
...8-1-118-08337-6

...cebook For Dummies,
... Edition
...8-1-118-09562-1

...m Blogging
...r Dummies
...8-1-118-03843-7

...itter For Dummies,
...d Edition
...8-0-470-76879-2

...rdPress For Dummies,
... Edition
...8-1-118-07342-1

## ...siness

...sh Flow For Dummies
...8-1-118-01850-7

...esting For Dummies,
... Edition
...8-0-470-90545-6

## Cooking & Entertaining

Job Searching with Social
Media For Dummies
978-0-470-93072-4

QuickBooks 2012
For Dummies
978-1-118-09120-3

Resumes For Dummies,
6th Edition
978-0-470-87361-8

Starting an Etsy Business
For Dummies
978-0-470-93067-0

## Cooking & Entertaining

Cooking Basics
For Dummies, 4th Edition
978-0-470-91388-8

Wine For Dummies,
4th Edition
978-0-470-04579-4

## Diet & Nutrition

Kettlebells For Dummies
978-0-470-59929-7

Nutrition For Dummies,
5th Edition
978-0-470-93231-5

Restaurant Calorie Counter
For Dummies,
2nd Edition
978-0-470-64405-8

## Digital Photography

Digital SLR Cameras &
Photography For Dummies,
4th Edition
978-1-118-14489-3

Digital SLR Settings
& Shortcuts
For Dummies
978-0-470-91763-3

Photoshop Elements 10
For Dummies
978-1-118-10742-3

## Gardening

Gardening Basics
For Dummies
978-0-470-03749-2

Vegetable Gardening
For Dummies,
2nd Edition
978-0-470-49870-5

## Green/Sustainable

Raising Chickens
For Dummies
978-0-470-46544-8

Green Cleaning
For Dummies
978-0-470-39106-8

## Health

Diabetes For Dummies,
3rd Edition
978-0-470-27086-8

Food Allergies
For Dummies
978-0-470-09584-3

Living Gluten-Free
For Dummies,
2nd Edition
978-0-470-58589-4

## Hobbies

Beekeeping
For Dummies,
2nd Edition
978-0-470-43065-1

Chess For Dummies,
3rd Edition
978-1-118-01695-4

Drawing For Dummies,
2nd Edition
978-0-470-61842-4

eBay For Dummies,
7th Edition
978-1-118-09806-6

Knitting For Dummies,
2nd Edition
978-0-470-28747-7

## Language &
## Foreign Language

English Grammar
For Dummies,
2nd Edition
978-0-470-54664-2

French For Dummies,
2nd Edition
978-1-118-00464-7

German For Dummies,
2nd Edition
978-0-470-90101-4

Spanish Essentials
For Dummies
978-0-470-63751-7

Spanish For Dummies,
2nd Edition
978-0-470-87855-2

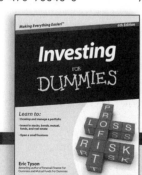

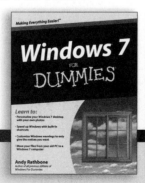

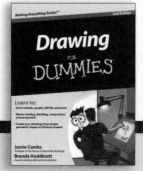

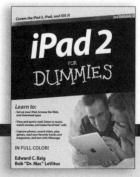

## Math & Science

Algebra I For Dummies,
2nd Edition
978-0-470-55964-2

Biology For Dummies,
2nd Edition
978-0-470-59875-7

Chemistry For Dummies,
2nd Edition
978-1-1180-0730-3

Geometry For Dummies,
2nd Edition
978-0-470-08946-0

Pre-Algebra Essentials
For Dummies
978-0-470-61838-7

## Microsoft Office

Excel 2010 For Dummies
978-0-470-48953-6

Office 2010 All-in-One
For Dummies
978-0-470-49748-7

Office 2011 for Mac
For Dummies
978-0-470-87869-9

Word 2010
For Dummies
978-0-470-48772-3

## Music

Guitar For Dummies,
2nd Edition
978-0-7645-9904-0

Clarinet For Dummies
978-0-470-58477-4

iPod & iTunes
For Dummies,
9th Edition
978-1-118-13060-5

## Pets

Cats For Dummies,
2nd Edition
978-0-7645-5275-5

Dogs All-in One
For Dummies
978-0470-52978-2

Saltwater Aquariums
For Dummies
978-0-470-06805-2

## Religion & Inspiration

The Bible For Dummies
978-0-7645-5296-0

Catholicism For Dummies,
2nd Edition
978-1-118-07778-8

Spirituality For Dummies,
2nd Edition
978-0-470-19142-2

## Self-Help & Relationships

Happiness For Dummies
978-0-470-28171-0

Overcoming Anxiety
For Dummies,
2nd Edition
978-0-470-57441-6

## Seniors

Crosswords For Seniors
For Dummies
978-0-470-49157-7

iPad 2 For Seniors
For Dummies, 3rd Edition
978-1-118-17678-8

Laptops & Tablets
For Seniors For Dummies,
2nd Edition
978-1-118-09596-6

## Smartphones & Tablets

BlackBerry For Dummies,
5th Edition
978-1-118-10035-6

Droid X2 For Dummies
978-1-118-14864-8

HTC ThunderBolt
For Dummies
978-1-118-07601-9

MOTOROLA XOOM
For Dummies
978-1-118-08835-7

## Sports

Basketball For Dummies,
3rd Edition
978-1-118-07374-2

Football For Dummies,
2nd Edition
978-1-118-01261-1

Golf For Dummies,
4th Edition
978-0-470-88279-5

## Test Prep

ACT For Dummies,
5th Edition
978-1-118-01259-8

ASVAB For Dummies,
3rd Edition
978-0-470-63760-9

The GRE Test For
Dummies, 7th Edition
978-0-470-00919-2

Police Officer Exam
For Dummies
978-0-470-88724-0

Series 7 Exam
For Dummies
978-0-470-09932-2

## Web Development

HTML, CSS, & XHTML
For Dummies, 7th Edition
978-0-470-91659-9

Drupal For Dummies,
2nd Edition
978-1-118-08348-2

## Windows 7

Windows 7
For Dummies
978-0-470-49743-2

Windows 7
For Dummies,
Book + DVD Bundle
978-0-470-52398-8

Windows 7 All-in-One
For Dummies
978-0-470-48763-1

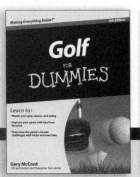

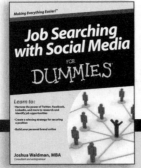

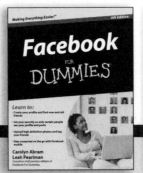

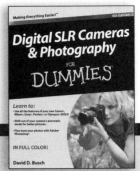

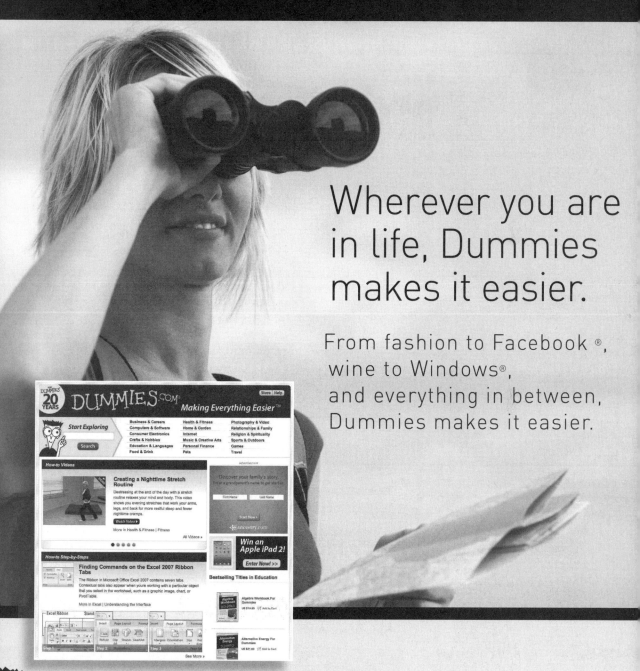

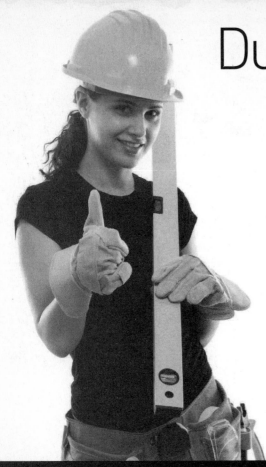
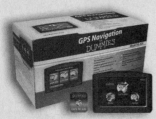
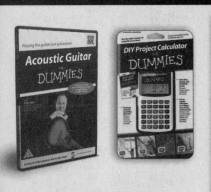
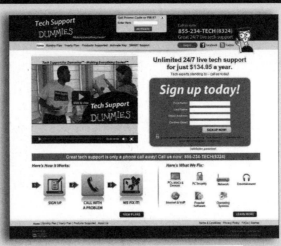
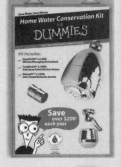
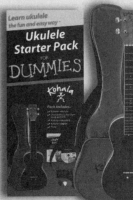
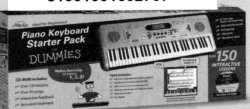
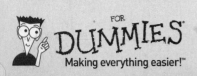